Pediatric Dermatopathology

Clinical and Pathologic Correlations

Pediatric Dermatopathology

Clinical and Pathologic Correlations

Bernett L. Johnson, Jr., M.D.
Vice Chairman and Professor of Dermatology
University of Pennsylvania School of Medicine
Philadelphia, Pennsylvania

Paul J. Honig, M.D.
Professor of Pediatrics and Dermatology
University of Pennsylvania School of Medicine
Director, Pediatric Dermatology
Children's Hospital of Philadelphia
Philadelphia, Pennsylvania

Christine Jaworsky, M.D.
Assistant Professor of Dermatology
University of Pennsylvania School of Medicine
Philadelphia, Pennsylvania

Butterworth–Heinemann

Boston   London   Oxford   Singapore   Sydney   Toronto   Wellington

Library of Congress Cataloging-in-Publication Data

Johnson, Bernett L.
    Pediatric dermatopathology : clinical and pathologic correlations / by Bernett L. Johnson, Jr., Paul J. Honig, Christine Jaworsky.
        p.   cm.
    Includes bibliographical references and index.
    ISBN 0-7506-9264-2 (alk. paper)
    1. Pediatric dermatology—Atlases. 2. Skin—Histopathology—Atlases. 3. Skin—Diseases—Atlases. I. Honig, Paul J. II. Jaworsky, Christine. III. Title.
    [DNLM: 1. Skin Diseases—in infancy & childhood. 2. Skin Diseases—pathology. 3. Skin—pathology.   WS 260 J66p 1994]
RJ511.J64   1994
618.92′5—dc20
DNLM/DLC
for Library of Congress   93-43543
                                                                                        CIP

British Library Cataloguing-in-Publication Data

A catalogue record for this book is available from the British Library.

Butterworth-Heinemann
313 Washington Street
Newton, MA 02158-1626

10 9 8 7 6 5 4 3 2 1

Printed in the United States of America

Contents

Preface

Pediatric Dermatopathology: Clinical and Pathologic Correlations was born of the natural tendency and enthusiasm of dermatologists to relate clinically discernible changes to microscopic findings. This text is a blend of many cumulative years of patient experience at the Children's Hospital of Philadelphia and the Naval Hospital, Philadelphia, and of material available at the University of Pennsylvania, Dermatopathology Laboratories. Every effort was made to provide both clinical and histological examples of entities discussed in this correlative atlas. This material is intended for pediatricians, dermatologists, pathologists, and dermatopathologists confronted with childhood diseases of the skin. Our aim was to make this text a practical and user-friendly reference with concise discussions and illustrative photographs enhanced with tables and charts. We hope that chapters such as "The Newborn," "Hair and Nails," "Lymphoproliferative Disorders," "Nevi, Melanoma, and Neural Tumors," and "Unclassified Disorders" add depth and breadth to materials available in other standard texts.

As with all undertakings requiring such a commitment of time and energy, this work represents many hours "borrowed" from our families. So, to Mary-Martha, Brian, Keith, Susanne, and Logan; Sharon, Karen, and Lisa; Julian, Alexander, and Stefan, we thank you for all your support, love, and understanding.

ACKNOWLEDGMENTS

We are indebted to all those who have taught us: teachers, colleagues, students, and children. We would like to thank our colleagues and the Pathology Department of Children's Hospital of Philadelphia, who eagerly shared their material with us. Finally, we would like to thank Margaret G. Wood, M.D., for her enthusiasm that sparked this project, her counsel, and her gracious wisdom.

Pediatric Dermatopathology

Clinical and Pathologic Correlations

1

Anatomy and Embryology

The anatomy of the skin and its components are well described and discussed (see references). It is our intent to describe the differences between skin of the newborn and child as compared to the skin of the adult. These observations assist in histological diagnosis of diseases in the pediatric age group (Tables 1-1-1 and 1-1-2).

1-1-1 Anatomic Differences of the Skin

Component	Newborn, Child	Adult
Epidermis	1–2 mm thick	1–2 mm thick; decreases with age
Melanocytes	Density greater per mm^2 than in adults	
Langerhans' cells	Density greater than in adults	
Dermis	More cellular	Less cellular
Glycosaminoglycan	Increased	Decreased
Sweat glands (eccrine)	Number high at birth, decreases with age; located in lower dermis	Located at dermal-subcutaneous junction or in subcutis
Sweat glands (apocrine)	Not well-developed until after puberty	Well-developed
Sebaceous glands	Developed in newborn, decreased size and function to age 8–9	Well-developed and large
Adipose tissue	Thin-walled cells, large and loose in appearance	Cell walls thicker, more uniform in arrangement

1-1-2 Embryology of the Skin

Structure	Gestational Age at Time of Development (in months)					
	0–1	2	3	4	5	6
Periderm	+ ----------	---------- +				
Stratification		+ ----------	----------	---------- +		
Desmosome	+					
Follicular keratinization			+			
Merkel's cell				18 wk		
Melanocyte			+			
Langerhans' cell		+				
Tooth buds			+			
Nail plate keratinizes				+ ----------	-- +	
Melanin granule transfer					+	
KF1 antigen				+		
Elastic fibers				+		
Adipose tissue				18 wk		
Sebaceous gland				16 wk		
Arrector pili				15 wk		
Apocrine gland function					20–24 wk	
Eccrine gland			+			
Eccrine gland function						+

REFERENCES

Hamada H: Age changes in melanocyte distribution of the normal epidermis. Jpn J Dermatol 1972; 82:223.

Holbrook KA: A histologic comparison of infant and adult skin. In Maibach HI, Boisits EK, eds: Neonatal skin. New York: Marcel Dekker, 1981:3.

Holbrook KA: Human epidermal embryogenesis. Int J Dermatol 1979; 18:329.

Pochi PE, Strauss JS, Downing DT: Age-related changes in sebaceous gland activity. J Invest Dermatol 1979; 73:108.

Smith LT, Holbrook KA: Development of dermal connective tissue in human embryonic and fetal skin. SEM 1982; 4:1745.

Stingl G, Tamaki K, Katz SI: Origin and function of epidermal Langerhans cells. Immunol Rev 1980; 53:149.

Zias N: Embryology of the human nail. Arch Dermatol 1963; 87:37.

2

Biopsy Technique

Contents

Textbooks of pathology often devote hundreds of pages to description of pathologic processes and only one or two pages to the technique of obtaining the specimen. Without precise and adequate sampling of the affected tissue, none of the following pages of this book would have been possible. The technique for biopsy is very simple: to remove the "classic lesion" expediently, leave the smallest defect possible, and preserve the tissue for immortality.

Biopsies can be performed relatively easily in children who are properly prepared. The child's age and developmental level determine how that child is handled (Table 2-1-1). The physician should give a step-by-step, age-appropriate explanation detailing the painful and pain-free parts of the procedure. Children who are well informed feel in control and are more likely to cooperate. Educational aids such as pictorial explanations or coloring books are very effective. Questions and concerns on the part of both parent and child should be addressed immediately, simply, and truthfully.

Also important is the child's previous experience, which may lead to preconceptions concerning what is about to occur. It is therefore advisable to elicit information concerning previous injuries, illnesses, and hospital or emergency room experiences, to anticipate and allay misconceptions and fears.

Skin biopsies can be obtained with a punch, curette, scissors, or scalpel. The latter can be used for elliptical excisions or shave biopsies. The choice of method will depend on the size, shape, and location of the lesion and the physician's level of skill with each instrument. The use of the curette is discouraged at all times, since the resulting specimens are often inadequate.

The most commonly used technique, the punch biopsy, is performed with disposable sharp circular punches. Biopsy punches are available in sizes from 2 mm to 6 mm in diameter, the most common size being 4 mm. Specimens smaller than 3 mm in diameter are discouraged because small tissue samples often yield little information.

The skin is prepared with povidone iodine (Betadine), alcohol, or another appropriate antiseptic. Anesthesia is obtained with 1% or 2% lidocaine (Xylocaine) with 1:100,000 epinephrine (for hemostasis during the procedure). Following anesthesia, the skin is drawn taut, perpendicular to the skin lines. The punch is twisted (rotated) until the dermis is penetrated to the subcutaneous fat. The specimen is removed by gently holding the epidermal edge, lifting, and cutting as deep into the fat as possible. The specimen is then placed in the proper fixative. The wound is closed with one or two sutures, and wound care instructions are given to the parents.

2-1 SPECIAL CIRCUMSTANCES

Following are technical considerations to ensure the best results in special circumstances.

Bullous Diseases—The specimen should include early new blisters and adjacent uninvolved skin (the latter especially for immunodiagnostic techniques).

Inflammatory Diseases—The specimen should not be taken from a crust. A new lesion and a fully evolved one (two punches) should be biopsied.

Follicular Lesions—The specimen should be parallel to the direction of the growth of the follicle and extend into the subcutaneous fat.

Palms and Soles—Ensure that the specimen is taken through the dermis and into the fat (most biopsies of palms and soles contain only keratin and superficial epidermis).

Pigmentary Disorders—The specimen should include normal skin, clearly marked so that the normal skin can be differentiated from the pigmentary disorder.

Melanocytic Lesions—The entire lesion should be removed if malignancy is suspected, when possible. Always ensure adequate excision or incision.

SPECIMEN PRESERVATION

Specimens for most routine histology are preserved in 10% buffered formalin. For immunofluorescence studies transport media is used; the specimen should not be placed in formalin. For electron microscopy glutaraldehyde or Karnovsky's medium is used. For evaluation of lipid-soluble materials within sections, fresh frozen tissue or formalin-fixed frozen tissue will produce the best results. Immunoperoxidase studies can be performed on formalin-fixed material. When using formalin fixation in temperatures below 32°F or 0°C, 95% ethyl alcohol should be added to the formalin to prevent freezing of the specimen, especially if the specimen is transported by mail. Another alternative is to fix the specimen overnight before mailing.

2-2 EXPECTATIONS FROM THE BIOPSY

The clinician expects specific answers from the biopsy specimen. The pathologist expects to render a precise diagnosis on each specimen. The patient expects a cure. Interpreting the histopathology is a union of the clinical and the histological. The better the clinical information, the better the histological interpretation. Descriptions of diseases that include site, age, color, duration, evolution, and information about the patient are invaluable in the pathological diagnosis. Histological examination of tissues in dermatology is a major tool in making an accurate diagnosis.

2-1-1 Developmental Profile and Its Clinical Implications for Procedures

Child	Mother	Clinical Application
Birth–6 mo		
Dependent	Nuturent	Anyone can examine baby but manner of handling (physically) important
Nonverbal cues	Baby-mother as a fused unit	Mother is person who must be pleased
Baby primary cue giver	Mother is cue reader ("knows baby")	Attitude toward baby taken personally by mother (i.e., good baby, etc.)
6 mo–1 y		
Stranger anxiety (8–9 mo)	Recognizes stranger anxiety	Examine baby in mother's arms or allow gradual approach through mother
Selective smiling response	Encourages and allows for brief separation	Engage baby
Seeks response from environment; to make things happen, baby laughs, initiates response	Reassurance of anxiety	Use mother to help with child
		Interest baby with objects
		Do not send mother out of examining room if at all possible
1–2 y		
Stranger and separation anxiety continues with attempts at mastery (begins to walk around or away from mother for period of time)	Greater expectations that may be unrealistic	Don't be discouraged if child is uncooperative and crying and rejects all efforts
	Issues of limit-setting, discipline	With help of mother, finish procedure
		Talk with child, engage in play with objects in office or objects of theirs (transitional objects)
		Anticipate mother's expectations of child to be "good for doctor"
		Acknowledge to mother how difficult this stage is
2–4 y		
Separation-individuation, panic reaction common	Allows for separation and reassurance	Talk directly with child
Imagination, imaginary companions, animals, etc.	Limit setting	Still using mother, important to get child to relate to you positively (must engage and interest child to accomplish this)
"Little fears"		Let child participate when possible in exam or procedure (i.e., hold object, blow light)
Peak exploration		Anticipate growing anxiety, no-no quality of response
Feelings for objects and people at extremes		Recognize panic reaction as it begins to develop from increasing anxiety
Testing limits		Use mother to support, reassure
4 y		
Social individual	Greater social expectations	Delightful if engaged
Concern for others	Concerns for learning	Same as age 2–3 but easier to examine
Can postpone or delay gratification		Don't promise unless you can comply
		Trust/mistrust: answer questions with honesty and in a way that child understands
5 y		
Beginning conscience	Growing expectation of home, school habits, attitude, relationship	More verbal interaction possible; listen to what child has to say
Good/bad feelings		Respect child's body during exam; may be shy or not (use sheet or have on hand)
Guilt		Don't exaggerate or take lightly child's shyness or need for privacy
Fears		

3

The Newborn

Contents

3-1 ACNE NEONATORUM

CLINICAL DESCRIPTION

Acne may be seen in the very young infant. It occurs in two forms: (1) acne neonatorum (onset two weeks to three months of life) and (2) infantile acne (onset over three months of age).

Etiology and Incidence

Neonatal acne is seen almost exclusively in boys, and is therefore thought to be secondary to unusual sensitivity to testosterone produced by both the testis and adrenal gland. Other unexplained hormonal influences may produce acne in infants over three months of age (male to female ratio, 1:1). Signs of sexual precocity should be sought, especially in girls who manifest acne before three months of age, but are rarely found.

Clinical Features

Most affected infants have comedones and inflammatory lesions on their cheeks (Figure 3-1-1), but other parts of the face may also be involved. Generally, the trunk is not involved. Most cases of acne clear in several months, but infantile acne may linger for up to three years or more.

Differential Diagnosis

Exposure to comedogenic chemicals
Frictional papules
Keratosis pilaris
Milia
Miliaria rubra or pustulosa
Precocious puberty

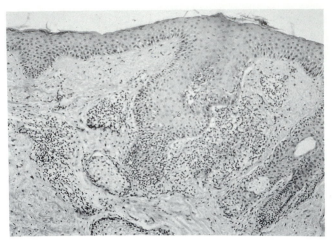

3-1-2 ACNE NEONATORUM: Low magnification shows several hair follicles with peri- and intrafollicular inflammation and hyperkeratosis at the follicular osteum. (100×)

HISTOLOGICAL DESCRIPTION

The histological features of acneiform eruptions seen in infants and children are similar to those seen in adults. There is follicular hyperkeratosis, perifollicular inflammation with lymphocytes and histiocytes, and, in some areas, polymorphonuclear leukocytes. The inflammatory cells produce intrafollicular as well as a perifollicular abscesses (Figures 3-1-2 and 3-1-3). Sebaceous glands (although in children relatively immature) are larger than one would expect for the age of the patient. The collagen is more loosely structured. There is no solar elastosis. Small follicular cysts (milial cysts) may also be seen (Figure 3-1-4).

Differential Diagnosis

Folliculitis

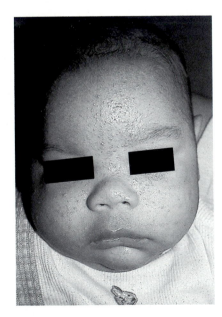

3-1-1 ACNE NEONATORUM (infantile acne): Discrete erythematous papules and pustules on the forehead, nose, cheeks, and chin of a three-month-old boy.

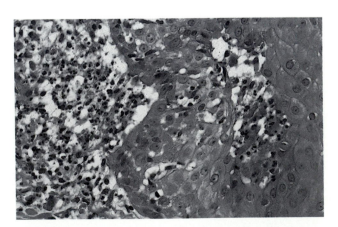

3-1-3 ACNE NEONATORUM: Neutrophilic abscess disrupting follicular epithelium. (400×)

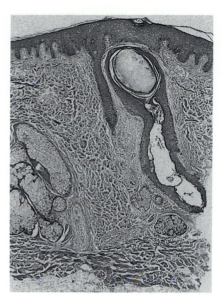

3-1-4 ACNE NEONATORUM: Follicular infundibulum is distended by a keratotic plug. There is also perifollicular fibrosis secondary to previous inflammation or rupture. (50×)

3-2 BRANCHIAL CLEFT CYST (FISTULA)

CLINICAL DESCRIPTION

Branchial cysts and fistulae are found in the neck anterior to the sternocleidomastoid muscle (SCM).

Etiology and Incidence

A genetic basis for this anomaly of the second branchial cleft has been hypothesized. One-third of fistulas occur bilaterally.

Clinical Features

External branchial fistulas are present at birth and can be found on physical examination (Figure 3-2-1). Branchial cysts may not be noticeable until after the neonatal period. The opening of the fistula is usually located anterior to the SCM in its lower third. A mucous secretion may be exuding from the opening.

Differential Diagnosis

Lymph node
Epithelial or keratinous cyst

HISTOLOGICAL DESCRIPTION

The histological features of the branchial cleft cyst (lympho-epithelial cyst) are a cyst lined by a thin, flattened layer of stratified squamous or respiratory epithelium and lymphocytic inflammatory infiltrates. The lumen may be filled with amorphous eosinophilic debris but is usually filled with keratin. Inflammatory cells, usually lymphocytes, may be noted within the luminal spaces, and a varying degree of inflammation may surround the cyst (Figure 3-2-2). The significant feature is organized lymphoid tissue that surrounds the cyst epithelial wall.

Differential Diagnosis

Keratinous cyst
Lymph node

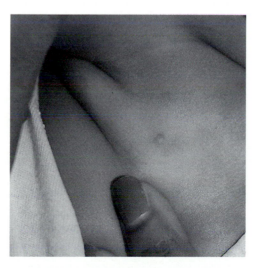

3-2-1 BRANCHIAL CLEFT CYST (fistula): A papule on the lower anterior neck with a central opening. There is mild surrounding erythema. (Courtesy of L. Robert Smith, M.D.)

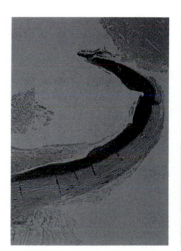 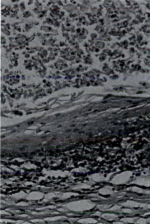

A   B

3-2-2 BRANCHIAL CLEFT CYST: **A** Low magnification shows a cystic structure containing keratin. Part of the cyst wall is surrounded by a dense inflammatory infiltrate. Peripheral to this fibrosis of the stroma is present. (12.5×) **B** The lining of the cyst is stratified squamous epithelium of variable thickness. It is surrounded and infiltrated by large numbers of lymphocytes admixed with histiocytes. (200×)

3-3 CUTIS MARMORATA TELANGIECTATICUM CONGENITA

CLINICAL DESCRIPTION

Cutis marmorata telangiectaticum congenita may be difficult to distinguish from physiologic mottling.

Etiology and Incidence

Cutis marmorata telangiectaticum congenita (CMTC) is a rare disorder that represents an anomaly of superficial capillaries and veins (i.e., ectasias). These vessels are dilated and very noticeable.

Clinical Features

Persistent reddish blue mottling in a lacelike pattern (Plate 3-3-1) is seen at birth and may be generalized or segmental. There may be extension with time; however, the condition improves as the child becomes older. On rare occasion the skin changes persist into adult life. Ulcerations and atrophic areas of skin may be seen. Other vascular and nonvascular anomalies may be associated with CMTC (e.g., port-wine stains, hemangiomas, varicosities, bony and soft tissue growth anomalies, glaucoma, mental retardation). CMTC may be a part of the Riley Smith syndrome.

Differential Diagnosis

Physiologic mottling
Livedo reticularis

HISTOLOGICAL DESCRIPTION

The histological features seen in CMTC are essentially normal stratum corneum, epidermis, and dermis. There is no significant inflammatory response, although there may be some dermal edema. Vessels do not appear to be altered but may appear telangiectatic (Figure 3-3-1).

Differential Diagnosis

Normal skin
Thin-walled angiomas

3-4 MILIARIA

CLINICAL DESCRIPTION

Miliaria is a heat-induced, benign condition that responds rapidly to lowering of ambient temperature.

Etiology and Incidence

Miliaria occurs secondary to obstruction of sweat ducts and trapping of sweat. When the process is very superficial, vesi-

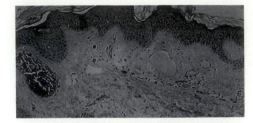
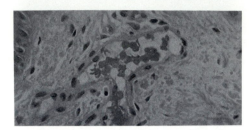

A

B

3-3-1 CUTIS MARMORATA TELANGIECTATICA CONGENITA: **A** Low magnification shows superficial vascular ectasia. (40×) **B** High magnification shows endothelial-lined vascular channels distended by erythrocytes. (200×)

cles, called sudamina, form. When the process is deeper, prickly heat (miliaria rubra) occurs. The condition occurs throughout childhood but is seen most frequently in the neonatal period because immature eccrine ducts are obstructed more easily.

Clinical Features

Superficial vesicles or erythematous papules (Plate 3-4-1) are seen on the scalp, neck, or any of the intertriginous regions. Skin surfaces covered with clothing are also especially susceptible. Lesions may be surrounded by a rim of erythema (Figure 3-4-1) but do not have hairs growing through them (i.e., are not associated with hair follicles).

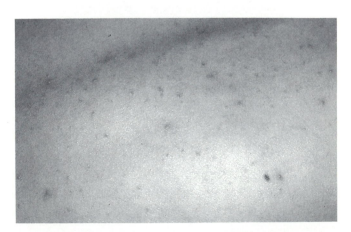

3-4-1 MILIARIA: Dusky erythematous (deeper-seated) papules of miliaria rubra. Note lack of association of lesions with hair follicles.

Differential Diagnosis

Erythema toxicum neonatorum
Folliculitis
Candida albicans
Infantile acne (when facial)

HISTOLOGICAL DESCRIPTION

On histological examination, two forms of miliaria may be identified: miliaria crystallina and miliaria rubra. In miliaria crystallina there is a subcorneal and/or intracorneal vesicle. Multiple sections reveal that this vesicle communicates with the underlying acrosyringium. Miliaria rubra is a spongiotic process in which there is intraepidermal spongiosis about the acrosyringium with associated exocytosis of lymphocytes. The intraepidermal spongiosis may lead to microvesicle formation within the epidermis. Periodic acid-Schiff-positive, diastase-resistant material may be seen within the lumen of the sweat duct.

Differential Diagnosis

Erythema toxicum neonatorum
Bullous impetigo

3-5 MONGOLIAN SPOTS
(see Chapter 8)

3-6 NASAL GLIOMA

CLINICAL DESCRIPTION

Nasal glioma is a congenital malformation seen protruding from between the eyes.

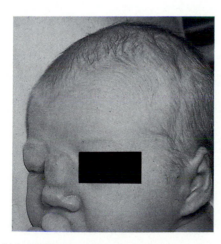

3-6-1 NASAL GLIOMA: A broad-based skin-covered nodule distorts the normal architecture of the nasal root. The nodule consists of ectopic neuroectodermal tissue.

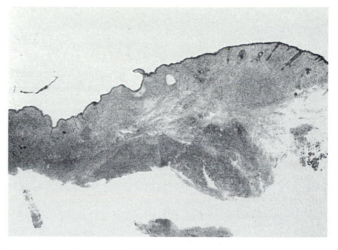

3-6-2 NASAL GLIOMA: Low-power view shows a deep-seated collection of eosinophilic cells within the dermis. On one edge, the process is present also within the upper dermis. The areas of involvement show a lack of appendiceal structures. (25×)

Etiology and Incidence

This congenital anomaly is rare. During gestation, incomplete invagination of the neural plate results in herniation of brain tissue. This herniation eventually loses its connection to the subarachnoid space. At birth, the ectopic brain tissue can be appreciated as a protuberance on the face between the eyes, near the nasal root.

Clinical Features

Nasal gliomas are skin-colored to reddish blue protrusions from the nasal bridge (Figure 3-6-1). They may be several centimeters wide and extend a similar distance from the skin surface.

Differential Diagnosis

Nasal dermoid
Encephalocele
Hemangioma

HISTOLOGICAL DESCRIPTION

The epidermis is usually normal but thinned overlying these tumors (Figure 3-6-2). The dermis has an intermingling of neural and collagen tissues. The neural tissue (glial cells, glial substance, or astrocytes) stain eosinophilic. Astrocytes have a finely fibrillar cytoplasm with ill-defined cell borders (Plate 3-6-1). Many of these cells appear in a syncytial arrangement. The nuclei are large and vesicular. There may also be dermal fibrosis with sparse inflammation, which when present is lymphohistiocytic in character. Calcification may occur within these tumors. Neurons may be rarely seen.

Differential Diagnosis
Encephalocele
Neural tumor
Granular cell tumor
Neurofibroma

3-7 SALMON PATCH

CLINICAL DESCRIPTION

Salmon patch lesions represent the most common vascular anomaly of infancy.

Etiology and Incidence
Salmon patch occurs in 30% to 50% of newborns and represents a persistence of fetal vessels rather than an overgrowth. The areas of involvement include the nape of the neck (22%), glabella (20%), upper eyelids (20%), and nasolabial regions.

Clinical Features
Macular erythema occurs on the regions described above. Telangiectasia is frequently seen within this patch of erythema. Most areas fade by one year, except for the lesions on the nape of the neck (50% fade) (Figure 3-7-1).

Differential Diagnosis
Early hemangioma
Port-wine stain

HISTOLOGICAL DESCRIPTION

The histological features of salmon patch are thin, mildly dilated superficial vessels in the papillary dermis not associated with inflammation. These vessels appear essentially as normal vessels that show some ectasia, not to the extent seen in angiokeratomas.

Differential Diagnosis
Port-wine stain
Early hemangioma
Essential telangiectasia

3-8 SEBACEOUS GLAND HYPERPLASIA

CLINICAL DESCRIPTION

Sebaceous gland hyperplasia is a transient phenomenon.

Etiology and Incidence
Sebaceous gland hyperplasia is thought to be due to stimulation of the glands by passively transferred maternal androgens. Since the hormonal influence is transient, the condition disappears after several weeks.

Clinical Features
Many very tiny white or yellow papules appear, mainly on the nose (Figure 3-8-1). Other involved areas include the upper lips and malar regions.

Differential Diagnosis
Epidermal inclusion cyst
Milia

HISTOLOGICAL DESCRIPTION

The histological features of sebaceous gland hyperplasia are enlarged sebaceous glands and/or sebaceous follicles (Figure

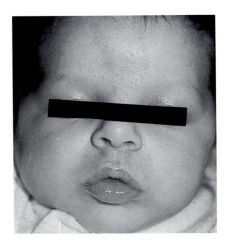

3-7-1 SALMON PATCH: Patches of erythema involving the forehead, medial upper eyelids, and infranasal area of a two-month-old child. These areas blanche with the application of pressure.

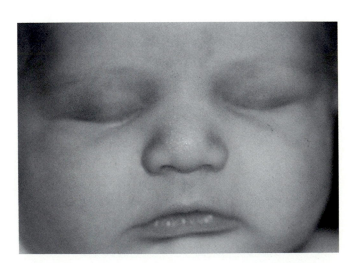

3-8-1 SEBACEOUS GLAND HYPERPLASIA: Grouped yellowish papules on the tip of the nose in a newborn. Also note the salmon patches of both upper eyelids and the forehead.

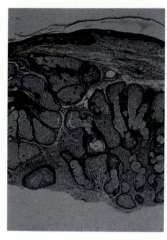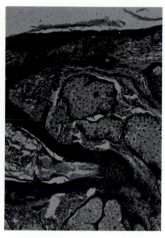

A   B

3-8-2 SEBACEOUS GLAND HYPERPLASIA: **A** Hyperplastic sebaceous lobules surround follicular canals and are placed high in the dermis. (100×) **B** Sebaceous lobules encroach on the papillary dermis as a result of their hyperplasia. There is lack of solar elastosis or atypia of keratinocytes, features observed in adult sebaceous hyperplasia. (400×)

3-8-2A). There is no invasion of sebaceous structures by inflammatory cells, but there is an associated sparse perivascular lymphohistiocytic reaction about dermal vessels. In contrast to adults, newborns with sebaceous hyperplasia have no solar elastosis or atypical changes within the epidermis (Figure 3-8-2B).

Differential Diagnosis
Acne vulgaris

3-9 THYROGLOSSAL DUCT CYST

CLINICAL DESCRIPTION

A rounded mass in the midline of the neck in the region of the hyoid bone is most likely a thyroglossal duct cyst.

Etiology and Incidence
Thyroglossal duct cyst is a remnant of the thyroid stalk, which extends from the foramen cecum to the thyroid. The lesion can therefore occur anywhere from the base of the tongue to the thyroid area. Seventy-five percent of these cysts present within the first five years of life.

Clinical Features
A midline mass (Figure 3-9-1) is usually seen between one and five years of age but may be present at birth. Frequently

the lesion is 1 cm in diameter and firm and moves up and down when the child swallows or sticks out the tongue. It is usually found over the hyoid bone, although it can be located over the thyroid cartilage or suprasternal area. At times, a sinus or fistula over the hyoid bone discharges mucus (thyroglossal duct sinus or fistula). Infrequently the cyst is found at the base of the tongue. In this location signs of obstruction may occur.

Differential Diagnosis
Lymph node (submental)
Epidermal inclusion cyst
Branchial cleft cyst
Lipoma
Fibroma
Lymphangioma
Hemangioma

HISTOLOGICAL DESCRIPTION
The histological features seen are a cystic structure in the dermis lined with pseudostratified columnar epithelium (Figure 3-9-2). The luminal cells are ciliated. Goblet cells are seen within the epithelium. There is often underlying chronic inflammation (Figure 3-9-3). Smooth muscle is not associated with this cyst as it is in bronchogenic cysts, although thyroid tissue (follicles) may be seen in adjacent areas.

Differential Diagnosis
Bronchogenic cyst
Branchial cleft cyst

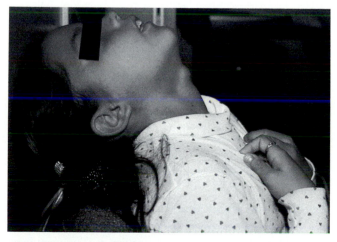

3-9-1 THYROGLOSSAL DUCT CYST: Hyperextension of the neck allows identification of a midline cystic structure with ease in this young girl.

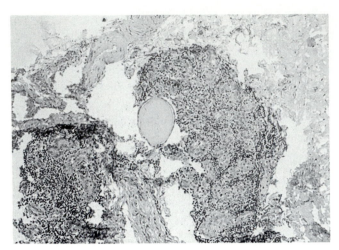

3-9-2 THYROGLOSSAL DUCT CYST: Surrounded by dermal stroma is a collection of glandular tissue. One glandular lumen is distended with homogeneous eosinophilic material. (50×)

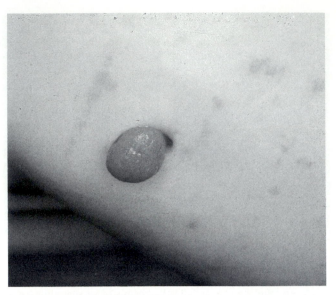

3-10-1 UMBILICAL GRANULOMA: An erythematous nodule with a partially eroded surface protrudes from the umbilicus.

Clinical Features

An umbilical granuloma is a grayish white (sometimes pink), nodular, firm, wet lesion (Figure 3-10-1). It will persist until treated.

Differential Diagnosis

Umbilical polyp
Umbilical sinus (a remnant of the omphalomesenteric duct)
Patent urachus

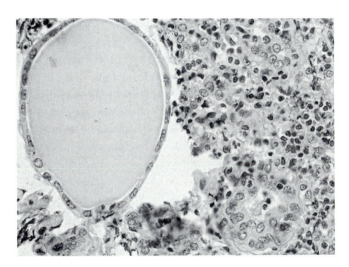

3-9-3 THYROGLOSSAL DUCT CYST: Cuboidal cells are arranged in one to two layers to form glands. One of these contains colloid. This aberrant thyroid gland tissue is surrounded and infiltrated by mononuclear cells. The variable distention of glandular lumina forms cysts. (200×)

3-10 UMBILICAL GRANULOMA

CLINICAL DESCRIPTION

Umbilical granuloma is seen frequently by pediatricians during routine well-baby care.

Etiology and Incidence

The exact incidence of umbilical granuloma has not been documented, but it occurs with regularity. The granuloma forms when complete healing does not occur following separation of the umbilical cord.

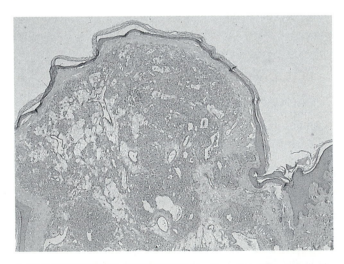

3-10-2 UMBILICAL GRANULOMA: Overview of an exophytic nodule surrounded by a collarette at the base. The rete ridge pattern of the epidermis is effaced and the epithelium is attenuated. The dermal stroma contains vascular spaces filled with erythrocytes. (25×)

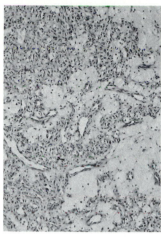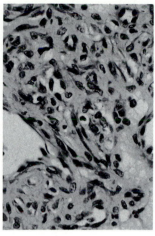

A   B

3-10-3 UMBILICAL GRANULOMA: **A** Numerous endothelial-lined vascular spaces are separated in areas by loose, edematous dermal stroma. (100×) **B** Plump endothelial cells without atypia protrude into the lumen. (400×)

HISTOLOGICAL DESCRIPTION

Umbilical granulomas are essentially pyogenic granulomas. The histological features are epidermal effacement and atrophy. The dermis is filled with a proliferation of endothelial cells, with the production of vascular lumina (Figures 3-10-2 and 3-10-3A). The lumina show plump endothelial cells without atypia (Figure 3-10-3B). The stroma is edematous and contains a lymphocytic infiltrate. When these tumors ulcerate the infiltrate contains acute inflammatory cells.

Differential Diagnosis

Capillary hemangioma
Granulation tissue
Kaposi's sarcoma
Angiosarcoma
Bacillary angiomatosis

REFERENCES

Acne Neonatorum
Lucky AW: Update on acne vulgaris. Pediatr Annals 1987; 16:29.
Plewig G: Morphologic dynamics of acne vulgaris. Acta Derm Venerol (Storkin) 1980; 89:9.

Branchial Cleft Cyst
Burge D, Middleton A: Persistent pharyngeal pouch derivatives in the neonate. J Pediatr Surg 1983; 18:230.
Gorlin RJ, Pindborg JJ: Syndromes of the head and neck. New York: McGraw-Hill, 1964.
Jaworsky C, Murphy GF: Cystic tumors of the neck. J Dermatol Surg Oncol 1989; 15:21.

Cutis Marmorata Telangiectaticum Congenita
Cohen PR, Zalar GL: Cutis marmorata telangiectaticum congenita: Clinicopathologic characteristics and differential diagnosis. Cutis 1988; 42:518.
Gelmetti C, Schianchi R, Ermacora E: Cutis marmorata telangiectatica congenita: 4 new cases and review of the literature. Ann Dermatol Venereol 1987; 114:1517.
Picascia DD, Esterly NB: Cutis marmorata telangiectaticum congenita: Report of 22 cases. J Am Acad Dermatol 1989; 6:1098.
Sandt DD, Jacobs AH: Cutis marmorata telangiectaticum congenita. J Pediatrics 1978; 93:944.

Miliaria
Holzle E, Kligman AM: The pathogenesis of miliaria rubra: Role of the resident microflora. Br J Dermatol 1978; 117:99.
Lowenthal LJA: The pathogenesis of miliaria. Arch Dermatol 1961; 84:2.
Shelley WB, Howath PN: Experimental miliaria in man. J Invest Dermatol 1950; 14:9.

Nasal Glioma
Paller AS, Renster JM, Tomita T: Nasal midline masses in infants and children. Arch Dermatol 1991; 127:362.

Salmon Patch
Lueng AK, Telmesani AMA: Salmon patches in Caucasian children. Pediatric Dermatol 1989; 6:185.
Maleville J, Taieb A, Roubaud E, et al. Immature cutaneous hemangiomas: Epidemiologic study of 351 cases. Ann Dermatol Venereol 1985; 112:603.

Sebaceous Gland Hyperplasia
De Villez RL, Roberts LE: Premature sebaceous gland hyperplasia. J Am Acad Dermatol 1982; 6:933.
Nauda A, Kaur S, Bhakoo ON, et al.: Survey of cutaneous lesions in Indian newborns. Pediatr Dermatol 1989; 6:39.

Thyroglossal Duct Cyst
Ambiavagar PC, Rosen Y: Cutaneous ciliated cyst on the chin: Probable bronchogenic cyst. Arch Dermatol 1979; 115:898.
Fraga S, Helwig EB, Rosen SH: Bronchogenic cyst in the skin and subcutaneous tissue. Am J Clin Pathol 1971; 56:230.
Hoffman MA, Schuster SR: The management of thyroglossal duct cysts. Resident and Staff Physician 1990; 36:19.

Umbilical Granuloma
Kliegman RM, Behrman RE: The umbilicus. In Behrman RE, Vaughan VC III, eds: Textbook of pediatrics. 13 ed. Philadelphia; W.B. Saunders, 1987; 415.

4

Hereditary Skin Disorders

Contents

4-1 ANGIOFIBROMA AND TUBEROUS SCLEROSIS

CLINICAL DESCRIPTION

Tuberous sclerosis is a neurocutaneous disorder defined by the criteria shown in Table 4-1-1. The classic triad includes seizures, mental retardation, and a variety of skin lesions: the ash-leaf macule, angiofibroma, and connective tissue nevus. However, there is extreme variability in expression, and the triad is not always completely present. At least two distinct genetic loci have been identified based on family linkage studies (chromosomes 9q and 16p).

Etiology and Incidence

Tuberous sclerosis occurs in 7 per 100,000 births. The disorder is inherited as an autosomal dominant trait, however greater than 60% of cases are new mutations (with unaffected parents).

Clinical Features

A valuable early marker is the ash-leaf macule; more than 80% of children with tuberous sclerosis manifest this sign. The ash-leaf macule may appear anywhere on the body. Less than 20% are ash leaf in shape: most are oval or round and vary greatly in size (Plate 4-1-1). Ash-leaf macules are often present at birth but can sometimes occur later in childhood, often persisting throughout life. However, ash-leaf macules, when few in number, may also be seen in normal children, without tuberous sclerosis. Other patterns of hypopigmenta-

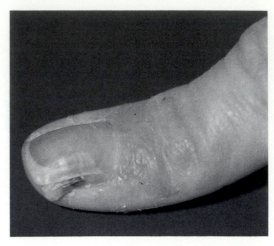

4-1-1 ANGIOFIBROMA: Periungual fibroma generally grows at lateral margin of nailplate.

tion are also seen in tuberous sclerosis: these include speckled 1 to 3 mm macules of leukoderma in a confetti-like pattern and poliosis (tufts of white hair).

Angiofibromas (previously erroneously called adenoma sebaceum) are also a characteristic and diagnostic skin finding in this disorder. The lesions occur in more than 70% to 80% of patients but usually do not appear until five years of age. Only 13% of children manifest this finding within the first year of life and some not until puberty. These appear as pink to red, 1 to 4 mm dome-shaped nodules with a smooth surface and are often seen with fine telangiectasias. They are characteristically observed in the nasolabial folds, cheeks, chin, forehead, and sometimes on the scalp (Plate 4-1-2).

Connective tissue nevi, or shagreen patches, which develop after two years of age in 20% to 50% of patients, are most frequently seen in the lumbosacral area as a flesh-colored or yellow/orange plaque. They may be singular or multiple.

The skin surface above this lesion is elevated and irregular (peau d'orange) (Plate 4-1-3). The margins are irregular and the skin thickened. They may occur in patients without tuberous sclerosis. Twenty percent of patients develop fibromas in the periungual (Figure 4-1-1) and subungual areas at puberty. Although less frequently seen than ash-leaf spots, they are more diagnostic of tuberous sclerosis and fulfill one of the major criteria for this disorder.

Other skin lesions include café-au-lait spots, skin tags, port-wine stains, mucosal fibromas, pretibial speckled leukoderma, poliosis, and pits in the permanent teeth.

Although seizures may be seen in about 75% or more of tuberous sclerosis patients and about 50% may have mental retardation, it is important to note that substantial numbers of these individuals may have completely normal cognitive function and that all manifestations vary greatly, even between members of the same family.

4-1-1   Criteria for Diagnosis of Tuberous Sclerosis

Definitive (One or More Features Present)	Presumptive (Two or More Features Present)
Cortical tuber	Infantile spasms
Subepidermal glial nodules	Myoclonic, tonic, or atonic seizures
Retinal hamartoma	Hypomelanotic macules
Facial angiofibroma (fibrous plaque of forehead or scalp)	Peripapillary retinal hamartoma
	Gingival fibromas
	Dental enamel pits
Ungual fibroma	Cardiac rhabdomyoma
Renal angiomyolipomas	Pulmonary lymphangiomyomatosis
	Wedge-shaped cortical or subcortical calcification
	Multiple subcortical hyperintense lesions in magnetic resonance scans of the head
	First-degree relative with tuberous sclerosis
	Shagreen patches
	Radiographic "honeycomb" lungs

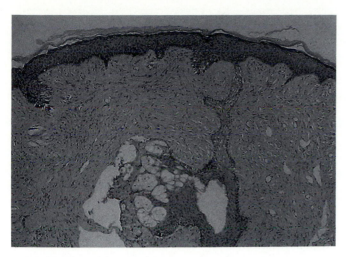

4-1-2 ANGIOFIBROMA: Epidermal effacement, vascular ectasia, and dermal fibrosis. (20×)

Other systemic features to be screened for include renal cysts and angiomyolipomas (which may grow throughout life), ocular hamartomas, osseous lesions (bone cysts and sclerosis), and visible CNS tubers and giant cell astrocytomas, even without clinical evidence of neurologic dysfunction.

Differential Diagnosis

Ash-Leaf Macule
Vitiligo
Leukoderma
Achromic nevus
Nevus anemicus
Partial albinism

Angiofibromas
Acne
Sarcoidosis

Periungual Fibroma
Verruca vulgaris

Shagreen Patch
Focal dermal hypoplasia
Other connective tissue nevi including Buschke-Ollendorff
    Syndrome
Pseudoxanthoma elasticum

HISTOLOGICAL DESCRIPTION

Angiofibroma
Angiofibromas show epidermal thinning with orthokeratosis. The papillary dermis has superficial vascular ectasia without significant inflammation (Figures 4-1-2 to 4-1-4). The striking feature is that of sclerotic collagen, perivascular as well as periadnexal, seen as concentric layers resembling the cross section of an onion. Sebaceous glands and follicular structures are usually atrophic. These tumors do not show significant cellular infiltrate, the main cell being that of a large plump and/or stellate fibroblast. Periungual and/or subungual fibromas (Figures 4-1-2 to 4-1-4) have similar features with or without associated capillary ectasia. Usually all have large stellate fibroblasts present.

Tuberous Sclerosis
Ash-Leaf Macule
The histological features of ash-leaf macule are those of normal-appearing skin on hematoxylin and eosin stain. There is no significant inflammation and the histologic features are normal for the site of the biopsy (Figure 4-1-5). If the biopsy

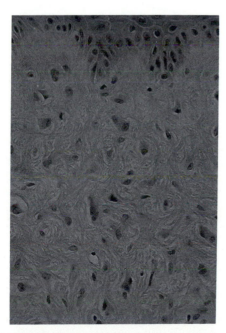

4-1-3 ANGIOFIBROMA: Glial-like fibroblasts in a fibrotic dermis. Small vascular structures are also seen. (100×)

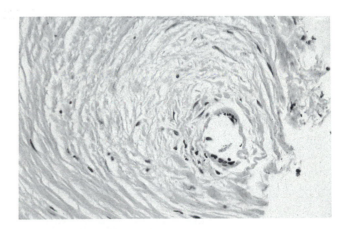

4-1-4 ANGIOFIBROMA: Perivascular fibrosis in an angiofibroma. (100×)

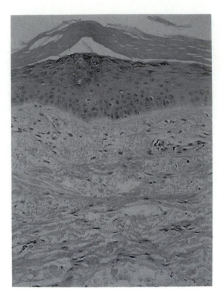

4-1-5 TUBEROUS SCLEROSIS (ash-leaf macule): The skin appears normal for this site. Only in comparison to normal skin can a decrease in the number of basilar melanocytes be appreciated. (50×)

specimen is taken through the area of hypopigmentation into normal skin, there is an apparent decrease in melaninization compared to the areas within the ash-leaf macule.

The number of melanocytes per square millimeter within the lesion is the same as that in adjacent areas. The reaction with dopa stain shows that melaninization occurs in the ash-leaf macule, but is deficient with a decrease in the size of melanosomes, and packaging of melanosomes.

Connective Tissue Nevi

Collagen or connective tissue nevi on small biopsy specimens are difficult to differentiate from normal skin. In larger specimens the usual finding is collagen sclerosis in the lower reticular dermis that resembles scleroderma and/or morphea (Figure 4-1-6). Broad bands of collagen may be seen in the dermis. Good clinical and histological correlation is important in making a diagnosis of connective nevus. Comparison of elastic tissue stains in the collagen nevus with that of adjacent normal skin reveals clumping, some fragmentation, and a decrease in elastic tissue within the collagen nevi (Figure 4-1-7).

Differential Diagnosis
Angiofibroma
Fibrous papule
Regressed nevus
Scar
Connective tissue nevus

Ash-Leaf Macule
Vitiligo
Partial albinism (piebaldism)

Connective Tissue Nevi
Morphea
Scleroderma

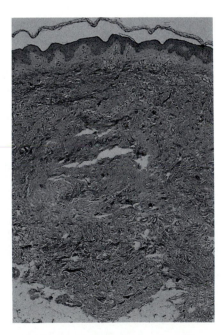

4-1-6 TUBEROUS SCLEROSIS (connective tissue nevus): There is only a suggestion of a stromal alteration in the midreticular dermis. (50×)

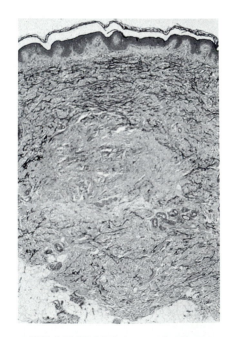

4-1-7 TUBEROUS SCLEROSIS (connective tissue nevus; elastic tissue stain): Elastic tissue stains show a discrete zone of elastic tissue loss in the midreticular dermis. (50×)

4-2 CUTIS LAXA

CLINICAL DESCRIPTION

Etiology and Incidence

This rare disorder occurs in four forms: (1) autosomal recessive (severe); (2) autosomal dominant (mild); (3) X-linked with deficiency of lysyl oxidase probably related to defective copper transport and (4) an acquired form. The X-linked form (also known as occipital horn syndrome and formerly called Ehlers-Danlos syndrome type IX) is probably allelic with the gene for Menkes' disease.

Clinical Features

In the genetic types, the skin manifestations are present at birth or shortly thereafter. The skin hangs in loose folds (Figure 4-2-1A), with the entire body involved, and is hyperextensible but does not spring back into place after releasing tension (Figure 4-2-1B). Affected children may have a hooked nose, ectropion, and long earlobes. Men with this disorder may be impotent. The skin changes become less obvious with age except for the autosomal recessive disorder where progression of the disease may occur with death from pulmonary emphysema or cardiovascular disease.

Other manifestations may include hernias, rectal prolapse, diverticulae of the bladder and gastrointestinal tract, hoarseness, emphysema, corneal clouding, mental retardation, athetosis, and bone abnormalities, in particular occipital horns and broad clavicles in the X-linked type. The acquired form may be associated with other illnesses and may follow a febrile episode, or allergic reaction, urticaria, drug eruption, or erythema multiforme. Some patients only have cutaneous involvement, but some also have internal manifestations.

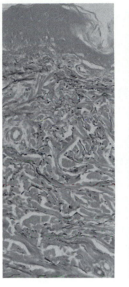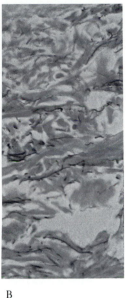

A   B

4-2-2 CUTIS LAXA: **A** Elastic tissue stains of cutis laxa, showing diminished papillary dermal elastic tissue. Some fibers in the dermis are thickened with fragmented ends. (20×) **B** Elastic tissue, showing elastic tissue thickening and fragmentation. (100×)

Differential Diagnosis

Ehlers-Danlos syndrome
Pseudoxanthoma elasticum
Geroderma osteodysplastica
De Barsy syndrome
Lenz-Majewski syndrome
Intrauterine exposure to penicillamine

HISTOLOGICAL DESCRIPTION

The histological features on hematoxylin and eosin-stained sections in cutis laxa are usually unimpressive. Sparse perivascular lymphohistiocytic inflammatory infiltrate without any other significant abnormalities may be seen.

The diagnostic changes in cutis laxa are seen in elastic tissue stains. Elastic tissue fibers may show thickening and have a distinctly granular appearance throughout their length (Figure 4-2-2). In some cases, there is diminution or complete absence of elastic tissue fibers. Fragmentation, shortening, or thinning of fibers may also be seen.

Cutis laxa of the acquired type may be preceded by an inflammatory and/or vesicular eruption. The vesicles in this condition are located in the subepidermal position and may have an infiltrate of neutrophils. Histological changes in the acquired type of cutis laxa are similar to those in the congenital type as well as to those in other postinflammatory anetodermas.

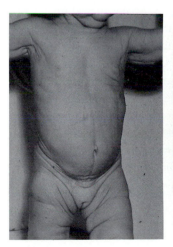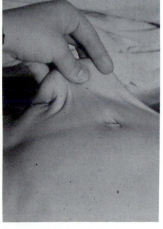

A   B

4-2-1 CUTIS LAXA: **A** Note hanging folds of skin in this patient with cutis laxa. **B** Hyperextensible skin.

Differential Diagnosis
Anetoderma
Dermatitis herpetiformis

4-3 ELASTOSIS PERFORANS SERPIGINOSA

CLINICAL DESCRIPTION

Elastosis perforans serpiginosa may be a marker of an underlying systemic disorder.

Etiology and Incidence
The disorder is generally seen in males over ten years of age. It is probably inherited as an autosomal dominant. The importance of its presence is its association with other systemic disorders in 44% of cases.

Clinical Features
Elastosis perforans serpiginosa appears on the face, neck, antecubital fossae, elbows, and knees and seems to be a marker of systemic disease (see Differential Diagnosis). Linear, arciform serpiginous arrangements of erythematous keratotic papules measuring up to 20 cm in length are present (Figure 4-3-1). These papules are asymptomatic.

Differential Diagnosis
Ehlers-Danlos syndrome
Down's syndrome
Osteogenesis imperfecta
Cutis laxa
Systemic sclerosis
Pseudoxanthoma elasticum
Rothmund-Thomson syndrome

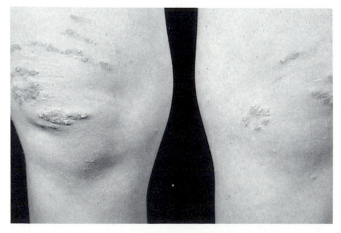

4-3-1 ELASTOSIS PERFORANS SERPIGINOSA: Typical erythematous keratotic papules arranged in an arciform distribution.

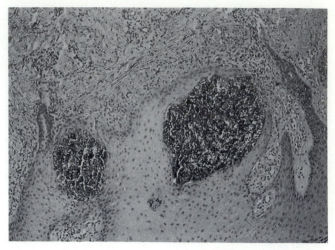

4-3-2 ELASTOSIS PERFORANS SERPIGINOSA: Several foci of altered elastic tissue in the papillary dermis and within intraepidermal channels. (40×)

Marfan's syndrome
Acrogeria
Penicillamine therapy
Renal disease

HISTOLOGICAL DESCRIPTION

The histological features of elastosis perforans serpiginosa on hematoxylin and eosin-stained sections often are a central, almost nodular area of epidermal hyperplasia within which intraepidermal collections of altered basophilic staining elastic tissue may be seen (Figure 4-3-2). This may occur within intraepidermal channels and may even appear to be part of a follicular structure. In the sites of altered tissue there is amorphous basophilic staining material as well as acute inflammatory cells, fragmented cells, and partially altered fibers that will stain eosinophilic. Adjacent to the areas of epithelial hyperplasia are chronic inflammation and elastic tissue that is increased in size and which has altered stainability. Elastic tissue stains confirm the presence of altered elastic tissue below, within, and on the epidermal surface (Plate 4-3-1).

The elastic tissue in elastosis perforans associated with genetic disorders is different than that seen in elastosis perforans secondary to penicillamine ingestion. The latter shows a greater number of enlarged or hyperplastic elastic fibers in the mid- and deep dermis that appear branched.

Differential Diagnosis
Reactive perforating collagenosis
Perforating folliculitis
Perforating granuloma annulare
Kyrle's disease

4-4 EPIDERMOLYSIS BULLOSA

CLINICAL DESCRIPTION

The mechanobullous disorders are a varied group of genetic diseases. Minimal trauma produces blistering in affected children. Classification of these entities is based on histologic, clinical, and genetic information. The three major categories of disease are simplex, junctional, and dystrophic. Table 4-4-1 lists many clinical variations of the disorder.

Etiology and Incidence

Epidermolysis bullosa simplex occurs in 1 birth per 50,000. The severe recessive dystrophic form is rarer, occurring in 1 birth per 500,000.

Remarkable progress has been made in understanding the molecular basis of two forms of epidermolysis bullosa. Studies in several EB families with Dowling-Meara form revealed point mutations of keratin genes for K5 and K14 on chromosome 12 or 17 respectively.

In dystrophic types, especially dominant dystrophic EB, the causative mutation appears to be on the gene encoding type VII collagen (COL7A1), the major component of anchoring fibrils. This gene is located at chromosome band 3p21. There is also evidence that mutations of this same gene underlie the defect in recessive dystrophic EB.

Abnormal and decreased hemidesmosomes are found in the junctional type.

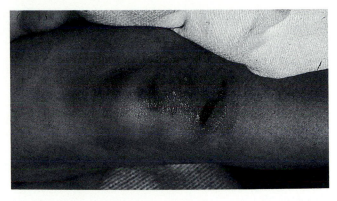

4-4-2 EPIDERMOLYSIS BULLOSA: Note herpetiform blisters milia on extremity.

Differential Diagnosis

Friction blisters
Epidermolytic hyperkeratosis
Staphylococcal scalded skin syndrome
Denudation secondary to herpes simplex virus infection
Dermatitis herpetiformis
Chronic bullous disease of childhood
Dyskeratosis congenita
E.D. aquisita

HISTOLOGICAL DESCRIPTION

The essential feature of all types of epidermolysis bullosa on hematoxylin and eosin-stained sections is a subepidermal blister without associated inflammation. Biopsy study of older lesions may show epidermal regrowth, which may be interpreted as an intraepidermal blister. Therefore, clinical correlation with the site and time of biopsy is important. The subepidermal

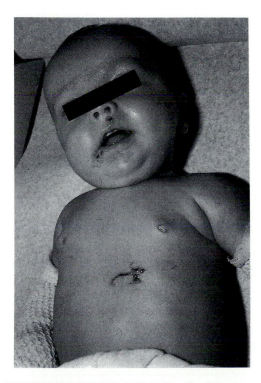

4-4-1 EPIDERMOLYSIS BULLOSA: Dowling-Meara type, in a child; note herpetiform blisters on trunk.

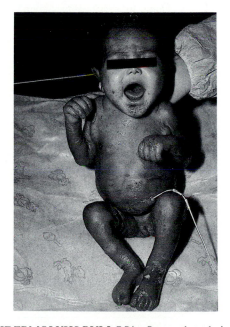

4-4-3 EPIDERMOLYSIS BULLOSA: Severe denudation and loss of nails in junctional type.

4-4-1   Epidermolysis Bullosa Types

Type	Inheritance	Level of Blister Formation	Clinical Features	Specific Structural Defect
Epidermolysis simplex	Dominant	Intraepidermal		
Localized (Weber Cockayne)			Blisters on hands and feet made worse by increased temperature; nails, mucous membrane, teeth spared; improves with age	Spinous cell cytolysis, K5, K14
Generalized (Koebner)			Same as localized; nails, mucous membrane, teeth may be involved	Basal cell cytolysis K5, K14
Dowling-Meara (Figs. 4-4-1, 4-4-2)			Herpetiform blisters; severe; involves oral mucous membranes and nails; hyperkeratosis of palms and soles; may clear with high fever	Tonofilament clumping K5, K14
Ogna			Similar to localized type; bruising tendency; onychogryphosis; linked to erythrocyte GPT locus (glutamic pyruvic transaminase)	Basal cell cytolysis
Mottled pigmentation			Like generalized; increase or decrease in pigmentation on trunk and extremities	Basal cell cytolysis
Junctional (Fig. 4-4-3)	Recessive	Within lamina lucida		Hemidesmosome defect
Gravis (Herlitz)			Severe; heals with granulation tissue; prominent perioral involvement; all MM involved; dysplastic teeth; nail loss	Hemidesmosome defect
Mitis			Same as gravis but milder; heals with atrophy; alopecia; improves with age	Hemidesmosome defect
Inversa			Same as mitis but blisters concentrated in flexures	Hemidesmosome defect
Progressiva			Onset at 5–8 years of age; worsening course	Hemidesmosome defect and amorphous deposits in lamina lucida
Dystrophic	Dominant (Plate 4-4-1)	Separation below B-M		Anchoring fibrils abnormal and decreased (type VII collagen defect)
Hypertrophic			Blisters localized to extremities; healing with scars and milia; nails lost or dystrophic; MM normal, teeth normal	Defect not found in nonblistered skin
Albopapuloidea			Same as hypertrophic; MM can be affected albopapuloid lesions on trunk	Defect in blistered skin
Dystrophic	Recessive	Separation below B-M		Absent or decreased anchoring fibrils (type VII collagen defect)
Gravis (Fig. 4-4-4, Fig. 4-4-5)			Severe; generalized blistering and scarring; severe MM involvement; chronic anemia; fusion of fingers and toes; esophageal stenosis	
Mitis			Essentially the same as gravis	
Localized			Essentially the same as gravis	
Inversa			Essentially the same as gravis	

B-M = basement membrane; MM = mucous membrane

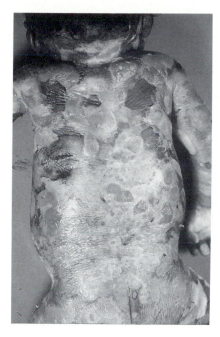

4-4-4 EPIDERMOLYSIS BULLOSA: Generalized blistering, denudation, and scarring seen in recessive dystrophic type.

blistering changes in this condition are often associated with small intraepidermal keratinous cysts (milia). This finding, combined with the features of extremity skin, is often helpful in the differential diagnosis of subepidermal blistering diseases.

Epidermolysis bullosa simplex develops secondary to degeneration of the basal cells. This change can be seen in early developing lesions of this condition or in skin that has been traumatized and biopsied within ten to fifteen minutes. The sites of separation, electron microscopic findings, and immunofluorescent patterns for the remaining types of epidermolysis bullosa are presented in Tables 4-4-2 and 4-4-3.

Differential Diagnosis
Porphyria cutanea tarda

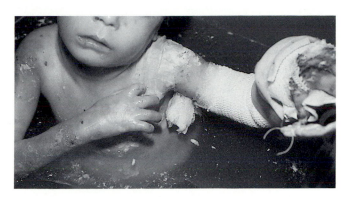

4-4-5 EPIDERMOLYSIS BULLOSA: Child in Figure 4-4-4 following surgery for fused digits.

4-4-2   Epidermolysis Bullosa

	Immunofluorescence
Epidermolysis bullosa simplex	
Generalized	BP antigen; Type IV collagen, laminin at the floor of the blister
Localized	BP antigen; Type IV collagen, laminin at the floor of the blister
Dowling-Meara	BP antigen; Type IV collagen, laminin at the floor of the blister
Ogna	BP antigen; Type IV collagen, laminin at the floor of the blister
Mottled pigmentation	BP antigen; Type IV collagen, laminin at the floor of the blister
Junctional	
Progressive	BP antigen at roof of blister; Type IV collagen, laminin at the floor of the blister
Dystrophic	
Dominant	BP antigen at roof of blister; Type IV collagen, laminin, bullous pemphigoid antigen at the roof of the blister

BP = bullous pemphigoid

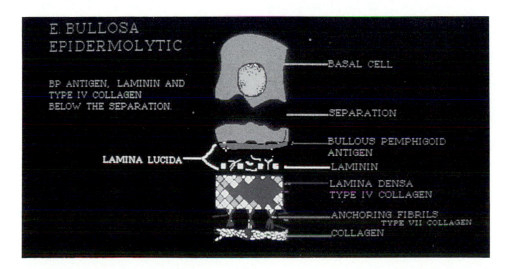

4-4-6 EPIDERMOLYSIS BULLOSA: Schematic drawing of simplex type. Note location of the split within the epidermis.

4-4-3   Histological Features of Epidermolysis Bullosa

	Light Microscopy	*Electron Microscopy*
Epidermolysis bullosa simplex (Fig. 4-4-6)		
Generalized	Basal cell swelling and degeneration (Fig. 4-4-7)	Cytolysis of basal cells, tonofilament lysis, cytolysis (Fig. 4-4-8)
Localized (recurrent bullous eruption of hands and feet)	Intraepidermal bulla in the upper stratum malpighii; dyskeratosis of epidermal cells	Epidermal cell cytolysis; tonofilament lysis
Dowling-Meara	Basal cell swelling and degeneration (Fig. 4-4-9)	Basal cell cytolysis; tonofilaments clumped and still attached to hemidesmosomes (Fig. 4-4-10)
Ogna	Basal cell cytolysis and degeneration are the earliest bullous changes.	Basal cell cytolysis; tonofilament lysis
Mottled pigmentation	Basal cell cytolysis and degeneration are the earliest bullous changes.	Basal cell cytolysis; tonofilament lysis
Junctional (Fig. 4-4-11)	Subepidermal blister; no inflammatory infiltrate	Separation in the lamina lucida; anchoring fibrils normal; hypoplasia of hemidesmosomes in nonblistered areas
Progressive	Subepidermal blister without inflammation	Depositions of amorphous material in the lamina lucida; separation in lamina lucida; hemidesmosomes normal
Dystrophic (Fig. 4-4-12)		
Dominant	Subepidermal blister (Figs. 4-4-13, 4-4-14)	Blister below basal lamina; anchoring fibrils absent in adjacent skin (Fig. 4-4-15)
Recessive	Subepidermal blister	Blister below basal lamina; absence of anchoring fibrils; collagenolysis

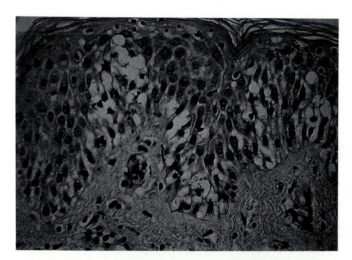

4-4-7 EPIDERMOLYSIS BULLOSA: Vacuolar degeneration in the basal cells without associated spongiosis or inflammation, in simplex type. This destruction will lead to a bulla. The reaction occurred five to ten minutes after injury with a pencil eraser. (200×)

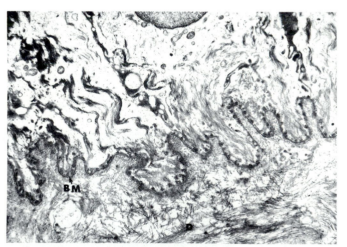

4-4-8 EPIDERMOLYSIS BULLOSA: Basal cell cytolysis. Anchoring fibers are still attached at the basal lamina. Hemidesmosomes are intact. BM, basement membrane; D, dermis. (1200×). (From Zelickson AS: Ultrastructure of normal and abnormal skin. Philadelphia: Lea and Febiger, 1967. Reprinted with permission.)

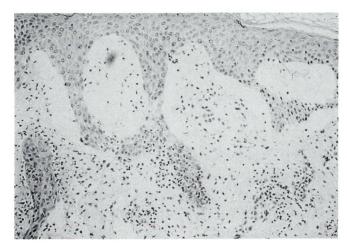

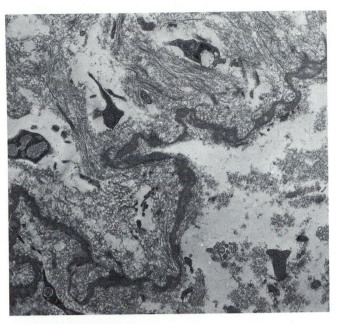

4-4-9 EPIDERMOLYSIS BULLOSA: Routine histological study of Dowling-Meara type shows prominent papillary dermal edema associated with basilar keratinocyte cytolysis. (40×)

4-4-10 EPIDERMOLYSIS BULLOSA: Electron microscopy of Dowling-Meara type shows clumped tonofilaments attached to desmosomes. (2500×)

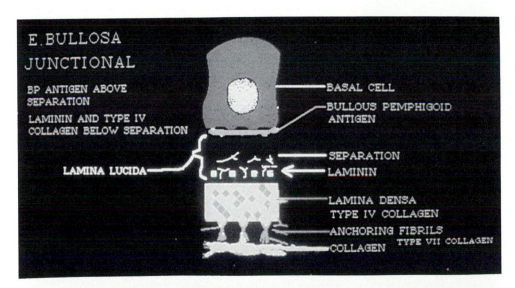

4-4-11 EPIDERMOLYSIS BULLOSA: Schematic drawing of junctional type. Note the level of separation within the lamina lucida.

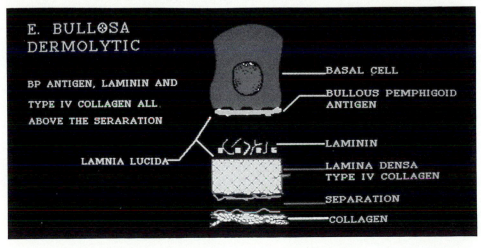

4-4-12 EPIDERMOLYSIS BULLOSA: Schematic drawing of dermolytic type. Note the level of separation within the dermis.

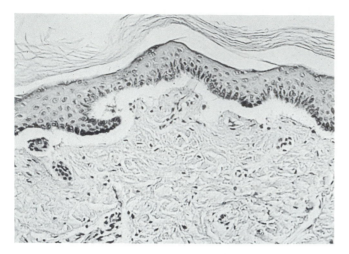

4-4-13 EPIDERMOLYSIS BULLOSA: Epidermolysis dermolytic type shows a subepidermal bulla. There is minimal dermal inflammation. (100×)

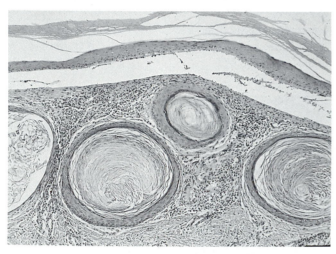

4-4-14 EPIDERMOLYSIS BULLOSA: Dermolytic type, showing many milia. (100×)

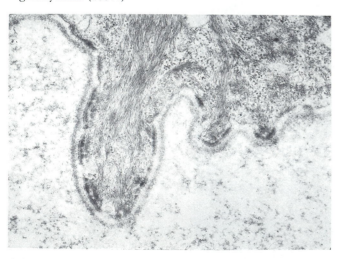

4-4-15 EPIDERMOLYSIS BULLOSA: The basal lamina is intact. The anchoring fibrils are lysed. (2000×). (From Zelickson AS: Ultrastructure of normal and abnormal skin. Philadelphia: Lea and Febiger, 1967. Reprinted with permission.)

4-5 ICHTHYOSIS

Two of the ichthyotic entities have specific histological findings and, therefore, will be discussed.

ICHTHYOSIS VULGARIS

CLINICAL DESCRIPTION

Etiology and Incidence

Ichthyosis vulgaris is the mildest and most common form, occurring at a rate of 1 in 250 to 1 in 1,000 persons. It manifests clinically after three months of age and is lifelong. The condition is inherited as an autosomal dominant trait.

Clinical Features

The extensors of the extremities are involved to a greater degree than the rest of the body, with the flexures usually spared (Figure 4-5-1). Frequently there is thickening and hyperlinearity of the palms and soles (Figure 4-5-2). Skin changes are characterized by small, fine scales, which may be larger over the legs. Keratosis pilaris, an associated finding, may be especially prominent on the arms and legs. The eruption is generally worse in winter and improves during the summer months. The condition is associated with atopy, especially atopic dermatitis.

Differential Diagnosis

Acquired ichthyosis
Chronic malnutrition
Lymphoma (especially Hodgkin's)
X-linked ichthyosis
Drugs that reduce cholesterol:
    Triparanol
    Nicotinic acid
    Dixyrazine
    Butyrophenones
Systemic lupus erythematosus

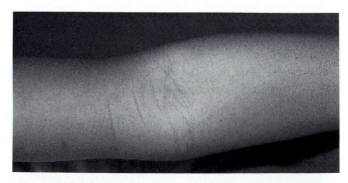

4-5-1 ICHTHYOSIS VULGARIS: Flexural sparing is seen in this patient.

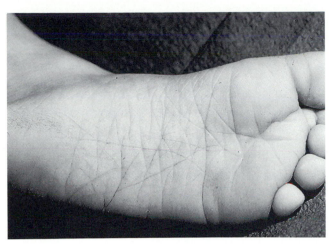

4-5-2 ICHTHYOSIS VULGARIS: Thickening and hyperlinearity of the sole.

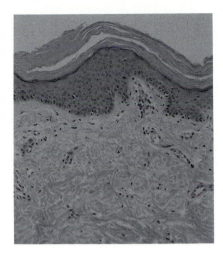

4-5-3 ICHTHYOSIS VULGARIS: Hyperkeratosis with a thinned granular cell layer. The dermis shows a few lymphocytes about dermal vessels. (40×)

HISTOLOGICAL DESCRIPTION

The histological features of ichthyosis vulgaris are absolute hyperkeratosis without associated hypergranulosis with a granular layer that is either thinned (one to two cells thick) or absent (Figure 4-5-3). Follicular hyperkeratosis may be associated in the overall hyperkeratotic process. The inflammatory response is absent to minimal, consisting mainly of a few perivascular lymphocytes.

Differential Diagnosis

Normal flexural skin
Aged skin
Keratosis pilaris

4-5-1 Classification of Ichthyosis

Type	Classical Appearance	Associated Features	Inheritance
X-linked ichthyosis	Dark large scales (dirty appearance); lateral face and neck involved; flexures variably involved; palms and soles normal	Corneal opacities (benign); steroid sulfatase deficiency; testicular seminoma (rare) may be part of a contiguous gene deletion syndrome with variable features of Kallmann syndrome, short stature, chondrodysplasia punctata, and/or mental retardation depending on extent of deletion	X-linked recessive (about 90% caused by gene deletion)
NBCIE* (lamellar ichthyosis)			
Classical	Dense, platelike, dark scale; generalized with all flexures involved; palms and soles involved	Prematurity; "collodion" membrane; ectropion; harlequin fetus	Autosomal recessive
Small scale	Finer, whiter scale; background erythema	Same as classical	Autosomal recessive
Bullous congenital ichthyosiform erythroderma (epidermolytic hyperkeratosis)	Erythroderma bullae and denudation in newborn period, later verrucous gray-brown scales over most of skin surface including flexural areas; keratosis palmaris et plantaris; no extropion usually; malodorous scale	Defects in K1 and K10	Usually autosomal dominant; some autosomal recessive

*Nonbullous congenital ichthyosiform erythroderma

4-5-2 Features of Ichthyosis

Ichthyosis	Clinical Appearance	Associated Features	Mode of Inheritance
Erythrokeratoderma variabolis	Transient migratory erythema; plaques of erythema; thickened palms and soles		Autosomal dominant; occasionally recessive
Ichthyosis linearis circumflexa (Netherton's syndrome)	Background erythema; polycyclic eruption with hyperkeratotic margin; flexures hyperkeratotic	Atopic diathesis; trichorrhexis invaginata; aminoaciduria	Unknown
Refsum's disease	Variable ichthyosis (nonspecific)	Polyneuritis; nerve deafness; retinitis pigmentosa; increased phytanic acid (serum); increased CSF protein	Autosomal recessive
Sjögren-Larsson syndrome	Mild nonbullous lamellar ichthyosis	Spastic paralysis; mental retardation; macular retinal degeneration; fatty alcohol oxidoreductase deficiency	Autosomal recessive
Rud's syndrome	Lamellar ichthyosis or X-linked ichthyosis	Gigantism or dwarfism; mental deficiency; hypogonadism; epilepsy; alopecia; nerve deafness; absent or hypoplastic teeth	Autosomal recessive or X-linked due to steroid sulfatase deficiency
Tay's syndrome	Red, scaly skin; sparse, brittle hair, keratoderma of palms and soles	Close-set eyes; beaked nose; sunken cheeks (progerialike); hair defects; pili torti or trichorrhexis nodosa; impaired intelligence; abnormal sulfur content of hair; one form with excision repair defect like xeroderma pigmentosum, group D	Autosomal recessive
BIDS	Brittle hair; short stature	Impaired intelligence; decreased fertility	Probable autosomal recessive
IBIDS	Ichthyosis and BIDS		
PIBID	Photosensitivity and IBIDS	Abnormal sulfur content of hair; one form with excision repair defect like xeroderma pigmentosum group D	
Conradi's disease (chondrodysplasia punctata)	Scaling of skin in whorl-like pattern; follicular atrophoderma; pigmentary changes; cicatricial alopecia; hyperkeratosis of palms and soles	Shortening of humerus and femur; lens opacities; other ocular changes; stippled epiphysis; asymmetric lesions in females with XD form; some forms associated with perioxosome abnormalities	Autosomal recessive; autosomal dominant, X-linked; recessive and X-linked dominant; some forms associated with perioxosome abnormalities; asymmetric in females with X-linked dominant form
CHILD syndrome	Unilateral ichthyosiform erythroderma	Congenital hemidysplasia; limb defects and other ipsilateral defects of internal organs and/or brain	X-linked dominant
KID syndrome	Fine, dry scales; follicular hyperkeratotic spines; hyperkeratosis of palms and soles	Keratitis; neurosensory deafness	Unknown
Neutral lipid storage disease		Cataracts; deafness; ataxia; droplets in many cells	Autosomal recessive
Multiple sulfatase deficiency	Like steroid sulfatase deficiency	Neurodegeneration; organomegaly; skeletal dysplasia (includes steroid sulfatase deficiency)	Autosomal recessive

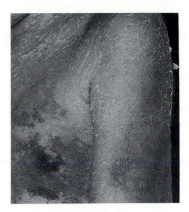

4-5-4 EPIDERMOLYTIC HYPERKERATOSIS: Note scales, erythema, and flexural involvement in this patient.

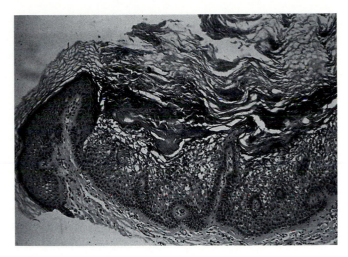

4-5-5 EPIDERMOLYTIC HYPERKERATOSIS: Marked vacuole change of the upper epidermis. The basal layer is intact and unaffected. There is also marked hyperkeratosis. (40×)

EPIDERMOLYTIC HYPERKERATOSIS

CLINICAL DESCRIPTION

Etiology and Incidence

Epidermolytic hyperkeratosis occurs at a frequency of 1 in 300,000 births. The condition is inherited as an autosomal dominant disorder. Several families with epidermolytic hyperkeratosis show linkage to chromosome 12 or 17 near the gene loci for the keratins. Defects in keratin genes (K1 and K10) are now known to be associated with this disorder. Mutations were found in the carboxy terminal of the rod domain of keratin 1 in one family, and the amino terminal of the rod domain of keratin 10 in two other families. Prenatal diagnosis is possible.

Clinical Features

The lower face is involved more than the upper face. The trunk and extremities are variably involved. The flexures are always involved, being moist and frequently odiferous (Figure 4-5-4). The palms and soles are usually affected. This type of ichthyosis may present in newborns, with extensive denudation of the skin (Plate 4-5-1) much like epidermolysis bullosa. More commonly, generalized erythema and scaliness appear in the first few weeks of life. Tiny vesicles or bullae begin to appear. Blistering diminishes with age, but does persist in 20% of patients. Coarse verrucous scales that are thick and brown are present, especially in the flexures. Pyogenic infections frequently occur. Severity varies greatly between families.

Differential Diagnosis

Epidermolysis bullosa
Herpes simplex virus
Urticaria pigmentosa
Staphylococcal scalded skin syndrome

HISTOLOGICAL DESCRIPTION

On routine sections there is well-defined hyperkeratosis of the orthokeratotic type. Underlying the hyperkeratosis there is vacuolar degeneration of the granular cell that includes the midspinous layer.

The basal cell layer is not involved in this vacuolar degenerative process (Figure 4-5-5). When this change is severe, intraepidermal bullae may occur. The granular cell layer in this process is thickened, with increased numbers of irregularly shaped keratohyaline granules (Plate 4-5-2, Figures 4-5-6 and 4-5-7). The mitotic rate in this portion of the epidermis is increased. The dermis shows an inflammatory infiltrate that varies in severity and consists of lymphocytes.

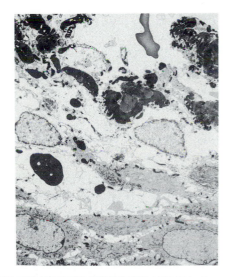

4-5-6 EPIDERMOLYTIC HYPERKERATOSIS: Large clumped keratohyaline granules. The desmosome connections are altered. Several cells over the surface show excessive tonofilament production. (1200×)

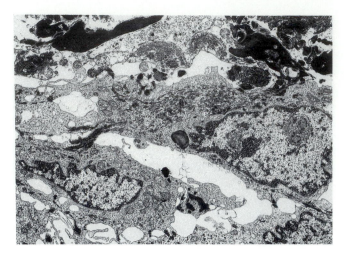

4-5-7 EPIDERMOLYTIC HYPERKERATOSIS: Excess tonofilament production associated with clumped keratohyaline granules. (200×)

Differential Diagnosis
Linear epidermal nevus
Darier's disease
Transient acantholytic dermatosis
Warty dyskeratoma
Seborrheic keratosis

4-6 FOCAL DERMAL HYPOPLASIA

CLINICAL DESCRIPTION

Focal dermal hypoplasia (Goltz syndrome) affects the skin, bones, eyes, nails, and teeth.

Etiology and Incidence
The inheritance of this rare disorder is most likely X-linked dominant with lethality in males or autosomal dominant with sex limitation.

Clinical Features
The skin changes are usually present at birth. They include linear areas of denudation erythema or pigmentation. Characteristic yellow, baggy herniations of fat occur through atrophic skin. Reticular cribriform hyper- or hypopigmentation occurs. Papillomas appear in or near the mouth, anogenital region, axillae, and inguinal region and around the umbilicus. Other features include partial alopecia, dystrophic nails, hypoplastic teeth, delayed eruption of teeth, syndactyly of the third and fourth fingers, skeletal defects (scoliosis, vertebral asymmetry, osteopathia striata on x-rays, syndactyly, cleft hand), ophthalmic abnormalities (strabismus, coloboma, microphthalmia), and short stature. Several females with deletions of the distal

short arm of the X (Xp.22.3-p.22.2) have recently been described who have overlapping features of this syndrome.

Differential Diagnosis
Ectodermal dysplasia
Incontinentia pigmenti
Poikiloderma congenitale
Linear scleroderma
Nevus lipomatosis cutaneous superficialis
Amniotic bands
Aplasia cutis congenita

HISTOLOGICAL DESCRIPTION

The striking histological feature is an absence of or marked thinning of the dermis. The remaining collagen is composed only of thin strands or fibers. The usual formation of collagen bundles is not seen. Adipose tissue replaces the dermis and in some areas may be in contact with the epidermis. The overlying epidermis is effaced but does not show other significant changes. There is a sparse perivascular infiltrate of lymphocytes.

Differential Diagnosis
Nevus lipomatosis

4-7 INCONTINENTIA PIGMENTI AND HYPOMELANOSIS OF ITO

CLINICAL DESCRIPTION

Incontinentia pigmenti and hypomelanosis of Ito are frequently associated with systemic findings.

Etiology and Incidence
Incontinentia Pigmenti
Incontinentia pigmenti is a hereditary disorder that affects the skin, central nervous system, eyes, and skeletal and immune systems. It is thought to be inherited as an X-linked dominant (lethal to males). The familial form of this disorder maps to Xq28 by linkage analysis. Several isolated cases of females with pigmentation similar to stage III of incontinentia pigmenti (see below) have had X-autosome translocations with breakpoints clustered in the proximal short arm of the X.

Hypomelanosis of Ito
Hypomelanosis of Ito is a pigmentary dyscrasia now known to be associated with chromosomal mosaicism in many cases. Often, this is detectable only in the skin. In a few families with recurrences (rare), autosomal dominant inheritance is possible, but the vast majority of cases are sporadic.

Clinical Features
Incontinentia Pigmenti

Ninety-six percent of patients with incontinentia pigmenti have lesions of the skin by six weeks of age. Most have the vesicular first stage. Linear crops of vesicles involve the trunk and extremities, especially the posterior legs. This phase lasts weeks to months and in 70% of cases is associated with peripheral eosinophilia. The second verrucous phase is seen in 70% of patients (Plate 4-7-1). Linear, warty lesions disappear spontaneously in several months. The third pigmentary stage is seen in almost all children. Swirling bands of brown to blue-gray pigmentation develop on most any skin surface, not necessarily previously affected areas (Figure 4-7-1). This pigmentation peaks at two years of age and then fades, at times completely by adulthood. The last stage is manifest by streaked hypopigmented lesions on the lower extremities. This finding may be the only clue in a female carrier of this disorder and is important for genetic counseling of families.

Other manifestations include alopecia, dystrophic nails, pegged or conical teeth (Figure 4-7-2), anodontia, microcephaly, seizures, less commonly mental retardation, progressive retinal changes, optic atrophy, blindness, and immunologic abnormalities (chemotactic defects).

Hypomelanosis of Ito

This pigmentation anomaly is noted at birth or shortly thereafter as asymmetric streaked or whorled hypopigmentation (Figure 4-7-3). Sometimes hyperpigmentation is also observed. The changes can be unilateral or bilateral. The scalp, palms, and soles are not involved. Unlike incontinentia pigmenti, there is no vesicular or warty stage.

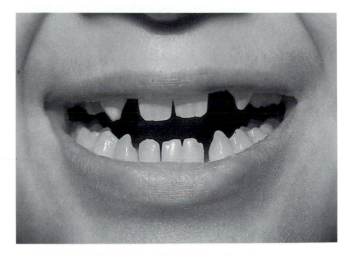

4-7-2 INCONTINENTIA PIGMENTI: Conical teeth.

Fifty percent of patients have associated systemic manifestations, including seizures, mental retardation, strabismus, nystagmus, microphthalmia, macrocephaly, skeletal changes, and scoliosis.

Differential Diagnosis
Incontinentia Pigmenti

Vesicular Stage:
Herpes simplex virus
Acropustulosis of infancy
Histiocytosis X
Eosinophilic pustular folliculitis
Erythema toxicum neonatorum
Epidermolysis bullosa
Bullous pemphigoid
Focal dermal hypoplasie of Goltz

Verrucous Stage:
Warts

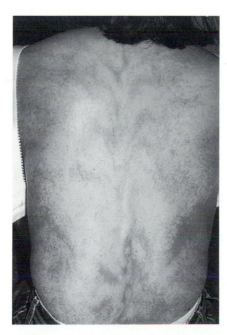

4-7-1 INCONTINENTIA PIGMENTI: Swirling pigmentation.

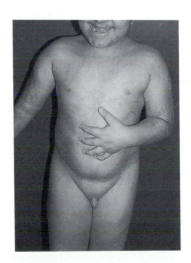

4-7-3 HYPOMELANOSIS OF ITO: Whorled hypopigmentation.

Pigmented Stage:
Franceschetti-Jadassohn syndrome
Conical teeth (in children with ectodermal dysplasia or
     syphilis)
Epidermal nevus

Hypomelanosis of Ito
Achromic nevus
Nevus anemicus

HISTOLOGICAL DESCRIPTION

Incontinentia Pigmenti
The histological features of incontinentia pigmenti vary, depending on the stage at which the biopsy specimen was taken. In the vesicular stage, hypokeratosis associated with acanthosis, eosinophilic spongiosis, and the presence of intraepidermal microvesicles filled with eosinophils (Figure 4-7-4) are seen. The epidermis in the nonvesicular areas shows occasional dyskeratotic cells as well as focal areas of swirl-like keratinization. The dermal reaction is that of a marked inflammatory infiltrate, the predominant cell being the eosinophil with an admixture of lymphocytes and histiocytes.

In the verrucous hyperkeratotic stage, hyperkeratosis, acanthosis, papillomatosis, and small focal individual, nodular areas of keratinization within the epidermis (Figure 4-7-5) are seen. These swirls of keratinocytes resemble the squamous eddies of inverted follicular keratoses. The dermal reaction is that of chronic inflammation in which there are numerous melanophages filled with pigment. The inflammatory infiltrate in the dermis is focally exocytotic to the epidermis and in these areas causes basal cell vacuolar degeneration. The

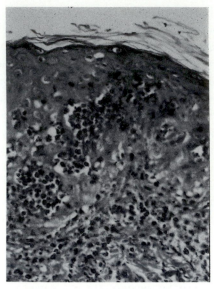

4-7-5 INCONTINENTIA PIGMENTI: Nonbullous form, showing marked eosinophil exocytosis into an acanthotic epidermis. (100×)

basal cell layer does not show increased pigment; the hyperpigmentation noted on clinical examination is produced by the presence of dermal melanin.

Hypomelanosis of Ito
The features of hypomelanosis of Ito seen on hematoxylin and eosin-stained sections are not diagnostic. On sections stained for melanin (Fontana-Masson and other silver precipitate stains) there is a decrease in melanin granules in the basal layer of the epidermis. In areas of hypopigmentation on fresh tissue using the Dopa staining technique, melanocytes are smaller and less dendritic than those in an affected area.

Differential Diagnosis
Incontinentia Pigmenti
Erythema toxicum neonatorum
Pre-bullous bullous pemphigoid
Bullous pemphigoid
Eosinophilic spongiotic dermatosis

Hypomelanosis of Ito
Vitiligo
Post inflammatory hypopigmentation

4-8 KERATOSIS FOLLICULARIS (DARIER'S DISEASE)

CLINICAL DESCRIPTION
Attentiveness to distribution of lesions and a good family history will often enable the diagnosis of keratosis follicularis (Darier's disease) during childhood.

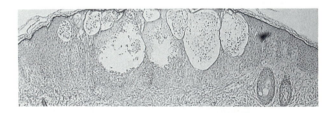

A

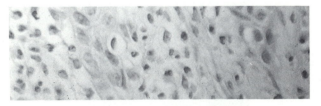

B

4-7-4 INCONTINENTIA PIGMENTI: This composite section shows the vesicular stage, with intraepidermal microvesicles filled with eosinophils. (20×) The lower panel shows eosinophils within the microvesicles. (200×)

Etiology and Incidence

Keratosis follicularis typically occurs between eight and sixteen years of age. The condition is inherited as an autosomal dominant with complete penetrance in adults. Up to one-third of cases may represent new mutations. The gene has recently been mapped to the long arm of chromosome 12. The disease prevalence is estimated to be 1 in 50,000 in the United Kingdom.

Clinical Features

Lesions begin on the seborrheic areas of the body and the flexures of the extremities as tiny, flesh-colored papules. A unilateral zosteriform distribution may be seen in 10% of cases. Greasy, crusted, yellow or brown follicular papules soon appear (Plate 4-8-1). Secondary infection and a foul smell follow. Other findings include acrokeratosis verruciformis of Hopf on the backs of the hands (Plate 4-8-2), punctate keratotic pits on the palms and soles, palmoplantar hyperkeratosis, verrucous white plaques on the mucous membranes, and nail abnormalities (longitudinal red or white streaks and distal subungual wedge-shaped hyperkeratosis) (Plate 4-8-3). Sun exposure seems to cause this condition to flare, while clearing occurs during the winter months.

Differential Diagnosis

Acanthosis nigricans
Ichthyosis vulgaris
Keratosis pilaris
Seborrheic keratosis
Warts
Hailey-Hailey disease

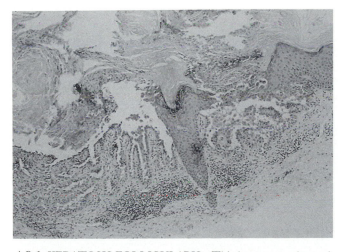

4-8-1 KERATOSIS FOLLICULARIS: This low-power photomicrograph shows hyperkeratosis with parakeratotic grains. There is suprabasilar acantholysis with formation of villi and several small lacunae. (40×)

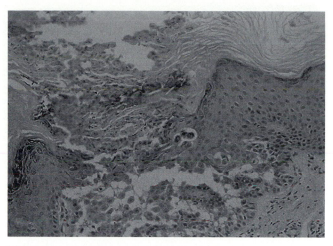

4-8-2 KERATOSIS FOLLICULARIS: High magnification shows corps ronds at the epidermal stratum corneum junction with overlying hyperkeratosis and a few grains in the stratum corneum. There is suprabasilar acantholysis. (400×)

HISTOLOGICAL DESCRIPTION

The histological features are suprabasilar acantholysis with focal midspinous acantholysis surmounted by hyper- and parakeratosis with the presence of dyskeratotic cells (Figure 4-8-1). Dyskeratotic cells are in the form of corps ronds characterized by a central basophilic pyknotic nucleus surrounded by a clear halo (Figure 4-8-2). These cells are usually larger than the cells in the superficial portion of the squamous cell layer where they are most commonly found. The grain type of dyskeratotic cell most closely resembles a small parakeratotic nucleus and can be found at the stratum corneum-epidermal junction, as well as in the areas of acantholysis. The small slitlike spaces that occur in a suprabasilar location, called lacunae, are a common finding in Darier's disease. Villous formation of the dermis may be prominent. The epidermal reaction is proliferative with associated papillomatosis and overlying hyperkeratosis. These changes occur in follicular as well as perifollicular locations. The reaction in the dermis is chronic inflammation with the presence of perivascular lymphocytes and histiocytes.

Differential Diagnosis

Warty dyskeratoma
Hailey-Hailey disease
Grover's disease

4-9 LIPOID PROTEINOSIS

CLINICAL DESCRIPTION

Lipoid proteinosis should be included in the differential diagnosis of a hoarse child.

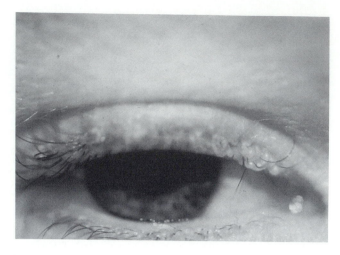

A

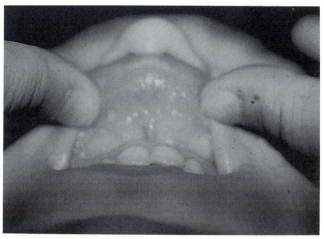

B

4-9-1 LIPOID PROTEINOSIS: **A** Pearly flesh-colored papules lining the upper eyelids. (Courtesy of Corrado Angelo, M.D.) **B** Similar pearly papules on the lower gingiva. (Courtesy of Corrado Angelo, M.D.)

Etiology and Incidence

The disorder is inherited as an autosomal recessive trait which is associated with abnormal deposits of hyaline material in the skin, mucosa, upper respiratory and gastrointestinal tracts, and other visceral organs.

Clinical Features

The first symptom of lipoid proteinosis, hoarseness, begins at birth or early infancy. Cutaneous and mucosal lesions follow. Children often manifest vesicles and pustules. Some lesions are mistaken for impetigo. Atrophic scars (thought to be secondary to impetigo) involve the face and proximal extremities. About 50% have characteristic pearly beadlike papules which involve the lid margins, causing thickened eyelids (Figure 4-9-1). Verrucous plaques are present on the elbows, knees, hands, and feet. Morphea-like plaques on the trunk

may also be seen. A thick, stiff tongue, producing difficulty in swallowing and extrusion of the tongue and eversion of the lips, occurs in adult life. Seventy percent of patients over ten years of age have asymptomatic central nervous system calcifications, and some have seizures. There may be alopecia of the scalp, eyebrows and lashes, hypohidrosis, hypertrichosis, hypoplasia or aplasia of permanent teeth, a yellow waxy appearance with diffuse skin thickening (especially in the flexures), parotid pain and swelling secondary to obstruction of Stensen's duct and impaired nail growth.

Differential Diagnosis
Limited

HISTOLOGICAL DESCRIPTION

The histological features are hyperkeratosis with follicular hyperkeratosis overlying an epidermis that shows atrophy and/or effacement. A striking feature is papillomatosis of the dermis in which there is an amorphous eosinophilic material primarily about the superficial dermal vessels. This material is oriented perpendicularly to the epidermis and extends into the midreticular dermis (Figure 4-9-2). This eosinophilic hyalin like material is noted about the sweat glands and in these areas, sweat glands become atrophic. A similar type of material can be found in the midreticular and lower dermis, usually more focal than in the upper portion of the dermis. The dermal cellular response consists of histiocytes, stellate-appearing fibroblasts, and occasional lymphocytes. The follicular adnexi are not spared in this hyalinizing process. They are often seen surrounded by this material and subsequent atrophy. The arrector pili muscle is invaded by eosinophilic hyalin.

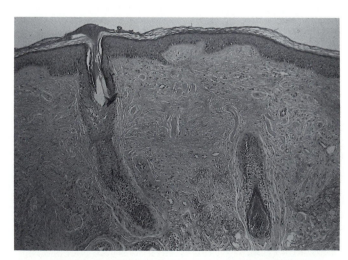

4-9-2 LIPOID PROTEINOSIS: Low magnification shows hyaline material around dermal blood vessels and follicles and in the dermis. (200×)

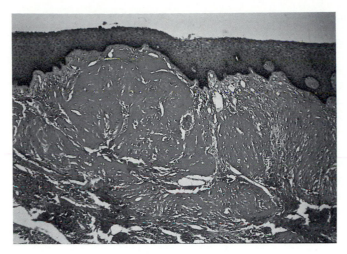

4-9-3 LIPOID PROTEINOSIS: Periodic acid-Schiff stain shows positive staining of the homogeneous material in the superficial dermis.

Special stains show this hyalinlike material to be periodic acid-Schiff–positive and diastase-resistant (Figure 4-9-3). It stains with Alcian blue at pH 2.9 but not at pH 0.7. Staining for lipids results in a positive reaction with Sudan black III. Oil red O stains for cholesterol are also positive. It is thought that this material is a noncollagenous glycolipoprotein.

Differential Diagnosis

Amyloid

Erythropoietic protoporphyria

4-10 MUCOPOLYSACCHARIDOSIS (HUNTER SYNDROME)

CLINICAL DESCRIPTION

Etiology and Incidence

Mucopolysaccharidosis is rare. See Table 4-10-1 for a description.

4-10-1 Mucopolysaccharide Storage Diseases with Skin Changes

Type	Inheritance	Skin Change	Associated Findings	Enzyme Defect	Urinary Findings
IH Hurler	Autosomal recessive	Hirsutism; thick, dry, pale, leathery, inelastic hard skin	Retardation; corneal clouding; hepatosplenomegaly; dyostosis multiplex; death in childhood	α-L-Iduronidase	↑ Dermatan sulfate, heparan sulfate
IS Scheie	Autosomal recessive	Hirsutism; carpal tunnel; bound-down skin over fingers; telangiectasias	Normal intelligence; corneal clouding; milder osteochondrodystrophy; aortic insufficiency; retinitis pigmentosa; normal face in childhood; normal lifespan	α-L-Iduronidase	↑ Dermatan SO_4 heparan SO_4
IH/S Hurler/ Scheie	Autosomal recessive	Intermediate phenotype	Intermediate phenotype	α-L-Iduronidase	Dermatan and heparan SO_4
II Hunter	X-linked recessive	See Hurler/Scheie; cutaneous papules ("pebbling") in reticular pattern over trunk, proximal extremities	Mild retardation; no corneal clouding; deafness; atypical retinitis pigmentosa; cardiovascular and pulmonary disease; slower progress than in Hurler	Iduronate sulfatase	↑ Dermatan sulfate, heparan sulfate
III Sanfilippo A, B, C, D subtypes	Autosomal recessive	Mild hypertrichosis and coarse hair	Severe retardation; mild somatic changes	Heparan N-sulfatase or N-acetyl-d-glucosaminidase	↑ Heparan SO_4
IV Morquio	Autosomal recessive	Skin loose but thickened, especially on extremities; telangiectasias on face	Normal intelligence; corneal clouding; dwarfism; severe orthopedic abnormalities; aortic regurgitation; odontoid hypoplasia	Galactosamine 6-sulfatase or β-galactosidase	↑ Keratan sulfate, chondroitin 6-sulfate

4-10-1   Mucopolysaccharide Storage Diseases with Skin Changes *(continued)*

Type	Inheritance	Skin Change	Associated Findings	Enzyme Defect	Urinary Findings
VI Maroteaux-Lamy	Autosomal recessive	Thickened subcutaneous tissues around fingers	Normal intelligence; dwarfism; hepato-splenomegaly; severe orthopedic changes; corneal clouding; severity and survival vary	Arylsulfatase B	↑ Dermatan SO_4
VII Sly	Autosomal recessive	Hirsutism, skin thickening	Dysostosis multiplex; organomegaly; progressive MR; variable course; cloudy corneas in one type; Hurler-like facies	β-glucuronidase	Dermatan SO_4, heparan SO_4, chondroitin 4-SO_4, chondroitin 6-SO_4

Clinical Features

Although many of the mucopolysaccharidoses have associated skin changes, including thickening and hypertrichosis, only children with Hunter syndrome have truly distinctive cutaneous findings. Before the age of ten years, symmetrically distributed lesions occur in the area from the angle of the scapula to the axillary line. These lesions are flesh-colored to ivory papules or ridges in a reticular pattern (Figure 4-10-1). These changes are also found on the pectoral ridges, neck, and/or upper arms and thighs.

Differential Diagnosis

Connective tissue nevus

HISTOLOGICAL DESCRIPTION

The mucopolysaccharidoses all show metachromatic granules within fibroblasts, causing the fibroblasts to resemble mast cells. Metachromatic material is also noted between collagen bundles and occasionally in some epidermal cells, as well as in eccrine gland and duct cells. These granules stain with alcian blue and colloidal iron. There is no other significant infiltrate in the dermis. Touch smears fixed in absolute alcohol and stained with toluidine blue can aid in office diagnosis (Plates 4-10-1 and 4-10-2).

Differential Diagnosis

Other mucopolysaccharidoses
Mast cell disease

4-11 POROKERATOSIS

CLINICAL DESCRIPTION

A diagnosis of porokeratosis is made easily and can be confirmed histologically.

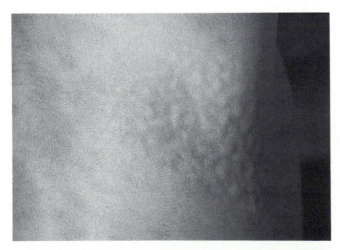

4-10-1 MUCOPOLYSACCHARIDOSIS: Irregular skin surface over lateral aspect of back.

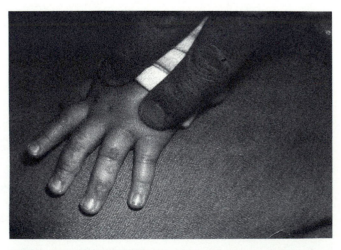

4-11-1 POROKERATOSIS: Note ridged lesions on fingers of this young child.

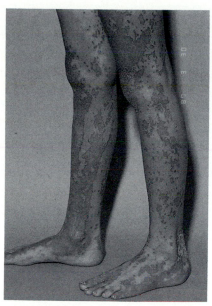

4-11-2 POROKERATOSIS: Systematized porokeratosis. Linear distribution on lower extremities.

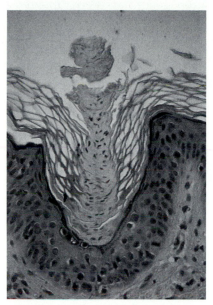

4-11-4 POROKERATOSIS: The cornoid lamella, consisting of stacked parakeratosis. The granular layer under the lamella is thinned. (400×)

Etiology and Incidence

Porokeratosis has an autosomal dominant mode of inheritance, with decreased penetrance in females. Lesions are believed to arise from an abnormal clone of cells with faulty keratinization. Chromosomal aneuploidy has sometimes been detected in lesional material.

Clinical Features

Onset occurs in early childhood. The condition seems to favor the extremities (especially the hands and feet; see Figure 4-11-1), face, neck, genitalia, and mucous membranes. A papule grows to form an annular or circinate lesion with an elevated firm ridge. A linear distribution (Figure 4-11-2) may cause confusion with a linear verrucous epidermal nevus.

Differential Diagnosis

Lichen planus
Lichen sclerosis et atrophicus
Verruca
Epithelial nevus
Granuloma annulare
Tinea corporis
Elastosis perforans serpiginosa

HISTOLOGICAL DESCRIPTION

The histological features are an area of stacked parakeratosis (cornoid lamellae) extending into an invagination of the epidermis; this parakeratosic stack is surrounded by hyperkeratosis (Figures 4-11-3 and 4-11-4). The granular cell layer underlying the cornoid lamella is absent. The cells in the midspinus layer of the epidermis may show a disorderly arrangement and early keratinization. The dermis may show early fibroplasia associated with chronic inflammation of the lymphohistiocytic type. There is no solar elastosis.

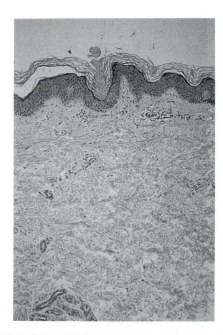

4-11-3 POROKERATOSIS: Low power shows a cornoid lamella in a delled (invaginated) epidermis. There is associated perivascular inflammation. (40×)

Differential Diagnosis

Disseminated porokeratosis

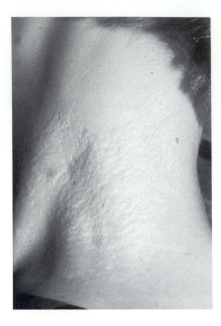

4-12-1 PSEUDOXANTHOMA ELASTICUM: Typical yellow-ish coalescent papules on neck.

4-12 PSEUDOXANTHOMA ELASTICUM

CLINICAL DESCRIPTION

Pseudoxanthoma elasticum is a rare syndrome that is difficult to diagnose in childhood.

Etiology and Incidence

Skin lesions occur in childhood but may be too subtle to be detected and the diagnosis may not be established until the second or third decade of life. The disorder has at least two autosomal recessive and two autosomal dominant forms. They differ in that the recessive and dominant type (type I) has flexural skin changes and significant systemic findings. The skin changes in type II, recessive form are generalized and without systemic changes. In type II of the dominant form there may be mild cardiovascular and retinal changes together with Marfanoid features (loose joints, high arched palate, blue sclerae). Some families assumed to be recessive may actually represent dominant forms of the disease with highly variable expression. Scar biopsy or biopsy of "normal" skin in predilection sites may be helpful in establishing the diagnosis in suspected cases.

Clinical Features

Lesions are frequently overlooked because of a lack of symptoms and their insignificant size. The areas most commonly affected are the neck (Figure 4-12-1) and axillae. The flexures, perineum, and thighs are also involved. Skin changes include soft, yellowish, coalescing papules that form polygonal plaques. Elastosis perforans serpiginosa may occur. Later, the skin is loose

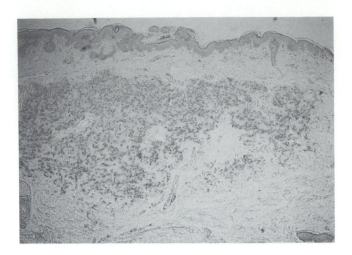

4-12-2 PSEUDOXANTHOMA ELASTICUM: Low power shows calcified swollen elastic tissue fibers in the middermis. Calcium stains reddish purple on hematoxylin and eosin sections. (40×)

and wrinkled. Eighty-five percent of affected adults have angioid streaks of the retina (also seen in sickle cell disease, Paget's disease of bone, ITP, acromegaly, Ehlers Danlos syndrome, and lead poisoning) which may lead to loss of vision. Calcification of vessels (coronary, gastric mucosal, and large peripheral vessels) also occurs.

Differential Diagnosis

Lichen sclerosis et atrophicus
Post-zoster scars
Scleroderma
Cutis laxa syndromes
Solar elastosis
Penicillamine therapy
Tumoral calcinosis

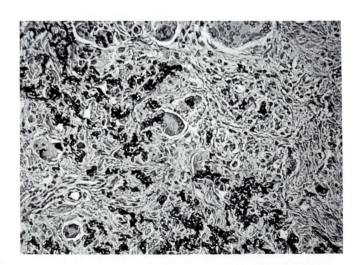

4-12-3 PSEUDOXANTHOMA ELASTICUM: Higher-power elastic tissue stains show elastic fibers to be clumped and calcified. (Movat, 400×)

Hypervitaminosis D
Elastosis perforans serpiginosa
Elastic tissue nevus

HISTOLOGICAL DESCRIPTION

Pseudoxanthoma elasticum is a disorder of altered elastic tissue of the skin, retina, and blood vessels. In the reticular dermis there are clumps of swollen, irregularly shaped, basophilic elastic tissue fibers (Figure 4-12-2). These areas of altered elastic tissue separate and push apart the normal-appearing collagen bundles. Elastic tissue not usually visible on routine sections is visible in this condition because of the altered state of the elastic fibers, such as increased size and the deposition of calcium on the altered elastic fibers (Figure 4-12-3).

In addition to the altered elastic tissue and calcification, there is an increase in an alcian blue- and colloidal iron-positive mucosubstance.

The altered elastic tissue stains intensify with orcein (black) or Alczaren red S (red), because of the calcification. Similar changes are seen in the elastic tissue of vessels and the retina.

Differential Diagnosis
Calcinosis cutis
Elastic tissue nevus

4-13 URTICARIA PIGMENTOSA

CLINICAL DESCRIPTION

Urticaria pigmentosa describes a group of conditions produced by dermal collections of mast cells.

Etiology and Incidence
Seventy-five percent of diseases characterized by a collection of mast cells in the skin occur in childhood. These disorders include solitary mastocytomas, urticaria pigmentosa, and diffuse cutaneous mastocytosis. Most often these are sporadic, but familial cases have been reported with both dominant and recessive inheritance patterns.

Clinical Features
The lesions are generally concentrated on the trunk but may appear anywhere. Typically the lesions are yellow-orange or hyperpigmented macules (Plate 4-13-1) or papules that urticate with stroking (Darier's sign). Blistering of these lesions may occur, especially before two years of age. Rarely, a diffuse involvement of the skin causes it to have a rippled, boggy, thickened appearance with doughy consistency (Plate 4-13-2). Pruritus, flushing attacks, fainting, diarrhea, gastrointestinal ulceration, respiratory distress, hematologic deficiencies, and death may occur. Childhood onset mastocytosis rarely has

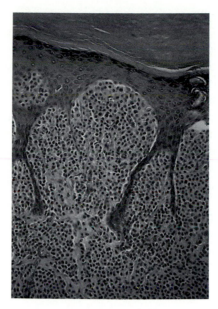

4-13-1 URTICARIA PIGMENTOSA: High power shows cuboidal mast cells with eosinophilic cytoplasm, which fill and distend the dermal papilla. The cells all have a uniform appearance. (200×)

serious systemic complications involving only 10 to 30% of affected children over 10 years and in less than 5% of children diagnosed before age 10. With advancing age, the symptoms and cosmetic changes disappear. Pigmentation remains when the skin lesions are extensive. If systemic involvement occurs, multiple organs may be affected (bones, liver, spleen, lymph nodes, peripheral blood, lung, kidney, GI tract, skeletal muscle, myocardium, etc.). Symptoms of systemic involvement include pruritus, urticaria, headache, flushing, tachycardia, GI symptoms, coagulation abnormalities, hypertension, and syncope. Solitary mastocytomas have the most favorable prognosis.

Differential Diagnosis
Xanthoma
Pigmented nevus
Juvenile xanthogranuloma
Impetigo
Blistering disorders

HISTOLOGICAL DESCRIPTION

Solitary mastocytomas, urticaria pigmentosa, and diffuse cutaneous mastocytomas all show infiltration of mast cells in the dermis. The nodular form presents a striking histologic picture of a dense infiltration of uniform cuboidal mast cells, filling the papillary dermis and extending into the reticular dermis and often into the fat (Figure 4-13-1). The epidermis shows focal acanthosis and basal layer hyperpigmentation, overlying the mast cell aggregates. The diffuse erythrodermic variety has a lichenoid infiltrate of mast cells in the upper dermis. Bullous lesions occur frequently in children. The bullae are subepidermal and are associated with papillary dermal edema.

The dermal infiltrate contains, in addition to mast cells, eosinophils and lymphocytes. The macular types of urticaria pigmentosa may demonstrate only a few mast cells about dermal vessels, where the mast cells are less cuboidal and more spindle-shaped. In this variety special stains are of value in confirming the diagnosis. Mast cell granules stain metachromatically with Giemsa and toluidine blue, and strikingly red with Leder's stain (Plate 4-13-3).

Differential Diagnosis

Dermal nevus
Histiocytosis X
Letterer-Siwe disease
Eosinophilic granuloma

4-14 APLASIA CUTIS CONGENITA

CLINICAL DESCRIPTION

Most physicians are familiar with these defects of the skin, most commonly seen on the scalp.

Etiology and Incidence

The etiology of aplasia cutis congenita is unknown. Most cases occur sporadically; however, syndromic, autosomal dominant and recessive forms exist.

Aplasia cutis congenita is usually present at birth. Sixty percent of lesions occur on the scalp, while other areas include the face, trunk, and extremities. Eighty percent of lesions are near the midline of the scalp, with 50% of these in the midline. Most infants have a single lesion, but 20% have two skin defects and 8% have three.

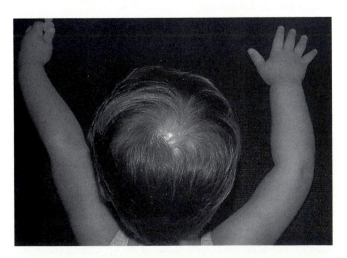

4-14-1 APLASIA CUTIS CONGENITA: Scarred defect on top of child's scalp.

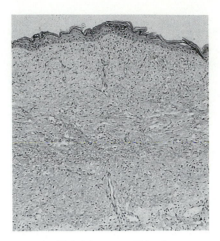

4-14-2 APLASIA CUTIS CONGENITA: Dermal stroma with normal cellularity for a newborn devoid of adnexal structures. (40×)

Clinical Features

The defect is usually a 1 to 2 cm ulcerated area initially, which then becomes scarred (Figure 4-14-1). Cleft lip and palate, neural tube defects, skeletal defects, hydrocephalus, and other defects have been associated with this disorder. Aplasia cutis congenita is also one of the cardinal features of trisomy 13, 4p-syndrome, and Bart's syndrome. It may also be a part of multiple conditions with more generalized ectodermal dysplasia or other malformation syndromes.

Differential Diagnosis

Birth trauma
Epidermolysis bullosa simplex
Forceps or electrode injury
Scalp infection
Congenital dermoid cysts
Sebaceous nevus

HISTOLOGICAL DESCRIPTION

The histological features are not specific. They may vary from those of an ulcer involving the entire thickness of the skin, including subcutaneous fat, to only thinning or fibrosis of the dermis. When there is an ulcer, the inflammatory response is much less intense than would be expected for the usual cutaneous ulcer. This lack of inflammation is a suitable clue to this diagnosis (Figure 4-14-2). Adnexal structures are absent in deep lesions, and there may be a complete deficit of all layers of the skin and subcutaneous tissues. There is no well-demarcated border between normal skin and the area of aplasia cutis, but there is usually an intermediate zone of skin in which dermal appendages are small or rudimentary.

Differential Diagnosis

Traumatic ulcer
Focal dermal hypoplasia
Nevus lipomatosis

4-15 ECTODERMAL DYSPLASIA

CLINICAL DESCRIPTION

Numerous variations of ectodermal dysplasias have been described; an entire book is devoted to the syndrome. This section describes the X-linked hypohidrotic type and the autosomal dominant hidrotic form, the most commonly seen forms.

Etiology and Incidence

Hypohidrotic (formerly called anhidrotic) ectodermal dysplasia is usually inherited as an X-linked recessive gene; however, variations with other inheritance patterns exist. The X-linked gene has been localized to Xq11-12 and flanking DNA markers are available for carrier detection and prenatal diagnosis in familial cases. The incidence is estimated to be 1 to 7 per 10,000. Hidrotic ectodermal dysplasia is inherited as an autosomal dominant disorder and is more common in areas settled by families of French descent carrying the gene (near Montreal and New Orleans).

Clinical Features

Hypohidrotic Ectodermal Dysplasia

This ectodermal dysplasia is characterized by partial or complete absence of sweat glands (resulting in heat intolerance secondary to reduced sweating), sparse hair, and dental abnormalities (delayed eruption, pegged or conical incisors and canines, and partial or complete anodontia). Children from different families with this disorder look more like each other than their nonaffected siblings (frontal bossing, hypoplastic central facies, prominent chin, thick lips, sparse hair, flat nasal bridge, and frequently periorbital pigmentation; Figure 4-15-1). Conjunctivitis, failure to thrive during infancy, episodic hyperthermia, and atopic dermatitis are frequently associated.

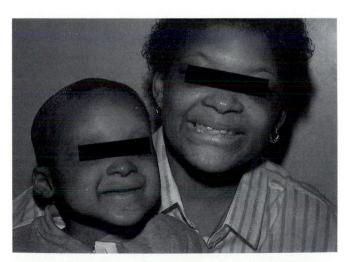

4-15-1 ECTODERMAL DYSPLASIA: Mother and child with hypohidrotic ectodermal dysplasia. Note mother's absent and pegged teeth. Periorbital hyperpigmentation is seen in both.

The maternal carrier of the gene frequently (approximately 70%) has partial anodontia and/or a reduced number of sweat glands. The nails in X-linked recessive ectodermal dysplasia are relatively unaffected. This feature and the severity of the dental defects are important differentiating features from the Clouston syndrome described below. Carriers may also demonstrate mammary hypoplasia and deficient lactation.

Hidrotic Ectodermal Dysplasia (Clouston syndrome)

The major features of this syndrome are sparse hair, hyperkeratosis of the palms and soles, and nail dystrophy (slow growth, thickening, striation, discoloration). Paronychial infections are common. Thirty percent of those affected show no defect other than nail dystrophy and the dentition is relatively normal, although dental caries may be present. Oral leukoplakia has been noted.

Differential Diagnosis

Other forms of ectodermal dysplasia
Congenital syphilis (nasal deformity and periorificial
    rhagades)

HISTOLOGICAL DESCRIPTION

Hidrotic and hypohidrotic ectodermal dysplasias show similar histological features. The epidermis is thinned (except for the palmar/plantar hyperkeratosis of Clouston syndrome), and there is no significant dermal infiltration. The significant features are those of hypoplasia of the adnexa, hair, and sebaceous and sweat glands. The sweat glands are more severely affected in the hypohidrotic variety and may be absent. Eccrine glands are generally diminished in number, even in areas where they are normally present in large numbers (palms and soles). When present, eccrine glands show only thin flat secretory cells and eccrine ducts have only one thin layer of cells. Similar changes occur in the apocrine gland; often the apocrine and eccrine glands are indistinguishable.

Differential Diagnosis

Normal skin
Other keratodermas (Clouston)/icthyoses

4-16 EHLERS-DANLOS SYNDROME

CLINICAL DESCRIPTION

Etiology and Incidence

This heterogeneous group of disorders is seen rarely. A frequency of 1:150,000 has been reported in the United Kingdom. A structural abnormality of connective tissue or enzyme defect has been described in several of the types (Table 4-16-1).

4-16-1   Ehlers-Danlos Disease

Type	Clinical Features	Inheritance	Biochemical Features
I Gravis	Severe	Autosomal dominant	Unknown
II Mitis	Mild	Autosomal dominant	Unknown
III Hypermobile	Joint findings severe; skin findings mild, minimal scarring	Autosomal dominant	Unknown
IV. Sack's ecchymotic	Visceral and large vessel rupture; thin skin; acrogeria	Autosomal dominant/ autosomal recessive	Defect of type III collagen (COL3A1 gene)
V X-linked	Skin hyperelasticity	X-linked	Unknown
VI Ocular	Retinal detachments; scoliosis	Autosomal recessive	Lysylhydroxylase deficiency
VII Arthrochalasis	Hypermobile joints; characteristic facies; short stature	Autosomal dominant	Structural mutation of type I collagen
VIII Periodontal	Periodontitis	Autosomal dominant	Unknown
IX Occipital horn syndrome (X-linked cutis laxa)	Bladder diverticula; lax skin may be limited to distal extremities	X-linked	Disorder of copper transport ↓ Lysyl oxidase (? allelic with Menkes)
X Fibronectin	Moderate skin extensibility; striae; joint hypermobility; aggregation defect of platelets	Autosomal recessive	Dysfunctional plasma fibronectin

Clinical Features

The characteristic features of this syndrome are hyperelasticity of the skin (Figure 4-16-1), hyperextensibility of joints (Figure 4-16-2), and fragility of the tissues and blood vessels. The most common skin changes include velvety texture, hyperextensibility, fragility (minor trauma produces gaping wounds), and poor healing (wide, parchment-thin "cigarette paper" scars). Fibrosis of hematomas results in subcutaneous nodules (spherules). There may be redundant skin and excessive wrinkling of the palms and soles of the feet. The patient's joints frequently dislocate and their mitral valves may prolapse. Vascular rupture is associated with type IV Ehlers-Danlos syndrome. There may also be associated GI and GU problems, periodontal disease, and pregnancy-related complications for both mother and child. Ten types have been described (Table 4-16-1).

Differential Diagnosis

Cutis laxa
Marfan's syndrome
Pseudoxanthoma elasticum
Osteogenesis imperfecta

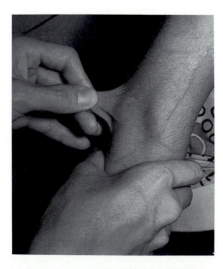

4-16-1 EHLERS-DANLOS SYNDROME: Hyperelasticity of skin.

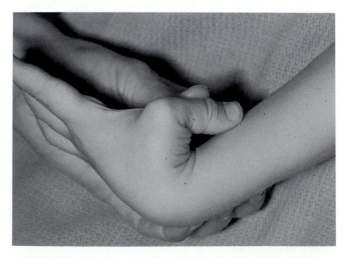

4-16-2 EHLERS-DANLOS SYNDROME: Hyperextensibility of joints.

HISTOLOGICAL DESCRIPTION

The histological features of all types of Ehlers-Danlos syndrome are not specific. There is no inflammatory response. There may be some suggestion of a decrease in collagen with a relative increase in elastic tissue volume. There is no alteration of the elastic tissue. Defects seen on electron microscopy are paucity or underdevelopment of rough endoplasmic reticulum, irregular outlining of collagen fibrils, and reduced lateral aggregation of fibrils into collagen bundles. Sites of hemorrhage show calcification, necrosis, and fibrosis. These changes are not specific but rather reflect response to injury. The pseudotumors at sites of hematomas may also show foreign body giant cells. The subcutaneous spherules consist of partially necrotic adipose tissue with areas of dystrophic calcification surrounded by a thick layer of dense collagen.

Differential Diagnosis

Normal skin

4-17 HYPERLIPIDEMIAS

CLINICAL DESCRIPTION

The hyperlipidemias that produce skin disease (xanthomas) in childhood are types I and II. The xanthomas commonly seen in these types are papuloeruptive, plane, and tendinous.

Clinical Features

Papuloeruptive xanthomas usually occur on the extensor surfaces of the arms, legs, and buttocks (Plate 4-17-1). Small yellow or red papules appear in crops. Plane xanthomas generally occur on the face, sides of the neck, upper trunk, in skin folds, elbows, knees, palmar creases, and scars. They are flat to elevated yellowish orange or yellow-brown intracutaneous plaques. Tendinous xanthomas favor the extensor surfaces of the fingers, elbows, or patellae. They are firm subcutaneous

nodules. Types I and II hyperlipoproteinemia are characterized in Table 4-17-1. Xanthelasma are slightly raised yellow soft plaques on the eyelids. They are frequent in type II and III hyperlipoproteinemia but may also be seen with normal lipoprotein levels. Tuberous xanthomas are large nodules or plaques most often seen on elbows, knees, fingers, and buttocks, and are seen in types II, III, and rarely IV.

Differential Diagnosis (conditions and syndromes associated with xanthomas)

Obstructive liver disease
Diabetes
Histiocytosis X
Nephrosis
Hypothyroidism
Pancreatitis
Tangier disease
Niemann-Pick disease
Juvenile xanthogranuloma
Alagille's disease

HISTOLOGICAL DESCRIPTION

All xanthomas have lipidized macrophages or histiocytes. The number of lesions and extent of lipidization may vary depending on the clinical presentation of the hyperlipemic state.

Papuloeruptive Xanthomas

Papuloeruptive xanthomas do not show as much macrophage lipidization as other types (tendinous, tuberous). The eruption may be distinctly angiocentric (Figures 4-17-1 and 4-17-2). Well-developed lesions (older) may contain numerous foamy histiomacrophages. The lipids are not doubly refractile with polarized light. There may also be nonfoamy cells (lymphocytes, histiocytes, neutrophils).

4-17-1 Hyperlipidemia Manifesting Skin Signs in Childhood

Type	Inheritance	Biochemical Changes	Clinical Features
I Familial hyperchylomicronemia (or Hyperlipoproteinemia)	Autosomal recessive	Deficiency of lipoprotein lipase; increased chylomicrons; increased fasting triglycerides; lactescent	Eruptive xanthomas (67%); hepatosplenomegaly (70%); foam cells in bone marrow; colicky abdominal pain (75%); no myocardial involvement
II Familial hypercholesterolemia hyperbetalipoproteinemia	Autosomal dominant	Defect in LDL receptor; normal triglycerides; normal VLDL; ↑ LDL, ↑ betalipoproteins, ↑ fasting cholesterol	50% xanthomas (tuberous, 15%); (tendinous only adulthood, 50%); coronary artery disease; arcus cornea (before 10 y)

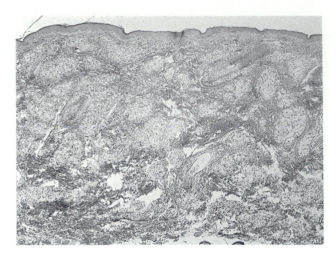

4-17-1 HYPERLIPIDEMIAS: Low power shows nodular aggregates of pale-staining cells in the dermis with an inflammatory response. (40×)

Plane Xanthomas

Plane xanthomas show foamy histiocytes on acral skin. Fibrosis may occur in the later stages of this process but is not a prominent feature. Lipids are doubly refractile with polarized light.

Tendinous Xanthomas and Tuberous Xanthomas

In tendinous xanthomas there are numerous foam cells. Touton giant cells may be present. An admixture of nonfoamy cells may be seen in these xanthomatous lesions, including lymphocytes, histiocytes, neutrophils, and rare eosinophils. The lipid in these tumors is doubly refractile with polarized light. Ultimately, collagen bundles replace the foam cells.

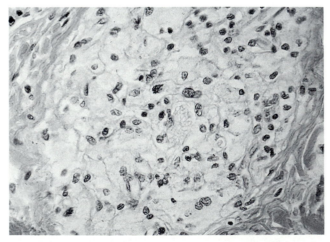

4-17-2 HYPERLIPIDEMIAS: High power shows that foamy histiocytes form the dermal nodules. These nodules are surrounded by compressed connective tissue. (100×)

Xanthelasmata differ from tuberous xanthomas by a more superficial localization of the foam cells and nearly complete absence of fibrosis.

Differential Diagnosis
Balloon cell nevus
Lepromatous leprosy
Granular cell tumor

4-18 KERATOSIS PALMARIS ET PLANTARIS

CLINICAL DESCRIPTION

Hyperkeratosis of the palms and soles includes a long list of rare diagnoses. Working through the various possibilities and arriving at a diagnosis can be difficult (Table 4-18-1). Recently the epidermolytic variant of keratosis palmaris et plantaris has been associated with mutations in keratin type 9, localized within the keratin gene cluster on chromosome 17q.

Differential Diagnosis
Ichthyosis
Chronic eczema
Psoriasis
Pityriasis rubra pilaris
Keratosis follicularis
Porokeratosis
Ectodermal dysplasia
Pachyonychia congenita
Tyrosinemia, type II

HISTOLOGICAL DESCRIPTION

There are several clinical varieties of keratosis palmaris et plantaris, but all have essentially similar histological features: hyperkeratosis, hypergranulosis, acanthosis, and mild perivascular lymphohistiocytic inflammatory infiltrate in the dermis. These changes of themselves are not specific, and since biopsy specimens are usually taken from an extremity the evaluation of hyperkeratosis is at some risk. Two varieties of the clinical forms of hyperkeratosis have distinctive histological features. Epidermolytic keratosis palmaris et plantaris demonstrates features similar to those described for epidermolytic hyperkeratosis (this chapter). The features in keratosis palmar-plantaris punctata are similar to those of other types of keratosis palmaris et plantaris, except that when the whole lesion and surrounding skin has been biopsied a very distinct central area of rather marked hyperkeratosis over a well-defined area is evident. In these latter two conditions, there is essentially no inflammatory infiltrate.

4-18-1 Keratosis Palmaris Et Plantaris

Type	Mode of Inheritance	Clinical Description	Associated Features
Keratosis palmoplantaris circumscripta of Unna-Thost	Dominant	Bilateral symmetrical hyperkeratosis; sharply demarcated with an erythematous rim; hyperhidrosis and fissuring, well-developed by 6–12 mo	Nails thickened, opaque, or curved; clinodactyly; clubbed fingers
Keratosis palmoplantaris linearis	Dominant	Keratosis composed of linear confluent streaks; onset at puberty	Buccal mucosa with papillomatous lesions; dotlike opacities of corneas
Keratosis palmoplantaris punctata	Dominant	Numerous yellow-brown discrete, hard, horny papules; pain from pressure; onset in 2nd to 3rd decade	Nail dystrophies
Keratosis palmoplantaris Progrediens	Dominant	Progressive thickening of palms and soles; extends to sides of hands and feet; arms and legs may be involved; onset during infancy	None
Keratosis palmoplantaris (Mal de Meleda type)	Recessive	Erythema early followed by hyperkeratosis; involves back of hands and feet, wrists, forearms, knees, other sites; hyperhidrosis, malodor, eczematization; brown-yellow plaques over joints of hands, knees, elbows, groin, axillae; onset during infancy	Koilonychia; subungual keratosis; short fingers; perioral plaques; physical and mental retardation
Papillon-Lefèvre syndrome	Recessive	Erythema and keratoderma extends to sides of hands, feet, achilles tendon, external malleoli, back of fingers and toes; hyperhidrosis; onset at 1–5 y	Premature loss of primary and secondary teeth following inflammation and swelling of gingiva; calcification of dura; sparse hair; dystrophic nails; mental retardation
Richner-Hanhart tyrosinemia II	Recessive	Small punctate lesions; partially striated keratosis; erosions; deficiency of hepatic tyrosine aminotransferase; onset at 12–15 y	Keratitis and corneal opacities; mental retardation

Differential Diagnosis

Clavus

Punctate porokeratosis

4-19 MUCOLIPIDOSIS

For a description of mucolipidosis, see Table 4-19-1.

ACKNOWLEDGMENT

Special thanks to Rhonda Schnur, M.D., for her editing and updating of this chapter.

REFERENCES

Tuberous Sclerosis

Fitzpatrick TB, Szabo G, Hori Y, et al.: White leaf-shaped macules. Arch Dermatol 1968; 98:1.

Nickel WR, Reed WB: Tuberous sclerosis: Special reference to the microscopic alterations in the cutaneous hamartomas. Arch Dermatol 1962; 85:209.

Cutis Laxa

Fitzsimmons JS, Fitzsimmons EM, Gulbert PR, et al.: Variable clinical presentation of cutis laxa. Clin Genet 1985; 28:284.

Goltz RW, Hult AM, Goldfard M, et al.: Cutis laxa. Arch Dermatol 1965; 92:373.

Kerl H, Berg G, Hoshimoto K: Fatal, penicillin-induced, generalized post-inflammatory elastolysis (cutis laxa). Am J Dermatopathol 1983; 5:267.

Reed WB, Horowitz RE, Beighton P: Acquired cutis laxa. Arch Dermatol 1971; 103:661.

Elastosis Perforans

Whyte HJ, Winkleman RK: Elastosis perforans (perforating elastosis). J Invest Dermatol 1960; 35:112.

Epidermolysis Bullosa

Anton-Lamprecht I, Schneider UW: Epidermolysis bullosa Dowling-Meara. Dermatologica 1982; 164:221.

Christiano AM, Uitto J: Polymorphism of the human genome markers for genetic linkage analysis in heritable diseases of the skin. J Invest Dermatol 1992; 99:519.

Epstein EH: Molecular basis of epidermolysis bullosa. Science 1992; 256:799.

4-19-1 Mucolipidosis

Type	Inheritance	Clinical Features	Skin Changes
Mucolipidosis I	Autosomal recessive	Mild Hurler-like dysostosis multiplex; cherry red macula spot—non–Hurler-like form; myoclonic seizures; decreased neuraminidase	
Mucolipidosis II I-cell disease	Autosomal recessive	Hurler-like syndrome; gingival hypertrophy; dysostosis multiplex; stiff joints; minimal corneal clouding; deficient uptake of lysosomal enzymes; (↓ N-acetylglucosamine phosphotransferase); early death	Tortuous veins around orbit; facial telangiectasias; rigid skin of ears, around eyes and neck
Mucolipidosis III	Autosomal recessive	↓ N-acetylglucosamine-1-phosphotransferase; mental retardation (mild); decreased joint mobility; mildly coarse facies; corneal clouding	
Mucolipidosis IV	Autosomal recessive	Corneal clouding; absence of facial coarsening and skeletal changes; increased frequency in Ashkenazi Jews	
Gangliosidoses	Autosomal recessive	Coarse facies; neurologic deterioration; cherry red spots; corneal clouding; kyphoscoliosis; dysostosis multiplex; hepatosplenomegaly; puffy eyelids; decreased β-galactosidase	
Fucosidosis	Autosomal recessive	Decreased α fucosidase; infantile form like other MPS syndromes; juvenile form like Fabry disease	Thickened skin in infantile form; increased sweat NaCl; angiokeratomas in juvenile form
Mannosidosis	Autosomal recessive	Decreased α mannosidase; corneal clouding; coarse facies; dysostosis multiplex	

Fine JB, Bauer EA, Briggaman RA, et al.: Revised clinical and laboratory criteria for subtypes of inherited epidermolysis bullosa: A consensus report by the subcommittee on diagnosis and classification of the national epidermolysis bullosa registry. J Am Acad Dermatol 1991; 24:119.

Fuchs E, Coulombe PA: Of mice and men: Genetic skin diseases of keratin. Cell 1992; 69:899.

Gamin WR, Briggaman RA, Woodley DT, et al.: Epidermolysis acquisita: A pemphigoid-like disease. J Am Acad Dermatol 1984; 11:820.

Gorlin RJ, Cohen MM: Craniofacial manifestations of Ehlers-Danlos syndromes, cutis laxa syndromes, and cutis laxa-like syndromes. Birth Defects:OAS 1990; 25:39.

Leigh IM, Lane EB: Mutations in the genes for epidermal keratins in epidermolysis bullosa and epidermolytic hyperkeratosis. Arch Derm 1993; 129:1571.

Pearson RW: The mechano bullous disease. In Fitzpatrick TB, Arndt KA, Clark WH Jr., et al. eds: Dermatology and general medicine. New York: McGraw-Hill, 1971: 621.

Vasser R, Coulombe PA, Degenstein L, et al.: Mutant keratin expression in transgenic mice causes marked abnormalties resembling a human genetic skin disease. Cell 1991; 64:365.

Ectodermal Dysplasias

Clarke A, Phillips DIM, Brown R, Harper PS: Clinical aspects of X-linked hypohidrotic ectodermal dysplesia. Arch Dis Child 1987; 62:989.

Freire-Maia N, Pinheiro M. Ectodermal dysplasias: A clinical and genetic study. New York: Alan R. Liss, 1984.

Ichthyosis

Ackerman AB: Histopathologic concept of epidermolytic hyperkeratosis. Arch Dermatol 1970; 102:253.

Frost P, Van Scott EJ: Ichthyosiform dermatoses. Arch Dermatol 1966; 94:113.

Rothnagel JA, Dominey AM, Dempsey LD, et al.: Mutations in the rod domains of keratins 1 and 10 in epidermolytic hyperkeratosis. Science 1992; 257:1128.

Williams ML: The ichthyosis—Pathogenesis and prenatal diagnosis: A review of recent advances. Pediatr Dermatol 1983; 1:1.

Focal Dermal Hypoplasia

Goltz RW, Henderson RR, Hitch JM, et al.: Focal dermal hypoplasia syndrome. Arch Dermatol 1970; 101:1.

Kilmer SL, Grix AW, Isseroff RR: Focal dermal hypoplasia: Four cases with varying presentations. JAAD 1993; 28:839.

Temple IK, MacDowell P, Baraitser M, Atherton AJ: Focal dermal hypoplasia (Goltz syndrome). J Med Genet 1990; 27:180.

Incontinentia Pigmenti

Carney RG: Incontinentia pigmenti: A world statistical analysis. Arch Dermatol 1976; 112:535.

Landy SJ, Donnai D: Incontinentia pigmenti (Bloch Sulzberger syndrome). J Med Genet 1993; 30:53.

Sulzberger MB: Incontinentia pigmenti (Bloch-Sulzberger). Arch Dermatol Syph 1938; 38:57.

Hypomelanosis of Ito

Glover MT, Brett EM, Atherton DJ: Hypomelanosis of Ito: Spectrum of the disease. J Pediatr 1989; 115:75.

Ritter CL, Steele MW, Wenger SL, Cohen BL: Chromosome mosaicism in hypomelanosis of Ito. Am J Med Genet 1990; 35:14.

Ruiz-Maldonado R, Toussaint S, Tamayo L, Laterza A, del-Castillo V: Hypomelanosis of Ito: Diagnostic criteria and report of 41 cases. Pediatr Dermatol 1992; 9:1.

Takematsu H, Soto S, Igarashi M, et al.: Incontinentia pigmenti et chromians (Ito). Arch Dermatol 1983; 119:391.

Darier's Disease

Beck AL, Finochio AF, White JP: Darier's disease: a kindred with a large number of cases. Br J Dermatol 1977; 97:335.

Buxton RS: Yet another skin defect, Darier's disease, maps to chromosome 12q. Hum Molec Genet 1993; 2:1763.

Gottlieb SK, Lutzner MA: Darier's disease. Arch Dermatol 1973; 107:225.

Lipoid Proteinosis

Aubin F, Blanc D, Badet JM, et al.: Lipoid proteinosis: Case report. Pediatr Dermatol 1989; 6:109.

McCusker JJ, Kaplan RM: Lipoid proteinosis (lipoglycoproteinosis). Am J Pathol 1962; 40:599.

Pierard GE, Van Cauwenberge D, Budo J, et al.: A clinical-pathologic study of 6 cases of lipoid proteinosis. Am J Dermatopathol 1988; 10:300.

Mucopolysaccharidosis

Freeman RG: A pathological basis for the cutaneous papules of mucopolysaccharidosis II (the Hunter syndrome). J Cutaneous Pathol 1977; 4:318.

Prystowksy SD, Maumenee IH, Freeman RG, et al.: A cutaneous marker in the Hunter syndrome. Arch Dermatol 1977; 113:602.

Porokeratosis

Mandojana RM, Katz R, Rodman OG: Porokeratosis plantaris discreta. J Am Acad Dermatol 1984; 10:679.

Shaw JC, White CR Jr: Porokeratosis plantaris palmaris et disseminata. J Am Acad Dermatol 1984; 11:454.

Pseudoxanthoma Elasticum

Goodman RM, Smith EW, Patton D, et al.: Pseudoxanthoma elasticum: A clinical and histopathological study (review). Medicine (Baltimore) 1963; 42:297.

Hausser I, Anton-Lamprecht I. Early preclinical diagnosis of pseudoxanthoma elasticum by specific ultrastructural changes of dermal elastic and collagen tissue in a family at risk. Hum Genet 1991; 87:693.

Lebwohl M, Phelps RG, Yannuzzi L, et al.: Diagnosis of pseudoxanthoma elasticum by scar biopsy in patients without characteristic skin lesions. N Engl J Med 1987; 317:347.

Strole WE, Margolis RJ: Pseudoxanthoma elasticum: Case 10-19198. N Engl J Med 1983; 308:579.

Viljoen DL, Pope FM, Beighton P. Heterogeneity of pseudoxanthoma elasticum: delineation of a new form. Clin Gen 1987; 32:100.

Urticaria Pigmentosa

DiBacco RS, DeLeo VA: Mastocytosis and the mast cell. J Am Acad Dermatol 1982; 7:709.

Mihm MC, Clark WH, Reed RJ, et al.: Mast cell infiltrates of the skin and the mastocytosis syndrome. Hum Pathol 1973; 4:231.

Aplasia Cutis

Deeken JH, Kaplan RM: Aplasia cutis congenita. Arch Dermatol 1970; 102:386.

Frieden I: Aplasia cutis congenita: A clinical review and proposal for classification. J Am Acad Dermatol 1986; 14:646.

Ehlers Danlos Syndrome

Beighton P, McKusick VA. Heritable disorders of connective tissue, 5th ed. St Louis, CV Mosby, 1993.

Wechsler HL, Fisher ER: Ehlers-Danlos syndrome. Arch Pathol 1964; 77:613.

Xanthomas

Crocker AC: Skin xanthomas in children. Pediatrics 1951; 8:573.

Keratosis Palmaris et Plantaris

Buchanan RN Jr: Keratosis punctata palmaris et plantaris. Arch Dermatol 1963; 88:644.

Torchard D, Blanchet Bardon C, Serova O, et al.: Epidermolytic palmoplantar keratoderma cosegregates with a keratin 9 mutation in a pedigree with breast and ovarian cancer. Nature Genetics 1994; 6:106.

Mucolipidosis
Aula P, Rapola J, Antio S, et al: Prenatal diagnosis and fetal pathology of I-cell disease (mucolipidosis II). J Pediatr 1975; 87:221.

Terashima Y, Katsuya T, Isomura S, et al: I-cell disease report of three cases. Am J Dis Child 1975; 129:1083.

5

Eczematous Eruptions in Childhood

Contents

5-1 ATOPIC DERMATITIS

CLINICAL DESCRIPTION

Any physician who sees children will have to diagnose and manage atopic dermatitis. Unfortunately, it is one of the most frustrating disorders to deal with. Many children are difficult to control. In addition, despite an enormous amount of research, its etiology remains an enigma.

Etiology and Incidence

Atopic dermatitis affects 3% of children and begins at one to two months of age. Sixty percent of affected children will acquire the disorder by one year of age and 90% by five years.

There is evidence that a combination of factors leads to the initiation and progression of atopic dermatitis. These factors include altered physiologic, pharmacologic, and immunologic mechanisms.

Clinical Features

The patient's age determines the distribution of skin lesions. During infancy the skin changes occur on the cheeks (Figure 5-1-1) and the extensor surfaces, frequently being generalized. More characteristic flexural involvement occurs at two years of age (Plate 5-1-1). During adolescence the distribution remains the same; however, there is also involvement of the face, neck, hands, and feet.

The skin changes are not characteristic enough to establish a diagnosis. An individual patient may exhibit erythema, edema, papules, vesicles, and crusting. Hyperpig-

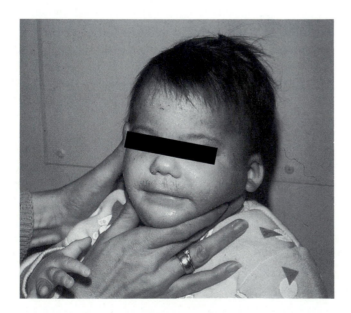

5-1-1 ATOPIC DERMATITIS: Young child with prominent eczematous facial changes of erythematous plaques involving the forehead, cheeks, skin, and area above the upper lip. Excoriations, secondary to pruritus, are apparent on the forehead.

5-1-1   Atopic Eczema

Major Criteria	Additional Features	Minor Features
Typical distribution Infancy: cheeks, extensor surfaces 2y to adolescence: flexural surfaces Adolescence: flexures, face, neck, hands, feet	Xerosis	Dennie-Morgan lines
Pruritus	Hyperlinear palms and soles	Cataracts
Chronically relapsing course	Follicular accentuation	Keratoconus
Personal or family history of atopic disease (80%)	Pityriasis alba	
	Scaling scalp Pseudo-tinea pedis Recurrent cutaneous infections Ichthyosis White dermographism	

mentation and lichenification are frequently present. Therefore, criteria were established to aid in the diagnosis of atopic eczema. Table 5-1-1 lists these criteria.

It is difficult to predict the course of an individual case. Thirty percent of those who develop atopic eczema during the first year continue to have the problem through childhood. Eighty to 90% of all children will clear by adolescence.

Differential Diagnosis

Contact dermatitis
Irritant dermatitis
Seborrheic dermatitis
Scabies
Many metabolic and immunologic disorders

HISTOLOGICAL DESCRIPTION

The histological features parallel the clinical course of this disorder. Early changes are inflammatory and exudative. With chronicity, epithelial and stromal alterations are more prominent and reflect repetitive trauma of rubbing and/or scratching. The microscopic changes thus permit classifying a lesion as acute, subacute, or chronic.

Acute Changes

Acute lesions are characterized by exudation of fluid and inflammation. Increased vascular permeability results in papillary dermal edema and accumulation of fluid within the

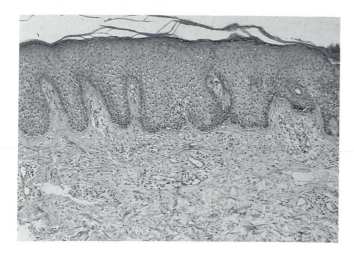

5-1-2 ATOPIC DERMATITIS: Low power shows pallor of the epidermis and dermis and a superficial dermal infiltrate. (100×)

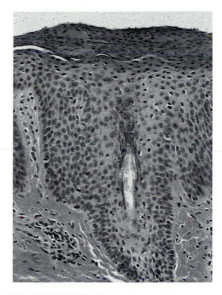

5-1-4 ATOPIC DERMATITIS: Subacute changes are evident: loculated serum in the scale, minimal spongiosis, acanthosis, and a less intense dermal infiltrate. (200×)

epidermis (Figures 5-1-2 and 5-1-3; Plate 5-1-2). The latter change may be appreciated as separation of keratinocytes and stretching of tonofilaments. Where these changes are marked, intraepidermal microvesicles form and may contain lymphocytes. Since keratinocyte maturation is disturbed, the associated scale frequently is parakeratotic. The inflammatory changes include a perivascular and interstitial infiltrate of lymphocytes, histiocytes, and rare eosinophils within the superficial dermis. The mid- to deep reticular dermis and subcutis are unaltered.

Subacute Changes

Histological changes in the subacute stage are less pronounced than in the acute stage. Spongiosis is spotty and minimal. Loculated serum may be seen in the parakeratotic scale and reflects elimination of earlier intraepidermal collections of fluid. Perivascular infiltrates are less prominent than

in the acute phase (Figure 5-1-4). While the exudative and inflammatory changes become less prominent, acanthosis indicates persistence of the lesion beyond the acute phase.

Chronic Changes

In the chronic stage, the epidermis is hyperplastic and surmounted by hyperkeratotic scale with zones of parakeratosis. The dermal edema and spongiosis of the acute phase and loculated serum in the scale of the subacute phase are no longer apparent. The inflammatory infiltrate is primarily perivascular

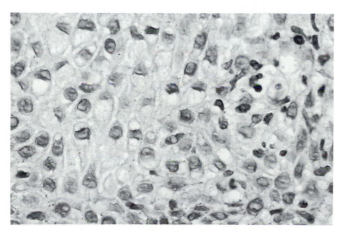

5-1-3 ATOPIC DERMATITIS: High power shows intercellular edema (spongiosis). The tonofilaments are stretched and outline individual keratinocytes. (400×)

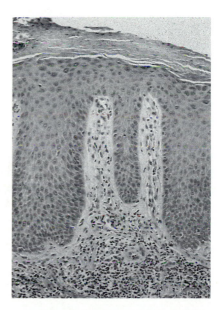

5-1-5 ATOPIC DERMATITIS: Chronic changes of hyperortho- and parakeratosis, acanthosis, and papillary dermal sclerosis. (200×)

and lymphocytic, admixed with a rare eosinophil. Acanthosis is accompanied by fibrosis of the papillary dermal collagen bundles, findings indicative of chronic trauma (Figure 5-1-5).

Differential Diagnosis
Dyshidrosis
Nummular dermatitis
Seborrheic dermatitis
Contact dermatitis
Dermatophytosis
Pityriasis rosea
Guttate parapsoriasis

5-2 CONTACT DERMATITIS

CLINICAL DESCRIPTION

The incidence of allergic contact dermatitis in childhood is approximately 1.5%; this is considerably less than the incidence in the adult population. Children less than one year old rarely develop a response to contactants.

Two steps are necessary to develop allergic contact dermatitis: (1) T lymphocytes must become sensitized to an antigen, and (2) the sensitized individual must be re-exposed to the same agent. Only after subsequent exposure do characteristic changes occur.

Clinical Features
Important clinical clues to the diagnosis of allergic contact dermatitis are the distribution, shape, and sharp demarcation of lesions. These characteristics reflect the limitation of skin changes to areas of contact with the offending substance (Plate 5-2-1). Lesions at affected sites have geometric or linear configurations and are characterized by erythema, edema, papules, and vesicles (Plate 5-2-2). Contact dermatitis is most often seen on the extremities, trunk, and face, and less often on the scalp, mucous membranes, palms, and soles.

The most common allergens inducing contact dermatitis in order of frequency, are rhus (poison ivy, oak and sumac), nickel, rubber compounds, dichromates, and paraphenyl diamine. Clinically apparent skin changes occur approximately 48 hours after re-exposure to the offending agent and may persist for one to 3 weeks.

Differential Diagnosis
Cellulitis
Atopic eczema
Irritant dermatitis
Blistering disorders
Factitial dermatitis

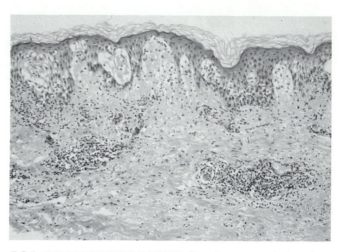

5-2-1 CONTACT DERMATITIS: Prominent spongiosis and papillary dermal edema give the epidermis a lacelike appearance. A superficial dermal inflammatory infiltrate is seen around blood vessels. (100×)

HISTOLOGICAL DESCRIPTION

Contact dermatitis demonstrates histological changes similar to those of atopic dermatitis, nummular eczema, dyshidrotic eczema, and seborrheic dermatitis. Early histological findings in common to these disorders include spongiosis, intraepidermal microvesiculation, variable acanthosis, and parakeratotic scale (Figure 5-2-1). Features that help to distinguish allergic contact dermatitis from other eczematous processes include: (1) intraepidermal nests of Langerhans cells (Langerhans cell microgranulomas) indicative of hyperplasia or nesting of antigen-presenting cells (Plate 5-2-3); (2) eosinophilic spongiosis or the presence of eosinophils individually distributed

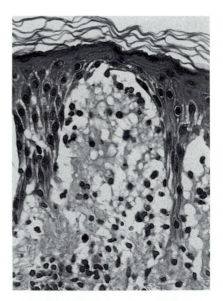

5-2-2 CONTACT DERMATITIS: Rete ridges are stretched by papillary dermal edema. Where keratinocytes are intact, spongiosis is prominent. (400×)

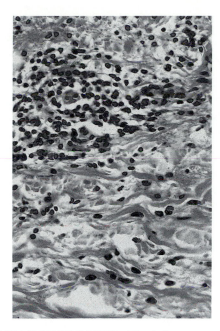

5-2-3 CONTACT DERMATITIS: The inflammatory infiltrate is composed of lymphocytes and large numbers of eosinophils. (400×)

within an edematous epidermis; and (3) the presence of eosinophils within the dermal inflammatory infiltrate (Figures 5-2-2 and 5-2-3). Where epidermal necrosis occurs, neutrophils may also be noted within the infiltrate. The subacute to chronic phases of contact dermatitis may be indistinguishable from the eczematous conditions listed above.

Differential Diagnosis
Atopic eczema
Nummular eczema
Dyshidrosis
Seborrheic dermatitis
Irritant dermatitis

5-3 DYSHIDROTIC ECZEMA

CLINICAL DESCRIPTION

Dyshidrotic eczema, or pompholyx, is a vesicular eruption of the hands and feet that is very difficult to manage clinically.

Etiology and Incidence
This type of eczema may occur at any age. Its etiology is still unknown.

Clinical Features
Dyshidrotic eczema appears as vesicles and bullae on the palms, soles, and lateral margins of fingers and toes (Figure 5-3-1). Vesicles often become pustules; both lesions eventu-

ally form hyperkeratotic crusts with or without secondary impetiginization. Symptoms of pruritus, burning, and stinging frequently precede but routinely accompany the eruption. The process may last several weeks, during which the symptoms and lesions may incapacitate the patient. Dyshidrotic eczema may wax and wane, becoming a constant source of frustration to the patient. This disorder is frequently associated with hyperhidrosis and atopic eczema.

Differential Diagnosis
Contact dermatitis
Pustular psoriasis
Fungal infection
"ID" reaction

HISTOLOGICAL DESCRIPTION

On histological study, dyshidrotic eczema most commonly shows acute or subacute changes of marked spongiosis associated with the formation of intraepidermal microvesicles (Figure 5-3-2). The vesicles are filled with lymphocytes in early phases and may accumulate polymorphonuclear leukocytes later in the disease. The stratum corneum is usually noticeably thick, reflecting the common site of occurrence of this disease on the palms or soles. In the dermis there is a perivascular lymphohistiocytic inflammatory infiltrate without eosinophilia. In a less acute stage, there is spongiosis without the formation of intraepidermal microvesicles and exocytosis of mononuclear cells (Figure 5-3-3). The acrosyringium remains unaltered.

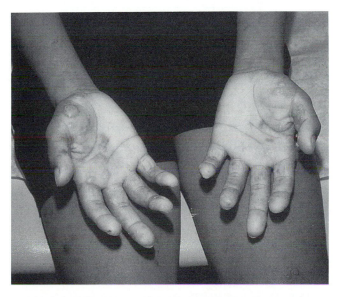

5-3-1 DYSHIDROTIC ECZEMA: Palms of a child, showing tense vesicles and bullae. Lesions extend to involve the lateral surfaces of the fingers. Hyperpigmentation from previous episodes can be seen as well.

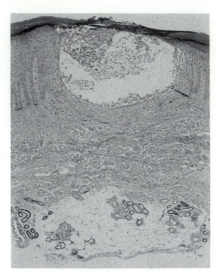

5-3-2 DYSHIDROTIC ECZEMA: Acral site (thick stratum granulosum, relatively thin dermis, many eccrine coils in subcutis) with large intraepidermal vesicle. (50×)

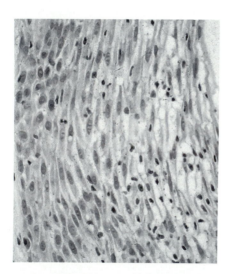

5-3-3 DYSHIDROTIC ECZEMA: High magnification shows epidermis adjacent to the vesicle. There is prominent spongiosis and exocytosis of lymphocytes with an occasional neutrophil. (400×)

Differential Diagnosis

Acute contact dermatitis
Nummular eczema
Atopic dermatitis
"ID" reaction

5-4 FIXED DRUG ERUPTION

CLINICAL DESCRIPTION

Sharply demarcated areas of hyperpigmentation that persist or recur at the same site raise the possibility of a fixed drug eruption.

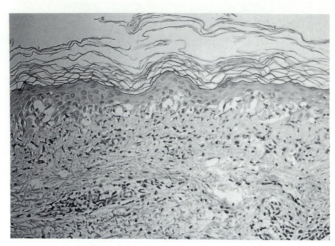

5-4-1 FIXED DRUG ERUPTION: Low power shows prominent necrosis of basilar keratinocytes and a superficial dermal lymphocytic inflammatory infiltrate. (100×)

Etiology and Incidence

Fixed drug eruptions are seen mostly in adolescence but can occur at any age. This problem is thought to represent a localized hypersensitivity reaction.

Clinical Features

The skin changes may be located on any part of the body. A localized, round or oval dermatitis recurs in the identical location with each exposure to the offending drug (Plate 5-4-1). The acute reaction (erythema and at times vesicles) disappears in seven to ten days after discontinuation of the drug, leaving behind varying shades of hyperpigmentation in its place. Lesions begin singly but frequently progress to involve multiple sites, including the lips, palms, soles, and glans penis. The discoloration may persist for months or years.

Differential Diagnosis

Erythema dyschromicum perstans
Lichen planus
Pinta

HISTOLOGICAL DESCRIPTION

The childhood and adult forms of fixed drug eruption have many histological features in common. In early lesions, a lymphocytic infiltrate admixed with occasional eosinophils is noted in the superficial dermis approximating the dermal-epidermal junction and infiltrating the lower portion of the epidermis. Lymphocytes can be found apposing individual keratinocytes, which then become necrotic (Figure 5-4-1). In more advanced lesions, homogeneous eosinophilic round bodies (Civatte bodies) can be found along the basilar region and in the papillary dermis; these are the remains of keratinocytes injured by the inflammatory infiltrate (Plate 5-4-2).

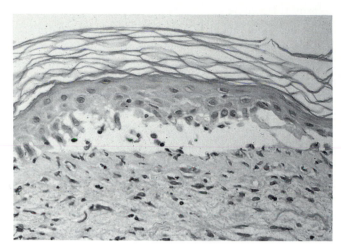

5-4-2 FIXED DRUG ERUPTION: An early bullous lesion, showing subepidermal separation beneath necrotic basilar keratinocytes. (200×)

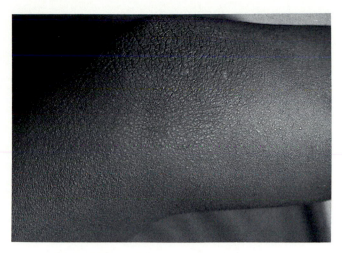

5-5-1 FRICTIONAL LICHENOID ERUPTION: Numerous discrete 1 to 2 mm papules grouped on the elbow of a young child.

In the resolving phases, a prominent feature is the presence of melanin in melanophages within the superficial dermis. The amount of pigment is much greater in this disorder than in other lichenoid processes, including erythema multiforme.

A notable difference in childhood fixed drug eruptions is the increased frequency of bullous reactions (Figure 5-4-2). The blisters are subepidermal and result from basal layer liquefaction degeneration and less well-developed epidermal attachments in young children.

In the resolving phase, only a sparse perivascular infiltrate composed of lymphocytes and papillary dermal collections of pigment remain. These findings correlate with the clinical findings of hyperpigmented patches without significant erythema.

Differential Diagnosis
Lichen planus
Drug-induced lichenoid eruption
Erythema multiforme
Erythema dyschromicum perstans

5-5 FRICTIONAL LICHENOID ERUPTION

CLINICAL DESCRIPTION

Children frequently play on their hands and knees, sometimes resulting in skin changes from trauma.

Etiology and Incidence
Frictional lichenoid eruption occurs mainly in four- to twelve-year-olds during the spring and summer. As the name implies, the changes are thought to be secondary to frictional forces.

Clinical Features
This dermatitis is distributed on the backs of the hands, elbows, and knees (Figure 5-5-1). The lesions consist of groups of flesh-colored to erythematous lichenoid papules 1 to 2 mm in diameter. Pruritus is variable. The eruption disappears with the return of indoor activities in fall and winter.

Differential Diagnosis
Keratosis pilaris
Lichen nitidus
Lichen planus
Follicular accentuation

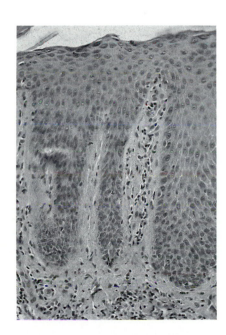

5-5-2 FRICTIONAL LICHENOID ERUPTION: Prominent acanthosis with slight thickening of the granular layer and papillary dermal sclerosis are accompanied by a moderate mononuclear inflammatory infiltrate. (200×)

HISTOLOGICAL DESCRIPTION

The histological findings in frictional lichenoid eruption are incongruous with the clinical appearance of a lichenoid process. There are changes secondary to chronic rubbing or irritation, consisting of acanthosis, follicular hyperkeratosis, and/or parakeratosis. The inflammatory infiltrate is composed of lymphocytes and histiocytes disposed about superficial dermal vessels. Hyperpigmentation of the basilar epidermal layer and pigment incontinence in the superficial dermis may be seen. In addition, sclerosis of papillary dermal collagen may be noted (Figure 5-5-2).

Differential Diagnosis

Eczematous dermatitides, chronic stage
Lichen simplex chronicus

5-6 HYPERIMMUNOGLOBULIN E SYNDROME

CLINICAL DESCRIPTION

Hyperimmunoglobulin E syndrome, an immunologic disorder, is characterized by four major features: recurrent pyogenic skin infections, extreme serum elevations of IgE, defective chemotaxis of neutrophils, and a personal or family history of atopy.

Etiology and Incidence

It has become clear that this rare disorder affects not only red-haired females who may have hyperextensible joints, but also males and females of any hair color. Hyper IgE syndrome is associated with a variable neutrophilic chemotactic defect. The basis for the recurrent infections is, however, still speculative.

Clinical Features

Hyper IgE syndrome may present at birth or shortly thereafter as a vesicular eruption (containing eosinophils) and a peripheral eosinophilia (25% to 75% at times). The vesicular, eczematous eruption may first start on the head and face (Figure 5-6-1) but then spreads to other areas of the skin. Immunoglobulin E levels are elevated in infancy and by early childhood are at least ten times normal (greater than 2,000 μ/ml). With increasing age, recurrent severe staphylococcal infections occur. Coarse facial features frequently develop. In addition to cutaneous infections, affected individuals may develop pneumonia, acute otitis media, osteomyelitis, pyogenic arthritis, and peritonitis.

Differential Diagnosis

Immune and metabolic disorders with eczematoid eruptions:

Ataxia-telangiectasia
Letterer-Siwe disease
Selective IgA deficiency
Severe combined immunodeficiency
X-linked agammaglobulinemia
Wiskott-Aldrich syndrome
Acrodermatitis enteropathica
Gluten-sensitive enteropathy
Hartnup disease
Histidinemia
Hurler syndrome
Phenylketonuria

HISTOLOGICAL DESCRIPTION

The histological features of hyper IgE syndrome reflect the stage at which the disorder is biopsied.

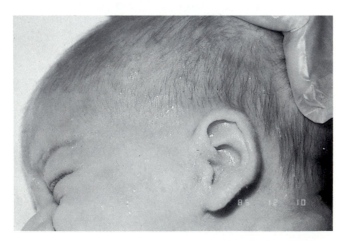

5-6-1 HYPERIMMUNOGLOBULIN E SYNDROME: Discrete and coalescent vesicles involving the face, ears, and scalp of a newborn. On the external ear crust formation is seen subsequent to vesicle rupture.

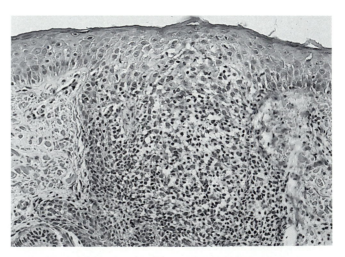

5-6-2 HYPERIMMUNOGLOBULIN E SYNDROME: Low-power view of a follicular infundibulum expanded by edema and inflammatory cells. (100 ×)

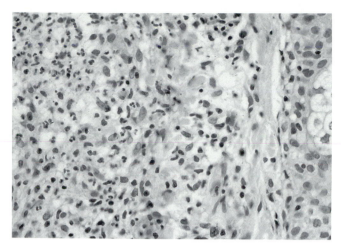

5-6-3 HYPERIMMUNOGLOBULIN E SYNDROME: High-power view of the area in Figure 5-6-2, showing large collections of neutrophils and eosinophils disrupting follicular epithelium. (400×)

Folliculitis and Dermal Abscesses

Cutaneous infections usually present as folliculitis and/or dermal abscesses. Folliculitis shows large aggregates of polymorphonuclear leukocytes permeating follicular epithelium, coalescing to form abscesses. Eosinophils may be prominent within the infiltrate, a finding likely related to the peripheral blood eosinophilia seen in most patients with this disorder. The dermis may show discrete areas of necrosis adjacent to the follicular and/or pustular areas (Figures 5-6-2 and 5-6-3).

If there is cellulitis, polymorphonuclear leukocytes may be seen distributed throughout the dermis and may extend into the subcutaneous fat, causing a superficial lobular panniculitis.

Atopic-like Dermatitis

The most common expression of this condition is chronic dermatitis of the type seen in atopic dermatitis. This may be manifested as an acute eruption in which there is spongiosis associated with acanthosis. In contrast to atopic dermatitis, numerous eosinophils are found in the inflammatory infiltrate. Eosinophils may also migrate into the overlying epidermis (Figures 5-6-4 and 5-6-5). These findings must be differentiated from Letterer-Siwe disease, infestations, and other causes of eosinophilic spongiosis.

The other inflammatory cells seen are lymphocytes and histiocytes. In the more chronic form of the disease, one sees acanthosis without much spongiosis and a mixed cellular inflammatory infiltrate of lymphocytes and histiocytes with occasional eosinophils. These findings may be interpreted as a chronic nonspecific dermatitis; occasionally a psoriasiform dermatitis may also be seen.

Differential Diagnosis

Eosinophilic pustular folliculitis
Fungal folliculitis
Letterer-Siwe disease
Parasitic infestation
Contact dermatitis

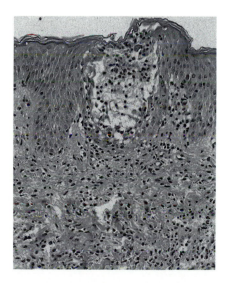

5-6-4 HYPERIMMUNOGLOBULIN E SYNDROME: In the epidermis there is a focus of spongiosis and exocytosis of eosinophils and lymphocytes. (125×)

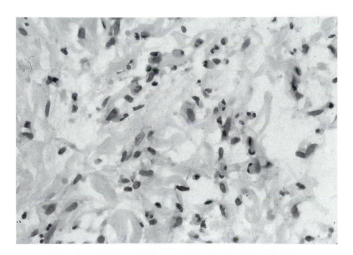

5-6-5 HYPERIMMUNOGLOBULIN E SYNDROME: The dermis shows separation of collagen fibers by edema and large numbers of eosinophils. (400×) (Courtesy of the Department of Pathology of Children's Hospital of Philadelphia.)

5-7 NUMMULAR ECZEMA

CLINICAL DESCRIPTION

Nummular eczema is one of the more frequently misdiagnosed dermatoses.

Etiology and Incidence

Nummular eczema occurs in all age agroups. Affected individuals usually do not have an atopic background, and IgE levels are generally not elevated. The disorder may be a manifestation of dry skin.

Clinical Features

Lesions occur in any location but especially in the extensor surfaces of the extremities. They begin as papules and vesicles that spread and then coalesce, typically forming coin-shaped erythematous, scaling, and crusted lesions (Figure 5-7-1). Pruritus is variable. The eruption is worse during the winter months. Affected individuals usually do not have a history of atopy. Most often the disorder is related to dryness of skin: it is worsened by overwashing, harsh soaps, and low humidity.

Differential Diagnosis

Atopic dermatitis
Contact dermatitis
Psoriasis
Tinea corporis
Pityriasis rosea
Granuloma annulare
Impetigo

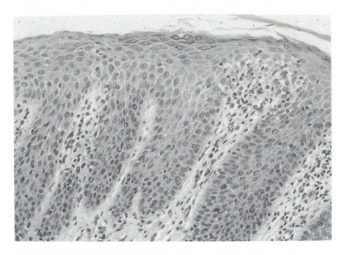

5-7-2 NUMMULAR ECZEMA: An established lesion of nummular eczema with prominent elongation or rete ridges and papillary dermal sclerosis of collagen bundles. Foci of spongiosis and exocytosis of lymphocytes may still be noted. (100×)

HISTOLOGICAL DESCRIPTION

Nummular eczema has many histological features in common with atopic dermatitis and thus closely resembles it. In the acute phase, spongiosis and exocytosis of lymphocytes are noted within a variably hyperplastic epidermis. Parakeratosis of the overlying scale is observed. Lymphocytes and histiocytes accompanied by occasional eosinophils are distributed about vessels in the subjacent dermis.

As lesions become chronic the epidermis becomes regularly hyperplastic and lacks the spongiosis of acute lesions (Figure 5-7-2). Similarly, parakeratosis is less noticeable. The inflammatory infiltrate becomes attenuated and is predominantly lymphocytic and angiocentric (Figure 5-7-3).

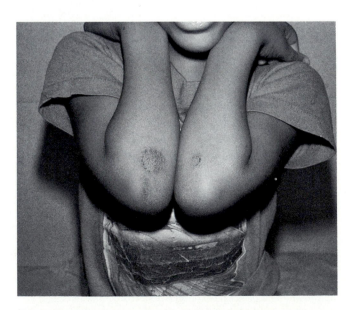

5-7-1 NUMMULAR ECZEMA: Coin-shaped plaques with crusted borders on the extensor surfaces of both arms.

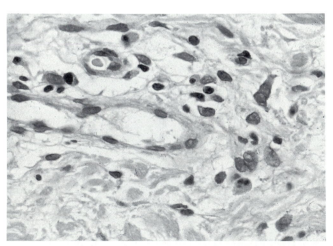

5-7-3 NUMMULAR ECZEMA: The infiltrate contains lymphocytes, histiocytes, and eosinophils. (400×)

Differential Diagnosis
Contact dermatitis
Atopic dermatitis
Pityriasis rosea
Frictional lichenoid dermatitis

5-8 SEBORRHEIC DERMATITIS

CLINICAL DESCRIPTION

It surprises some physicians that seborrheic dermatitis is not seen through most of the childhood years.

Etiology and Incidence

Seborrheic dermatitis is primarily seen in infants less than six months old and in adolescents. Although sebaceous gland dysfunction is frequently cited, the cause of this disorder has not been established.

Clinical Features

The areas of involvement during infancy are the scalp (cradle cap) and diaper area (Plate 5-8-1). Many times the eruption spreads to the locations more commonly seen during adolescence: the forehead, eyebrows, nasolabial creases, posterior auricular areas, neck, and axillae. Adolescents also exhibit involvement of the eyelid margins, sideburns, bearded area, mustache, anterior chest, and midback. Classic skin changes include salmon-colored patches covered with yellow, greasy scales. Generally the disorder does not cause irritability, and, in contrast to atopic eczema, pruritus may be absent. The prognosis is excellent during infancy; resolution usually occurs within several weeks to months. A more chronic situation may exist in adolescents (Plate 5-8-2).

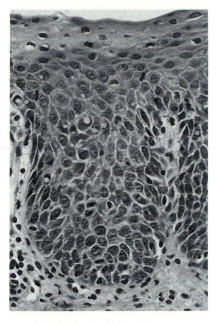

5-8-2 SEBORRHEIC DERMATITIS: The presence of spongiosis distinguishes seborrheic dermatitis from psoriasis. (200×)

Differential Diagnosis
Atopic eczema

HISTOLOGICAL DESCRIPTION

The histological features of seborrheic dermatitis are a cross between those of psoriasis and eczematous dermatitides. The epidermis is regularly acanthotic (Figure 5-8-1). Focal collections of neutrophils are seen within the overlying parakeratotic scale, especially at the shoulders of appendageal ostea. Within the papillary dermis a perivascular lymphohistiocytic infiltrate can be observed around ectatic vessels and is accompanied by edema. In addition, spongiosis is found in the epidermis (Figure 5-8-2). This latter finding allows discernment of seborrheic dermatitis from psoriasis.

Differential Diagnosis
Psoriasis
Subacute eczematous processes

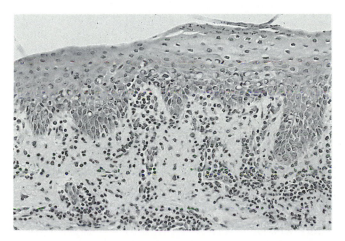

5-8-1 SEBORRHEIC DERMATITIS: Variable acanthosis and spongiosis. Exocytosis of neutrophils in the scale suggests psoriasis. (100×)

5-9 XEROTIC (WINTER) ECZEMA

CLINICAL DESCRIPTION

Xerotic eczema affects many children. The knowledgeable physician can easily curtail this process by prescribing good routine skin care.

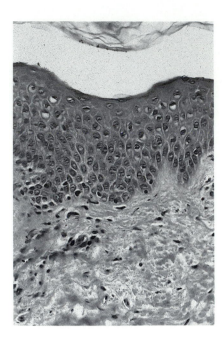

5-9-1 XEROTIC ECZEMA: Minimal epidermal alteration with a sparse dermal infiltrate. (100×)

Etiology and Incidence

Xerosis, or dry skin, may be seen in any age group. Family members frequently report the condition. The defect in the skin is unknown.

Clinical Features

The extremities and trunk are generally involved with rough, red, dry, scaling skin (Plate 5-9-1). Blacks often appear to have a hazy white color on their skin. The condition can be confused with atopic eczema, though pruritus may not be present. Nummular lesions may be seen. Low temperatures and low humidity will exacerbate the problem, hence the term *winter eczema*. Frequent bathing with harsh soap will unmask or exacerbate this condition.

Differential Diagnosis

Atopic eczema
Soap-and-water dermatitis

HISTOLOGICAL DESCRIPTION

The histological features of xerotic eczema are not specific. There may be flecks of parakeratosis overlying an epidermis that is somewhat acanthotic but lacks significant spongiosis or exocytosis. In the dermis there is a lymphohistiocytic perivascular infiltrate (Figure 5-9-1).

Differential Diagnosis

Normal skin
Minimally inflamed skin

5-10 WISKOTT-ALDRICH SYNDROME

CLINICAL DESCRIPTION

Etiology and Incidence

Wiskott-Aldrich syndrome is an X-linked recessive immunologic disorder.

Clinical Features

Onset is between birth and four months of age and occurs only in males. The distribution and appearance of the eruption is very similar to that of atopic eczema and is initially confused with this entity. One of the distinguishing features is a hemorrhagic skin component secondary to thrombocytopenia. Affected individuals are susceptible to infections (bacterial, viral, and fungal) because of defects in cell-mediated and humoral (decreased IgM, absent isohemagglutinins) immunity. The disease brings with it an increased risk for lymphoreticular malignancy and a poor prognosis.

Differential Diagnosis

Atopic dermatitis
Eczematous dermatitis accompanying other
    immunodeficiency states

HISTOLOGICAL DESCRIPTION

The histological features in Wiskott-Aldrich syndrome are similar to those seen in atopic dermatitis (Figure 5-10-1). There may be acute, subacute, and chronic changes similar to

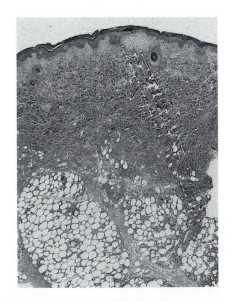

5-10-1 WISKOTT-ALDRICH SYNDROME: Low power shows papillary dermal pallor and alterations of subcutaneous adipose tissue. (25×) (Courtesy of the Department of Pathology of Children's Hospital of Philadelphia.)

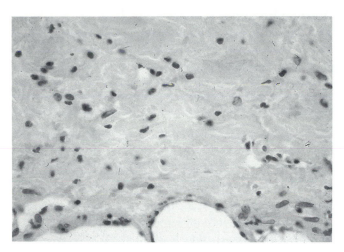

5-10-2 WISKOTT-ALDRICH SYNDROME: The reticular dermis shows prominent extravasation of erythrocytes and occasional mononuclear cells. (400×)

those in atopic dermatitis. Alternatively, there may be hyperkeratosis with focal parakeratosis, acanthosis without spongiosis, and a lymphohistiocytic perivascular inflammatory infiltrate. The one feature that may be present in Wiskott-Aldrich syndrome not usually seen in atopic dermatitis is a noninflammatory purpura: there is extravasation of erythrocytes in the papillary and/or reticular dermis not associated with an inflammatory reaction about the dermal vessels (Figures 5-10-2 and 5-10-3).

Differential Diagnosis
Atopic eczema
Other eczematous dermatitides
Noninflammatory purpuric processes

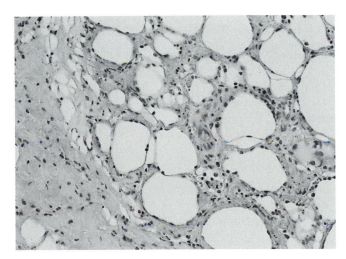

5-10-3 WISKOTT-ALDRICH SYNDROME: Variably sized spaces in the subcutis result from injury to adipocytes. Extravasation of erythrocytes in this case extends into fat lobules and is accompanied by a lymphohistiocytic inflammatory infiltrate. (200×)

REFERENCES

Atopic Dermatitis
Businco L, Zuruolo MG, Ferrara M, et al. Natural history of atopic dermatitis in childhood: An updated review and personal experience of a five-year follow-up. Allergy 1989; 44 (Suppl 9):70.

Mikon MC Jr, Soter NA, Dvorak HF, et al.: The structure of normal skin and the morphology of atopic eczema. J Invest Dermatol 1976; 67:305.

Rajka G: Natural history and clinical manifestations of atopic dermatitis. Clin Rev Allergy 1986; 4:3.

Sedlis E, Prose P: Infantile eczema with special reference to the pathologic lesion. Pediatrics 1959; 23:802.

Contact Dermatitis
Dvorak HF, Mikon MC Jr., Dvorak AM: Morphology of delayed type hypersensitivity in man. J Invest Dermatol 1976; 67:391.

Kuiters GR, Smitt JH, Cohen EB, Bos JD: Allergic contact dermatitis in children and young adults. Arch Dermatol 1989; 125:1531.

Rademaker M, Forsyth A: Contact dermatitis in children. Contact Dermatitis 1989; 20:104.

Dyshidrotic Eczema
Mehara M, Ofugi S: The morphogenesis of pustulosis palmaris et plantaris. Arch Dermatol 1974; 109:518.

Fixed Drug Eruption
Korkij W, Soltani K: Fixed drug eruption: A brief review. Arch Dermatol 1984; 120:520.

Sehgal VN, Gangwani OP: Fixed drug eruption: Current concepts. Int J Dermatol 1987; 26:67.

Frictional Lichenoid Eruption
Waisman M, Sutton RL: Frictional lichenoid eruption in children: Recurrent pityriasis of the elbows and knees. Arch Dermatol 1966; 94:592.

Hyperimmunoglobulin E Syndrome
Leung DY, Geha RS: Clinical and immunologic aspects of the hyperimmunoglobulin E syndrome. Hematol Oncol Clin North Am 1988; 2:81.

Saurat JH: Atopic dermatitis-like eruptions in primary immunodeficiencies. In Hopple R, Grosshands E, eds: Pediatric dermatology: Advances in diagnosis and treatment. New York: Springer-Verlag, 1987; 96.

Stanley J, Perez D, Gigli I, et al.: Hyperimmunoglobulin E syndrome. Arch Dermatol 1978; 114:765.

Nummular Eczema

Ackerman AB: Histologic diagnosis of inflammatory skin lesions: A method by pattern analysis. Philadelphia: Lea and Febiger, 1978: 227.

Braun-Falco O, Petry G: Feinstruktur der Epidermis bei chronischem nummularem Ekzem. Arch Klin Exp Dermatol 1965; 222:219 and 1966; 224:63.

Seborrheic Dermatitis

Allen HB, Honig PJ: Scaling scalp diseases in children. Clin Pediatr (Phila) 1983; 22:374.

Fox BJ, Odom RB: Papulosquamous diseases: A review. J Am Acad Dermatol 1985; 12:597.

Pinkus H, Mehregan AH: The primary histologic lesion of seborrheic dermatitis and psoriasis. J Invest Dermatol 1966; 46:109.

Xerotic Eczema

Hurwitz S: Clinical pediatric dermatology: A textbook of skin disorders of childhood and adolescence. Philadelphia: W.B. Saunders, 1981:58.

Wiskott-Aldrich Syndrome

Bean SF, South MA: Cutaneous manifestations of immunogenetic deficiency disorders. J Invest Dermatol 1973; 60:503.

Rosen FS: The primary immunodeficiencies: Dermatologic manifestations. J Invest Dermatol 1976; 67:402.

Shabalov NP: Wiskott-Aldrich syndrome (literature review). Vopr Okhr Materin Det 1975; 20:50.

Standen GR: Wiskott-Aldrich syndrome: New perspectives in pathogenesis and management. J R Coll Physicians Lond 1988; 22:80.

6

Papulosquamous Diseases and Related Disorders

Contents

6-1 PSORIASIS

CLINICAL DESCRIPTION

Psoriasis is a chronic papulosquamous disease frequently encountered in children. There is a predisposition for involvement of the scalp, perineum, and extensor surfaces of the body, particularly the elbows and knees.

Etiology and Incidence

Of adults with psoriasis, 37% experience onset in childhood or adolescence, 12% before ten years of age, and 25% between ten and nineteen years of age. There is a familial incidence with a polygenetic mode of inheritance. The major human leukocyte histocompatibility antigens (HLA) are important genetic markers of psoriasis. Of these, HLA-B13 and HLA-BW17 are associated with early onset disease. HLA-B13 is associated with a milder, more controllable psoriasis, often with a history of antecedent streptococcal infections. HLA-BW17 is more commonly identified with extensive skin involvement and a strong familial incidence. In childhood, there is a 2:1 female to male distribution of psoriasis.

Clinical Features

In children, the onset of psoriasis may take one of three forms: guttate, erythrodermic, or pustular. Any or all of these may eventuate into the chronic, plaque-type psoriasis (Figure 6-1-1). Guttate psoriasis is the most common form occurring in childhood. Guttate or droplike erythematous papules are scattered over the body. The characteristic silvery scale is only minimally expressed and the lesions may appear quite red. The eruption is often preceded by a streptococcal or acute upper respiratory infection. The antistreptolysin (ASO) titer is usually elevated.

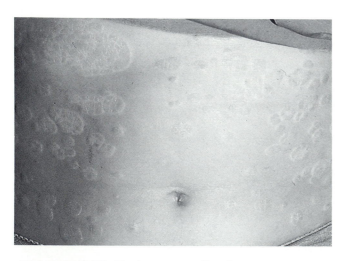

6-1-1 PSORIASIS: Erythematous scaling plaques.

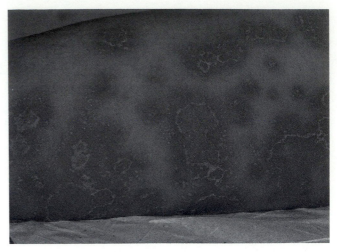

6-1-2 PUSTULAR PSORIASIS: A six-year-old girl with marked erythematous psoriatic lesions on the thigh, studded with pustules.

Erythrodermic psoriasis is less common and more severe (Plate 6-1-1). Onset may be abrupt or gradual with a diffuse erythema and severe desquamation. In the growing child there may be associated failure to thrive.

Pustular psoriasis is rare and the least frequently occurring form of psoriasis seen in children. This most severe form of psoriasis may not be associated with or preceded by typical psoriasis but is often associated with fever and leukocytosis. Varying sized sterile and superficial pustules develop on an erythrodermic background. Characteristic small, pitted lesions are frequently seen on the nails (Plate 6-1-2).

Differential Diagnosis

Pityriasis rosea
Secondary syphilis
Pityriasis rubra pilaris
Drug reactions
Lupus erythematosus

HISTOLOGICAL FEATURES

The classical histological features of psoriasis are parakeratotic mounds to confluent parakeratosis, hypogranulosis, acanthosis of the rete ridges with thinning of the suprapapillary plates, hyperproliferation of the rete cells, an intact basal layer, papillary capillary dilatation with an associated lymphohistiocytic infiltrate, and neutrophils passing from the papillary capillaries through the interstitial spaces of the rete and aggregating in the stratum corneum (Munro's abscess). As in adults, the classical features of psoriasis may be present in children, but often they are absent or poorly expressed in early, rapidly developing or late regressing lesions (Figures 6-1-2 and 6-1-3).

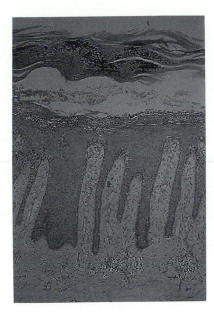

6-1-3 PSORIASIS: Low magnification shows a large parakeratotic scale and acanthosis of the epidermis with fusion of thickened rete. The dermis is papillomatous with mononuclear infiltrate of lymphocytes. (25×)

Guttate psoriasis frequently is difficult to diagnose on histological findings alone and may present with little beyond acanthosis and chronic inflammation. However, usually there is some diminution of the granular layer, sparse parakeratosis, and suggestively proliferative rete.

Erythrodermic psoriasis usually presents with a diagnostic histopathology demonstrating well-developed Munro's abscesses and other classical features, but may also demonstrate a deceptive subepidermal chronic lymphohistiocytic infiltrate.

Pustular psoriasis may also show considerable subepidermal inflammation but is recognized by the hallmark of this disease, the spongiform pustule. The latter consists of collections of polymorphonuclear leukocytes within the epidermis, involving viable epidermal cells and extending into the stratum corneum. The localized form of pustular psoriasis usually shows a clearly recognizable unilocular superficial pustule. In the generalized form, the spongiform pustule may occupy almost the entire epidermis, and only the margin of this massive infiltration of polymorphonuclear leukocytes will reveal the recognizable pattern of the spongiform pustule. In both the localized and generalized forms the epidermis may be uniformly thickened, and it is only as the lesions resolve that the classical features of psoriasis are revealed.

Differential Diagnosis

Seborrheic dermatitis
Chronic eczematous dermatitis
Nummular dermatitis
Atopic dermatitis

6-2 PARAPSORIASIS

CLINICAL DESCRIPTION

Etiology and Incidence

Parapsoriasis occurs infrequently in the pediatric patient. When it does occur it is usually a chronic condition that is very resistant to therapy. The etiology is unknown.

Clinical Features

The most common areas of skin involvement are the trunk and extremities; occasionally the face, palms, and soles show skin changes. Those changes include round or oval slightly scaling patches that may be brown, erythematous, yellow and hyper- or hypopigmented (Plates 6-2-1 and 6-2-2). The lesions are generally mildly pruritic. Unlike the disorder in adults, in childhood parapsoriasis is not a premalignant condition. The skin changes of parapsoriasis clear spontaneously after varying periods of time.

Differential Diagnosis

Atopic eczema
Psoriasislike dermatitis
Secondary syphilis

HISTOLOGICAL DESCRIPTION

The histological features of parapsoriasis are not in themselves diagnostic. In the dermis there is a mild perivascular lymphohistiocytic inflammatory infiltrate. Overlying the dermal inflammatory infiltrate there are focal areas of spongiosis and exocytosis. The epidermis may be thinned, normal, or focally acanthotic. One feature frequently consistent is that of discrete areas of parakeratosis, usually overlying the areas of spongiosis and exocytosis (Figure 6-2-1). Atypical cells are not seen in the childhood variety of this condition.

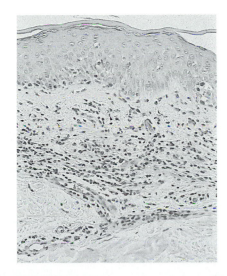

6-2-1 PARAPSORIASIS: Discrete exocytosis and a diffuse cellular infiltrate in the dermis. The cells show some variation in size. (200×)

Differential Diagnosis
Chronic dermatoses

6-3 PITYRIASIS ROSEA

CLINICAL DESCRIPTION

Etiology and Incidence
Pityriasis rosea has its peak incidence in adolescence. However, the disorder may be seen at any age. Pityriasis rosea is thought to be of viral origin.

Clinical Features
Seventy to 80% of children initially manifest a herald patch—a large oval, scaling patch with raised borders (Figure 6-3-1). After five to ten days, a more generalized eruption occurs. The lesions are oval, with the long axis parallel to skin lines. On the trunk the pattern of long, oval lesions in skin lines resembles the orientation of the branches of a Christmas tree (Figure 6-3-2). The individual lesions may be vesicles, pustules, papules, purpura, or urticaria. Pruritus is variable and may be severe in some children. Pityriasis rosea usually lasts six to twelve weeks.

Differential Diagnosis
Tinea corporis
Nummular eczema
Drug eruption
Viral exanthema
Guttate psoriasis
Mucha-Habermann disease
Secondary syphilis

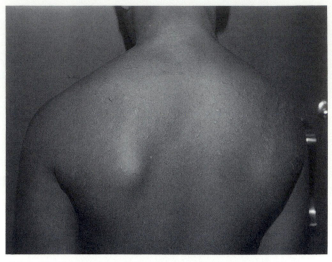

6-3-2 PITYRIASIS ROSEA: Note papulosquamous lesions arranged in "Christmas tree" distribution on this child's back.

HISTOLOGICAL DESCRIPTION

The histological changes in pityriasis rosea vary from subacute and/or vesicular dermatitis to chronic inflammation. The acute reactions are seen in the herald patch and consist of marked spongiosis, exocytosis of mononuclear cells, and papillary dermal edema with small focal areas of hemorrhage within the papillary dermis. The remainder of the dermis shows a chronic inflammatory infiltrate of lymphocytes and histiocytes; in some cases eosinophils may be seen. In this variety of pityriasis rosea, a parakeratotic scale is usually seen overlying the edematous epidermis (Figures 6-3-3 and 6-3-4). Other lesions of pityriasis rosea show a variable picture of chronic to subacute inflammation.

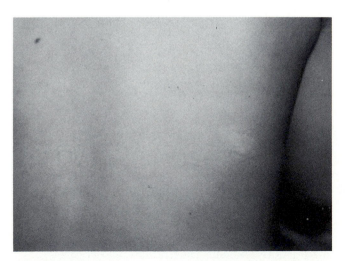

6-3-1 PITYRIASIS ROSEA: Herald patch. Note lesion on right side of child's back.

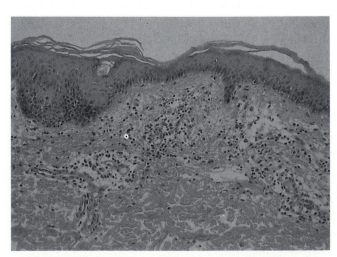

6-3-3 PITYRIASIS ROSEA: A thin ortho- and parakeratotic scale overlying a focally acanthotic epidermis. There is an infiltrate of lymphocytes about dermal vessels. (40 ×)

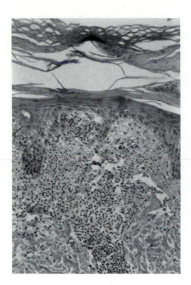

6-3-4 PITYRIASIS ROSEA: Parakeratosis with discrete epidermal thinning. The infiltrate is dense about dermal vessels. There is papillary dermal edema and scattered hemorrhage. (40×)

Differential Diagnosis
Atopic dermatitis
Parapsoriasis
Eczematous dermatitis
Pityriasis lichenoides acuta

6-4 PITYRIASIS RUBRA PILARIS

CLINICAL DESCRIPTION

Etiology and Incidence
The clinical course of pityriasis rubra pilaris, a rare condition in childhood, is variable but usually chronic. The etiology is unknown, although it is a disorder of keratinization.

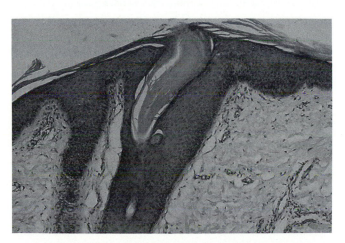

6-4-1 PITYRIASIS RUBRA PILARIS: Follicular hyper- and parakeratosis. The dermis does not show a significant infiltrate. (200×)

Clinical Features
There is a gradual onset of the disease, beginning in the scalp and spreading to involve the face and ears. The skin is generally salmon-colored and scaling. As the eruption progresses, it surrounds islands of normal skin (Plate 6-4-1). There is hyperkeratosis of the palms and soles. Acuminate follicular papules with keratotic plugs occur on the back of the fingers, side of the neck, and extensors of the extremities (Plate 6-4-2). Two variations of the condition have been described: familial, which has its onset in infancy and childhood, and acquired, which occurs in individuals fifteen years of age or older.

Differential Diagnosis
Psoriasis
Lichen planus
Vitamin A deficiency

HISTOLOGICAL DESCRIPTION

Hyperkeratosis, follicular hyperkeratosis, and follicular parakeratosis are the most significant histological features in pityriasis rubra pilaris (Figure 6-4-1). The dermal reaction is that of a mononuclear, lymphohistiocytic, perivascular inflammatory infiltrate.

The features seen in pityriasis rubra pilaris are not diagnostic. A helpful finding is surface parakeratosis extending into hyperkeratotic follicles (Plate 6-4-3). The epidermis shows essentially no other changes other than mild acanthosis.

Differential Diagnosis
Chronic dermatitis (atopic, nummular, neurodermatitis)
Pityriasis rosea
Parapsoriasis

6-5 LICHEN PLANUS

CLINICAL DESCRIPTION

Etiology and Incidence
Lichen planus is occasionally seen in pediatric patients as a chronic or pruritic eruption. The etiology is unknown.

Clinical Features
The distribution of the disease generally includes the flexors of the wrist, forearms, and legs, especially the dorsum of the foot and ankles. The lesions are characterized as small, violaceous, shiny, flat-topped polygonal papules (Plate 6-5-1). The surface of these papules may have white cross-hatching (Wickham's striae). Lesions may occur in sites of trauma or injury (Koebner's phenomenon). The scalp may be involved

and often results in a scarring alopecia (pseudopelade). The buccal mucous membrane is involved as a reticulated or lace-like pattern of white papules or streaks. The nails are frequently pitted, dystrophic, or ridged. The lesions in lichen planus in children are frequently vesicular or bullous. Hypertrophic and linear lesions occur but are less common. Frequently, persistent severe postinflammatory hyperpigmentation occurs, especially in blacks. Two-thirds of pediatric patients clear within eight to fifteen months.

Differential Diagnosis
Scabies
Pediculosis corporis
Pityriasis rubra pilaris
Pityriasis rosea
Guttate psoriasis
Graft vs. host reaction
Lichenoid syphilid
Drug reaction
Mucha-Habermann disease

Scalp
Systemic lupus erythematosus

Mucous Membranes
Systemic lupus erythematosus
Candidiasis
Traumatic stomatitis

HISTOLOGICAL DESCRIPTION
Hyperkeratosis, irregular hypergranulosis, irregular acanthosis (saw toothing), and a dense bandlike infiltrate of mononuclear cells that obscure the dermal-epidermal interface are the

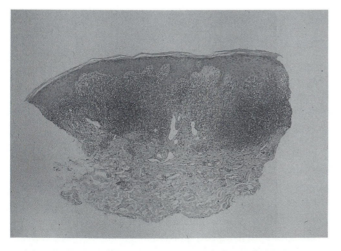

6-5-1 LICHEN PLANUS: Hyperkeratosis, focal hypergranulosis, acanthosis, and a basal-like papillary dermal infiltrate of lymphocytes. (40×)

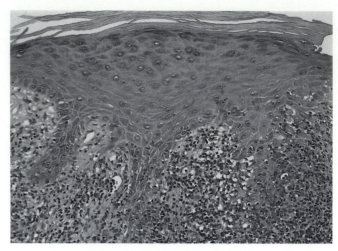

6-5-2 LICHEN PLANUS: The lichenoid infiltrate obscures the dermal-epidermal interface and is exocytotic to the lower epidermis. Some parakeratosis is present in the mucosal biopsy. (200×)

usual features of lichen planus (Figures 6-5-1 and 6-5-2). Parakeratosis and the presence of plasma cells are not usual features but if occasionally seen do not preclude the diagnosis.

Eosinophilic homogeneous round hyalinelike bodies (Civatte) may be seen in the upper dermis. These have on their surface immunoglobulins and are PAS-positive and diastase-resistant with the periodic acid-Schiff stain. Dermal-epidermal separation may be seen in lichen planus. These are small, slitlike spaces that result from the large areas of liquefaction degeneration. This separation occurs frequently in children, and often the histology is that of a subepidermal bulla.

There are several variations of lichen planus, included here for completeness. Lichen planopilaris is lichen planus that involves the follicles. The inflammatory infiltrate involves the upper third of the follicle, usually leading to destruction and scarring alopecia. Lichen planus pemphigoides (bullous lichen planus) demonstrates characteristic histology of lichen planus and bulla. The bulla may arise in nonlichen planus areas, and subepidermally with eosinophils in the dermis. Immunofluorescence studies show C3 and IgG at the basement membrane zone, with IgM, IgG, and C3 on the Civatte bodies. In contrast to bullous pemphigoid, the immunoglobulins are located on the floor of the bulla. Hypertrophic lichen planus shows essentially the same features as typical lichen planus, except that there is marked epidermal hyperplasia. This form is uncommon in children.

Differential Diagnosis
Lupus erythematosus
Lichen planus-like drug eruption
Secondary syphilis
Halo nevus
Lichen nitidus

6-6 LICHEN NITIDUS

CLINICAL DESCRIPTION

Etiology and Incidence
Lichen nitidus is a common disorder of childhood and is seen especially in African Americans. The etiology is unknown.

Clinical Features
Lichen nitidus involves the abdomen, genitalia, and extremities, with tiny, flat-topped, flesh-colored papules. Frequently these lesions are closely grouped and linear. Koebner phenomenon often occurs in lichen nitidus (Figure 6-6-1). The lesions are generally nonpruritic. The course is variable.

Differential Diagnosis
Follicular accentuation in atopic eczema
Keratosis pilaris
Lichen planus

HISTOLOGICAL DESCRIPTION

Lichen nitidus is a papular eruption. Each papule is composed of a granulomatous inflammatory infiltrate occupying one or two papillae. The granulomatous infiltrate is surrounded by an acanthotic (clawlike) epidermis, which has been described as a ball being clutched by a claw (Figure 6-6-2). The inflammatory infiltrate in the dermis is granulomatous in nature and consists of lymphocytes, histiocytes, and multinucleated giant cells. There is some extension to the overlying epidermis, with focal basal layer degeneration. The epidermis in this area is covered by a parakeratotic scale.

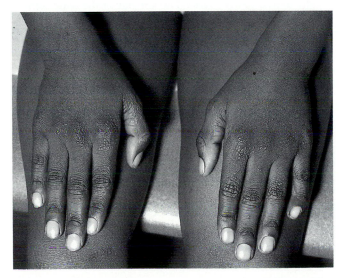

6-6-1 LICHEN NITIDUS: Flesh-colored tiny papules on back of hands. Note Koebner's phenomenon (linearly arranged papules) at base of thumb of child's left hand.

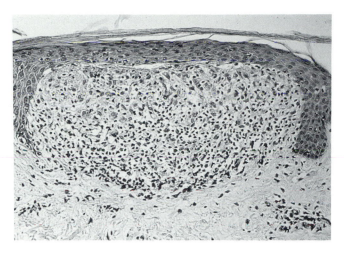

6-6-2 LICHEN NITIDUS: Histiocytes and lymphocytes in the infiltrate. (200×)

Differential Diagnosis
Lichen planus
Lichenoid keratosis
Halo nevus

6-7 LICHEN STRIATUS

CLINICAL DESCRIPTION

Etiology and Incidence
Lichen striatus occurs commonly in young children. There is a female predominance, with a female to male ratio of 2.5:1. The etiology is unknown.

Clinical Features
The lesions generally involve the extremities but can be seen on the face, neck, and trunk. The individual lesions are pink or flesh-colored, flat-topped, and lichenoid papules that are grouped and eventually coalesce to form a linear band, which may be continuous or interrupted (Figure 6-7-1). The band appears hypopigmented in African Americans. The eruption is usually asymptomatic, but pruritus may occur and may be severe. The course of lichen striatus may be several years from the initial skin change to total resolution of the disorder. On average, lichen striatus disappears after six to eighteen months without treatment.

Differential Diagnosis
Nevus unius lateris
Linear inflammatory epidermal nevus
Linear lichen planus
Linear lichen nitidus
Psoriasis
Verruca plana
Ichthyosis hystrix

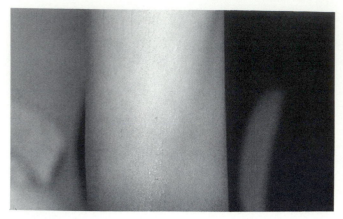

6-7-1 LICHEN STRIATUS: Band of linearly arranged, flesh-colored papules on patient's extremity.

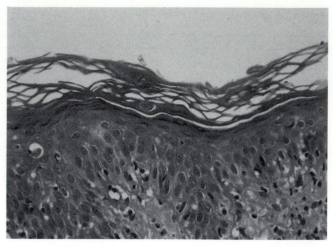

6-7-3 LICHEN STRIATUS: Dyskeratotic cells in the stratum corneum and stratum granulosum. Exocytosis of lymphocytes into the epidermis. (400×)

fused with lichen planus. The latter does not show dyskeratotic cells within the upper epidermis.

Differential Diagnosis
Inflammatory linear nevus
Lichen planus

6-8 LINEAR INFLAMMATORY EPIDERMAL NEVUS
CLINICAL DESCRIPTION

Etiology and Incidence
Linear inflammatory epidermal nevus (inflammatory linear verrucous epidermal nevus) has its onset early in childhood. There is a 4:1 female to male ratio. The left side of the body is more frequently involved than the right. The etiology is unknown.

Clinical Features
The lesions are generally red, scaling, severely pruritic verrucous papules arranged in one or more lines (Plate 6-8-1). Skeletal and other abnormalities have been associated with linear inflammatory epidermal nevi. The condition is persistent and refractory to treatment.

Differential Diagnosis
Nevus unius lateris
Linear inflammatory epidermal nevus
Linear lichen planus
Linear lichen nitidus
Psoriasis
Verruca plana
Ichthyosis hystrix
Linear Darier's disease

HISTOLOGICAL DESCRIPTION
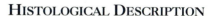

Lichen striatus shows chronic inflammatory changes characterized by a dense dermal infiltrate about the subpapillary vessels, extending into deeper dermis (Figure 6-7-2). This infiltrate consists of lymphocytes with the presence of histiocytes. The epidermis has an overlying parakeratotic scale, also showing spongiosis and exocytosis. The exocytotic cells are mononuclear. The distinguishing feature in this condition is the presence of altered keratinocytes, which are large, eosinophilic, and dyskeratotic. They may resemble the dyskeratotic cells seen in Darier's disease but are smaller in size (Figure 6-7-3). Older lesions of lichen striatus can be con-

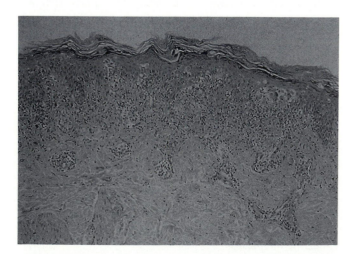

6-7-2 LICHEN STRIATUS: A lichenoid and deep perivascular infiltrate. The dermal infiltrate obscures the dermal-epidermal interface. (40×)

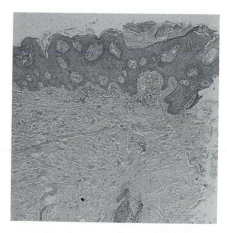

6-8-1 LINEAR INFLAMMATORY EPIDERMAL NEVUS: Hyperkeratosis overlying a hyperplastic epidermis. There is a sparse inflammatory dermal infiltrate. (40×)

HISTOLOGICAL DESCRIPTION

The histological features of inflammatory linear verrucous epidermal nevus are not specific. The changes seen are focal parakeratosis and acanthosis with localized spongiosis. In some cases there is noted alternating hyper- and parakeratosis with underlying hyper- and hypogranulosis. In the dermis there is a lymphohistiocytic perivascular inflammatory infiltrate (Figures 6-8-1 and 6-8-2). The features of this disorder are similar to those seen in lichen striatus, although dyskeratotic cells are not seen in the inflammatory linear verrucous epidermal nevus.

Differential Diagnosis
Lichen striatus

6-9 ACROPUSTULOSIS OF INFANCY

CLINICAL DESCRIPTION

Acropustulosis of infancy is a recently described entity characterized by acral papules, vesicles, and pustules.

Etiology and Incidence

The disorder is seen most commonly in black skin and has its onset from birth to twelve months of age. Intermittent exacerbations occur every two or three weeks, with lesions lasting three to fourteen days. Episodes decrease in frequency, usually disappearing when the child is between two and four years of age. All diagnostic procedures, including cultures and scraping for fungi or scabies, are negative. There is no known etiology for this disorder.

Clinical Features

The individual lesions are 1 to 3 mm vesicopustules that erupt in crops. The lesions evolve from an erythematous papule to a pustule over the course of twenty-four hours and are found primarily on the distal extremities, including the palms and soles (Figure 6-9-1), however they can be seen on other parts of the body.

Differential Diagnosis
Scabies
Impetigo
Candidiasis
Erythema toxicum neonatorum
Transient neonatal pustular melanosis
Dyshidrotic eczema
Pustular psoriasis

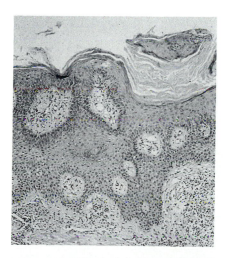

6-8-2 LINEAR INFLAMMATORY EPIDERMAL NEVUS: Mononuclear lymphocytic infiltrate about the dermal vessels and extending into the dermis. The epidermis shows patchy spongiosis and exocytosis. (200×)

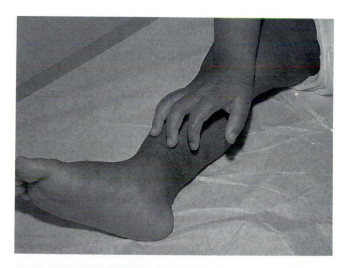

6-9-1 ACROPUSTULOSIS OF INFANCY: Papules and pustules on patient's hands and feet.

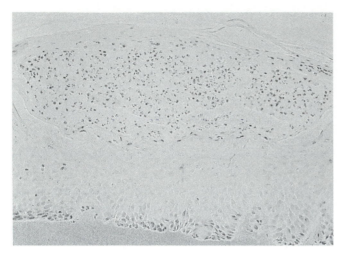

6-9-2 ACROPUSTULOSIS OF INFANCY: Subcorneal abscess of polymorphonuclear leukocytes. The epidermis shows minimal change in spite of the overlying inflammation. (20×)

HISTOLOGICAL DESCRIPTION

The histological picture of acropustulosis of infancy may vary from a subcorneal pustule to an intraepidermal pustule, both containing polymorphonuclear leukocytes (Figure 6-9-2). The difference in the described locations of the pustule is a reflection of the time of the biopsy. The initiating event is exocytosis of polymorphs, in response to a stimulus. The result of the marked exocytosis is an intraepidermal and later a subcorneal pustule.

There is associated parakeratosis, overlying the involved epidermis. There is in the dermis a mixed inflammatory infiltrate with associated vascular ectasia.

Differential Diagnosis

Subcorneal pustular dermatosis
Impetigo
Pustular psoriasis
Transient neonatal pustular melanosis

6-10 PAPULAR ACRODERMATITIS OF CHILDHOOD SYNDROME

CLINICAL DESCRIPTION

Etiology and Incidence

Papular acrodermatitis of childhood (Gianotti-Crosti syndrome) occurs in children six months to twelve years of age, with peak incidence generally between one and four years of age.

Clinical Features

The eruption is concentrated on the face (Figure 6-10-1), buttocks, and extremities (Figure 6-10-2). The exanthem is a

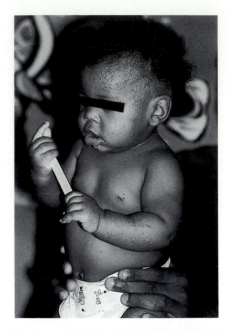

6-10-1 PAPULAR ACRODERMATITIS OF CHILDHOOD: Papular eruption on the face and arms in a young black child. Note sparing of trunk.

papular, lichenoid eruption that lasts two to eight weeks. Koebner's phenomenon is frequently seen. The disorder was first described by Gianotti in association with hepatitis B virus infection (subtype AYW). This classic type is seen in Italy, Japan, and Mediterranean countries. In the United States, papular acrodermatitis of childhood is usually associated with Epstein-Barr virus parainfluenza virus, coxsackie virus A-16, respiratory syncytial virus, and other viral infections. This

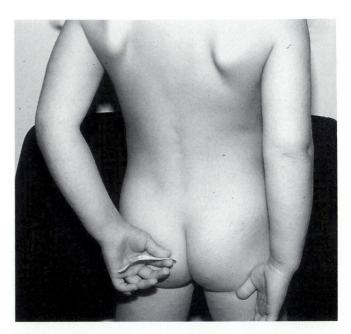

6-10-2 PAPULAR ACRODERMATITIS OF CHILDHOOD: Papular eruption on the buttock of a Caucasian child.

is probably due to the fact that hepatitis B virus infection (subtype AYW) is unusual in the pediatric population in this country.

Differential Diagnosis

Lichen planus
Inverse papular pityriasis rosea
Drug eruption

HISTOLOGICAL DESCRIPTION

The histological features in papular acrodermatitis are a dense papular perivascular infiltrate of lymphocytes and histiocytes. There is exocytosis of this infiltrate, with associated liquefaction degeneration of the basal layer. The epidermis is focally acanthotic, with spongiosis and hyperkeratosis. The dermal vessels may show endothelial swelling but there is no true vasculitis or invasion of vessel walls by inflammatory cells. These features are not of themselves diagnostic.

Differential Diagnosis

Parapsoriasis
Eczematous dermatitis

6-11 MUCHA-HABERMANN DISEASE

CLINICAL DESCRIPTION

Etiology and Incidence

Mucha-Habermann disease (pityriasis lichenoides et varioliformis acuta) occurs as an acute or chronic skin disease. The etiology is unknown.

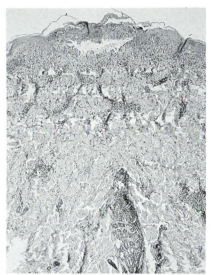

6-11-1 MUCHA-HABERMANN DISEASE: Parakeratosis, exocytosis, and a dense perivascular mononuclear cell infiltrate. There is incipient focal necrosis. (40×)

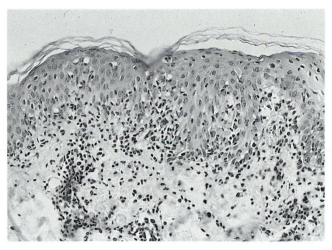

6-11-2 MUCHA-HABERMAN DISEASE: Lichenoid and perivascular infiltrate of lymphocytes. Marked exocytosis and papillary dermal hemorrhage. (200×)

Clinical Features

The lesions are found in greater numbers on the trunk and proximal extremities. The palms, soles, and mucous membranes are usually not involved. Mucha-Habermann disease is a polymorphous eruption consisting of yellowish or brown macules, papules, or papulovesicles that develop central necrosis, ulcerate, crust, and become hemorrhagic (Plate 6-11-1). Postinflammatory hypo- or hyperpigmentation occurs, as does scarring. The eruption lasts weeks to months; frequently, recurring crops of lesions continue over a two- to three-year period.

Differential Diagnosis

Varicella
Vasculitis
Impetigo
Lymphomatoid papulosis
Papular urticaria (insect bites)
Rickettsial disease

HISTOLOGICAL DESCRIPTION

The histological features in Mucha-Habermann disease are a wedge-shaped inflammatory infiltrate that extends from the papillary dermis into the reticular dermis. There is a dense perivascular mononuclear cell infiltrate involving the papillary dermal vessels. The inflammatory infiltrate may simulate that of a vasculitis, although this is not a leukocytoclastic vasculitis. There is exocytosis of mononuclear cells as well as focal red cell exocytosis. The overlying epidermis has a parakeratotic crusted scale with underlying spongiosis (Figures 6-11-1 and 6-11-2). The red cell exocytosis is secondary to focal hemorrhage within the papillary dermis. Epidermal necrosis may occur, especially when inflammation is severe. Occasional large reactive mononuclear cells may be seen in the inflammatory infiltrate.

There is a chronic variety of this condition—pityriasis lichenoides chronica variety of Juliusberg—in which there is a less intense perivascular mononuclear cell, inflammatory infiltrate. Small focal areas of red cell exocytosis are also present. Parakeratosis and spongiosis may be observed, but epidermal ulceration is rare. There is essentially no difference in histological findings in this condition between children and adults.

Differential Diagnosis
Eruptions due to drugs
Inflammatory pityriasis rosea
Eczematous dermatitis

6-12 MUCOCUTANEOUS LYMPH NODE SYNDROME

CLINICAL DESCRIPTION

Etiology and Incidence
Mucocutaneous lymph node syndrome (Kawasaki's disease) is a recently defined multisystemic disease affecting infants and young children. It most frequently affects children younger than five years of age, with more than half being less than two and one-half years old. The disease occurs more often in Japanese children but does occur in Caucasians and blacks. A genetic susceptibility is suspected: there is an increased incidence of HLA-BW22 and HLA-BW22J2 in affected patients. Other suspected causes include infections (rickettsial, viral, etc.), toxins (rug shampoo, mercury), and collagen vascular disease. Laboratory findings include an elevated sedimentation rate, leukocytosis, thrombocytosis, anemia, proteinuria, pyuria, elevated IgE levels, cerebrospinal fluid pleocytosis, and electrocardiographic changes. The etiology of this disorder is unknown.

Clinical Features
The principal signs include (1) fever for more than five days (95%); (2) palmar and plantar erythema (90%), edema of the hands and feet (75%), and desquamation of the fingertips (fourteen to twenty days after the onset of the syndrome (95%); (3) polymorphous exanthem, including pustules; (4) conjunctival inflammation (90%); (5) reddened, cracked lips (90%), strawberry tongue (75%), and intense erythema of the mucous membranes; and (6) nonsuppurative cervical lymphadenopathy (70%) (Plate 6-12-1).

Other significant findings include cardiovascular abnormalities (arrhythmias, murmurs, pericardial effusions, coronary aneurysms, and myocardial infarction). Patients frequently have vomiting, diarrhea, and abdominal pain and have

also been noted to have coughing and rhinorrhea, arthritis, seizures, facial palsies, and transverse nail grooves (Beau's lines). On rare occasion, hydrops of the gallbladder has been described. A desquamative diaper eruption may appear early in the course of the disease.

Differential Diagnosis
Erythema multiforme
Stevens-Johnson syndrome
Viral exanthems
Scarlet fever
Drug reaction
Infantile periarteritis nodosa
Staphylococcal scalded skin syndrome
Systemic lupus erythematosus
Acrodynia

HISTOLOGICAL DESCRIPTION

The usual histological features are a chronic inflammatory process in which there is only a perivascular infiltrate of lymphocytes and histiocytes with minimal epidermal involvement (Figure 6-12-1). In some instances the changes may be more acute, resembling those of the dermal-epidermal variety of erythema multiforme. A rather dense perivascular infiltrate of lymphocytes and histiocytes, associated with small areas of vacuolar degeneration of the basal cells and histiocytes may be observed. The reaction is associated with vacuolar degeneration of the basal cells and necrotic keratinocytes in the epidermis.

Differential Diagnosis
Erythema multiforme

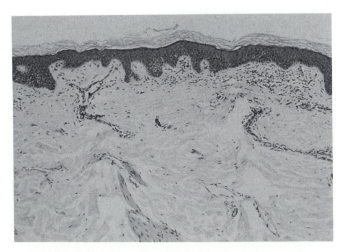

6-12-1 MUCOCUTANEOUS LYMPH NODE SYNDROME: Lymphocytic inflammatory infiltrate about the dermal blood vessels. Superficial vascular ectasia. (100 ×)

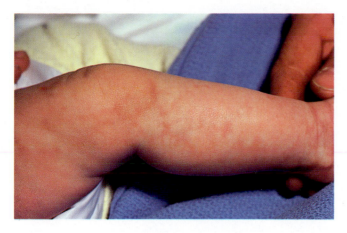

Plate 3-3-1 CUTIS MARMORATA TELANGIECTATICA CONGENITA: A lacelike pattern of dull erythema on the leg of a young child.

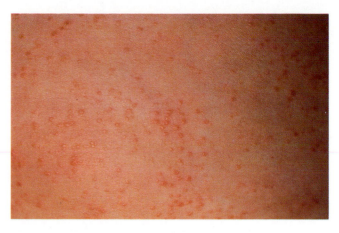

Plate 3-4-1 MILIARIA: Discrete vesicles and erythematous papules in large numbers on the abdomen.

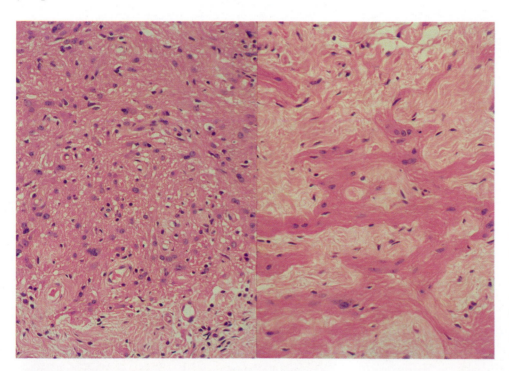

Plate 3-6-1 NASAL GLIOMA: **A** (left) Embedded in an eosinophilic matrix are cells with ovoid nuclei and prominent nucleoli. Some cells display stellate processes and are glial cells (astrocytes). Adjoining normal dermal stroma is shown. (250×) **B** (right) Interlacing bundles of fibrous and neural tissue. (400×)

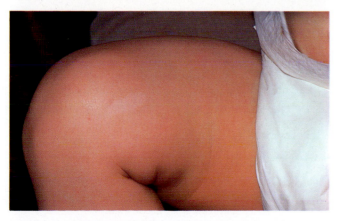

Plate 4-1-1 TUBEROUS SCLEROSIS (ash-leaf macule): Hypopigmented leaf-shaped macule on an infant's distal thigh.

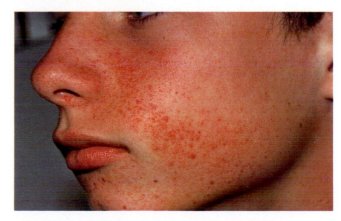

Plate 4-1-2 TUBEROUS SCLEROSIS (angiofibroma): Erythematous papules on a child's face.

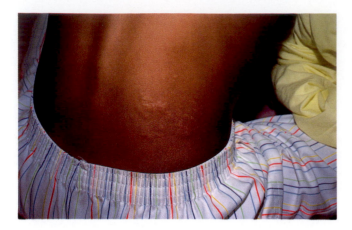

Plate 4-1-3 TUBEROUS SCLEROSIS (**connective tissue nevus**): Connective tissue nevus on flank. Note irregular skin surface.

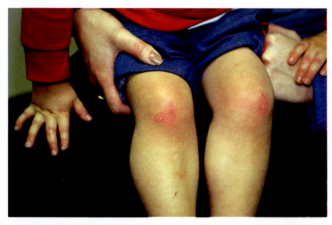

Plate 4-4-1 EPIDERMOLYSIS BULLOSA: Milia and scars on the hands and knees of child with dominant dystrophic type.

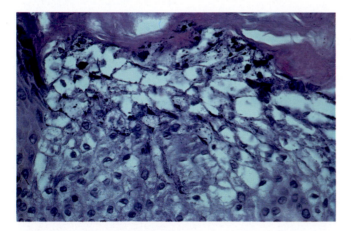

Plate 4-5-2 EPIDERMOLYTIC HYPERKERATOSIS: High power, showing large irregular keratohyaline granules and vacuolization of the epidermis. (400×)

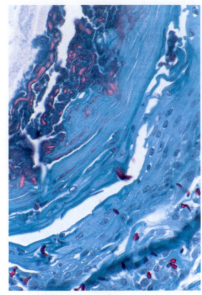

Plate 4-3-1 ELASTOSIS PERFORANS SERPIGINOSA: Elastic tissue stain (aldehyde fuchsin), showing altered elastic tissue in the papillary dermis and in the dermis. (40×)

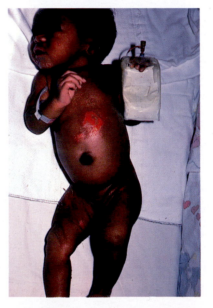

Plate 4-5-1 EPIDERMOLYTIC HYPERKERATOSIS: Denudation in newborn.

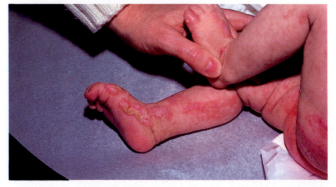

Plate 4-7-1 INCONTINENTIA PIGMENTI: Verrucous stage (note side of foot). Also note linear distribution of erythematous papules and vesicles on back of leg in this child.

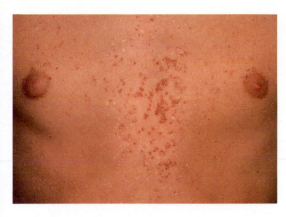

Plate 4-8-1 KERATOSIS FOLLICULARIS: Follicular brown papules on the chest.

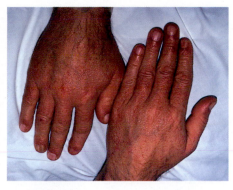

Plate 4-8-2 KERATOSIS FOLLICULARIS: Acrokeratosis verruciformis of Hopf on the back of hands. (Courtesy of Allen Gaisen, M.D.)

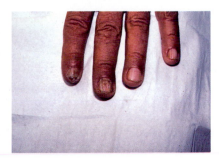

Plate 4-8-3 KERATOSIS FOLLICULARIS: Nails of patient. Note pterygium formation on index finger and red streaks on fifth digit.

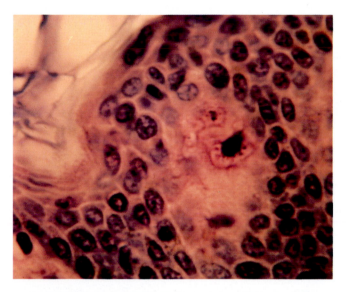

Plate 4-10-1 MUCOPOLYSACCHARIDOSIS: Metachromatic granules within a fibroblast seen in the dermal papillae. (Alcian blue stain, 100 ×)

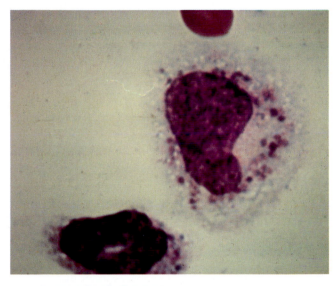

Plate 4-10-2 MUCOPOLYSACCHARIDOSIS: Touch smear, showing a fibroblast with metachromatic granules. (Toluidine blue stain, 200 ×)

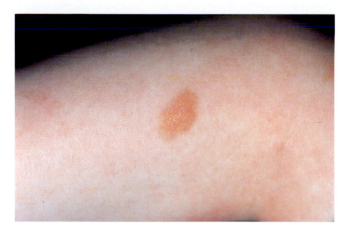

Plate 4-13-1 URTICARIA PIGMENTOSA: Yellow-orange mastocytoma.

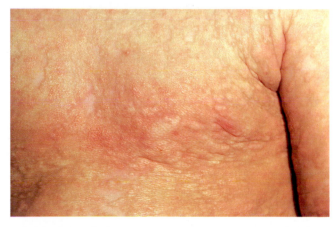

Plate 4-13-2 URTICARIA PIGMENTOSA: Diffuse mastocytosis. Note rippled, boggy, thickened appearance of skin.

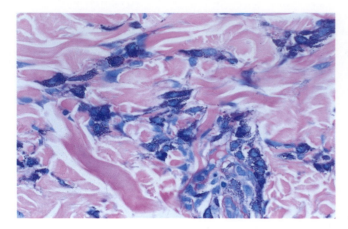

Plate 4-13-3 URTICARIA PIGMENTOSA: Giemsa stain of macular urticaria pigmentosa, demonstrating the metachromatic granules in the mast cells in the dermis and about dermal vessels. (200×)

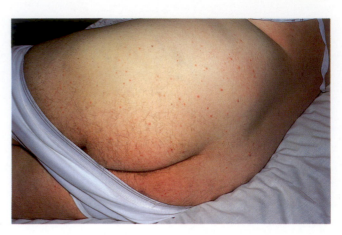

Plate 4-17-1 HYPERLIPIDEMIAS: Eruptive papular xanthomas on buttocks.

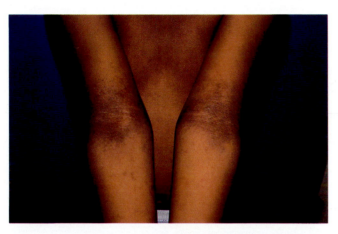

Plate 5-1-1 ATOPIC DERMATITIS: Characteristic involvement of antecubital fossae (flexures) with eczema. The hyperpigmented plaques show accentuation of skin markings, indicating chronicity of this process.

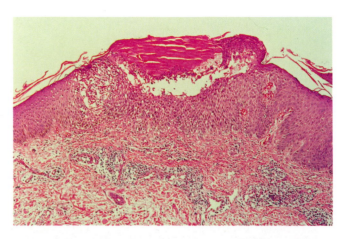

Plate 5-1-2 ATOPIC DERMATITIS: Spongiosis and intraepidermal vesiculation. Within the dermis, the infiltrate contains lymphocytes and histiocytes. (100×)

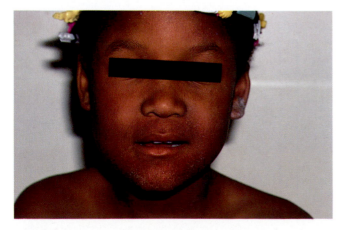

Plate 5-2-1 CONTACT DERMATITIS: Erythema, crusting, and vesiculation of the chin with slight extension onto the cheeks in this young black child.

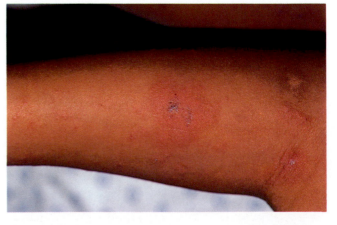

Plate 5-2-2 CONTACT DERMATITIS: The arm of the child in Plate 5-2-1, with an erythematous plaque and erythematous linear streaks. The latter finding is characteristic of contact dermatitis to rhus (poison ivy). Healing excoriations or erosions can also be seen.

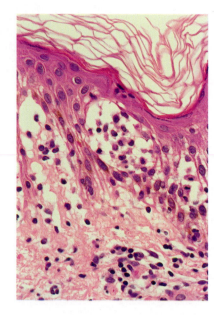

Plate 5-2-3 CONTACT DERMATITIS: Nested antigen-presenting cells in the epidermis (Langerhans' cell granuloma). (400 ×)

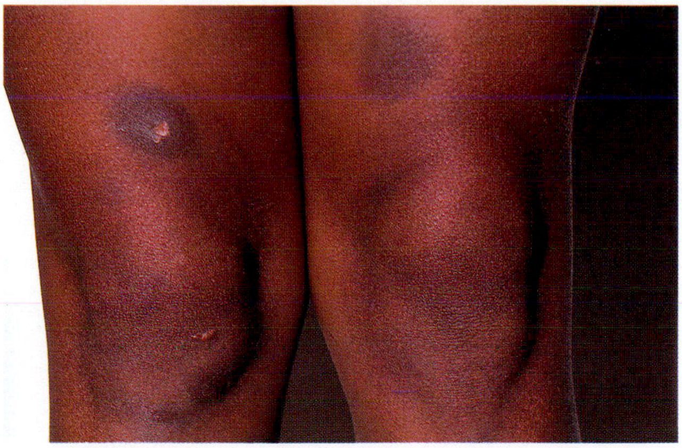

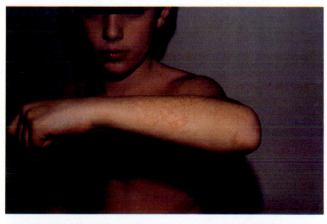

Plate 5-4-1 FIXED DRUG ERUPTION: Sharply demarcated hyperpigmented patches and plaque (one with excoriation) above the knees secondary to phenolphthalein.

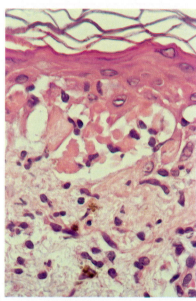

Plate 5-4-2 FIXED DRUG ERUPTION: High power shows collections of necrotic basilar keratinocytes with lymphocytes and prominent collections of melanin in superficial dermal macrophages. (400 ×)

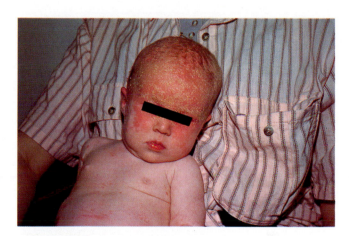

Plate 5-8-1 SEBORRHEIC DERMATITIS: Erythematous plaques with yellowish scale, accentuated in hair-bearing areas (scalp, eyebrows, and eyelashes) and extending onto the cheeks and midchest.

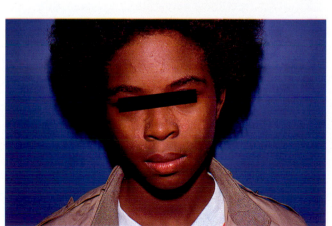

Plate 5-8-2 SEBORRHEIC DERMATITIS: Hypopigmented patches and plaques with scaling in the nasolabial folds of an adolescent.

Plate 5-9-1 XEROTIC ECZEMA: The extensor aspects of the arms, with annular patches with erythematous borders and scaling.

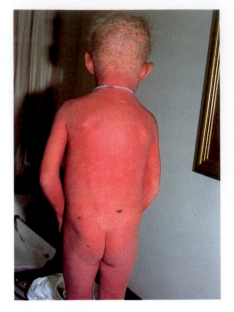

Plate 6-1-1 PSORIASIS: Erythrodermic psoriatic patient.

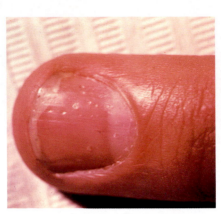

Plate 6-1-2 PSORIASIS: Pitted nail in a child.

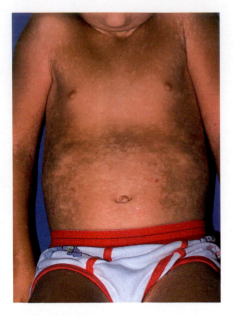

Plate 6-2-1 PARAPSORIASIS: Papulosquamous lesions in child with parapsoriasis.

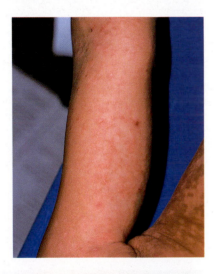

Plate 6-2-2 PARA-PSORIASIS: Arm of the child shown in Plate 6-2-1.

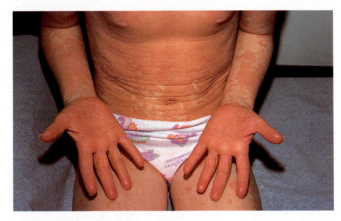

Plate 6-4-1 PITYRIASIS RUBRA PILARIS: Erythroderma with islands of spared skin. Child also has palmar hyperkeratosis.

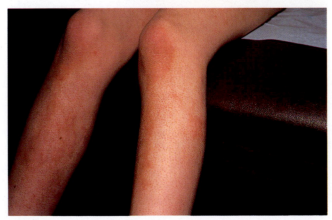

Plate 6-4-2 PITYRIASIS RUBRA PILARIS: Same child as in Plate 6-4-1, with follicular prominence.

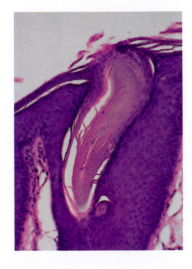

Plate 6-4-3 PITYRIASIS RUBRA PILARIS: Parakeratosis extends from the epidermal surface into the follicular canal, the hallmark of pityriasis rubra pilaris. (400×)

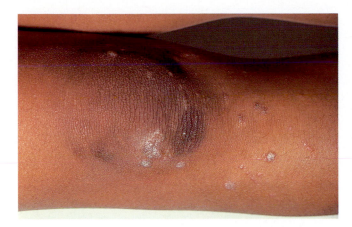

Plate 6-5-1 LICHEN PLANUS: Violaceous papules on patient's knee.

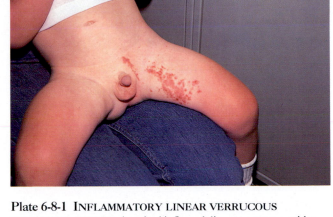

Plate 6-8-1 INFLAMMATORY LINEAR VERRUCOUS EPIDERMAL NEVUS: Acquired inflamed, linear verrucous epidermal nevus on child's leg.

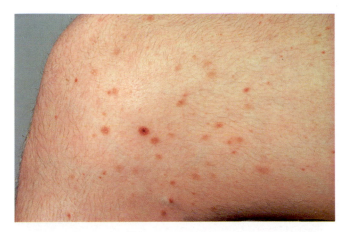

Plate 6-11-1 PLEVA: Erythematous and necrotic lesions.

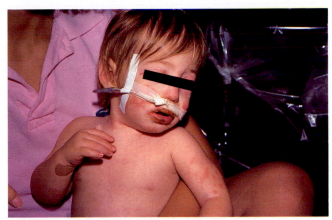

Plate 6-12-1 MUCOCUTANEOUS LYMPH NODE SYNDROME: There is involvement of eyes, lips, and hands.

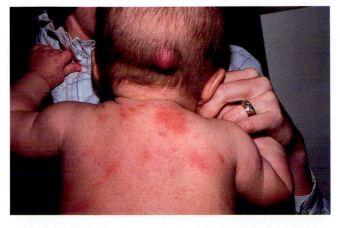

Plate 7-1-1 ERYTHEMA TOXICUM NEONATORUM: Individual and clustered pustules surrounded by erythema on infant's back. Note hemangioma on occiput.

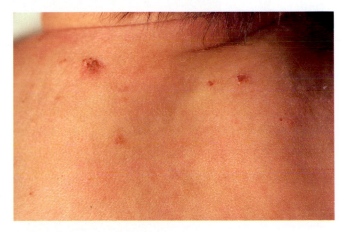

Plate 7-1-2 TRANSIENT NEONATAL PUSTULAR MELANOSIS: Vesicopustules surmounted by a crust on a neonate's back.

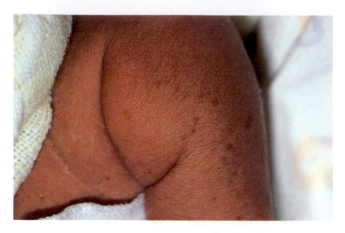

Plate 7-1-3 TRANSIENT NEONATAL PUSTULAR MELANOSIS: Hyperpigmented macules on the legs indicate previous sites of involvement.

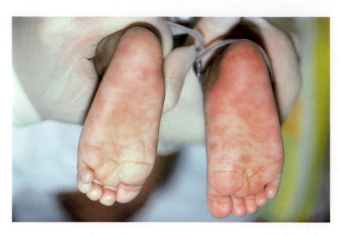

Plate 7-2-1 CONGENITAL SYPHILIS: Ham-colored macules on the plantar surface of a newborn's feet.

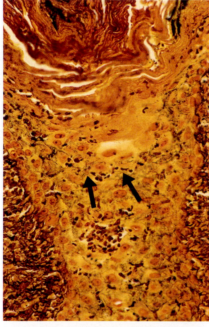

Plate 7-2-2 CONGENITAL SYPHILIS: Dieterle stain highlights the presence of corkscrew *Treponemes.* (400×)

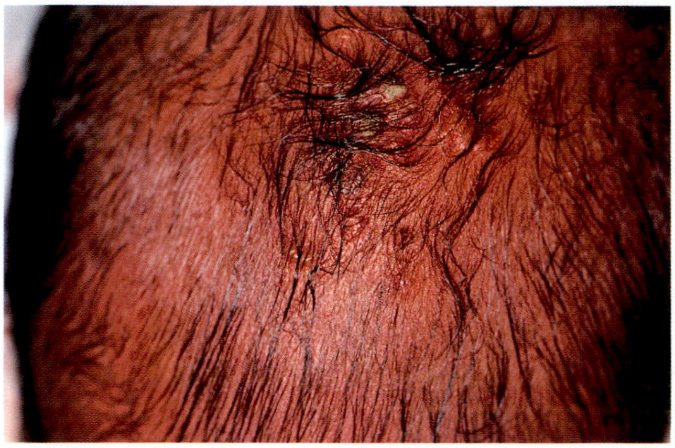

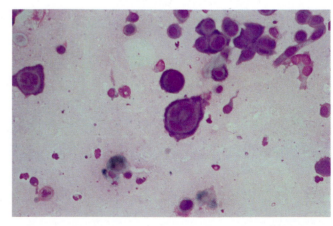

Plate 7-2-3 HERPES SIMPLEX: Scalp of a newborn with characteristic grouped vesicles.

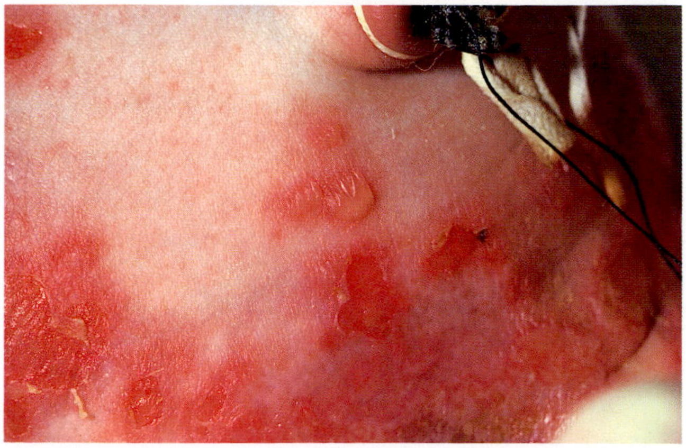

Plate 7-2-4 HERPES SIMPLEX: Abdomen of a newborn with grouped vesicles and bullae on an erythematous base.

Plate 7-2-5 HERPES SIMPLEX: Tzank preparation with multinucleated epithelial viral giant cells.

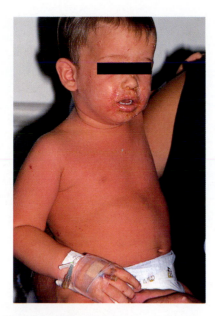

Plate 7-2-6 STAPHYLOCOCCAL SCALDED SKIN SYNDROME: Characteristic periorificial blisters, crusting, and fiery red skin.

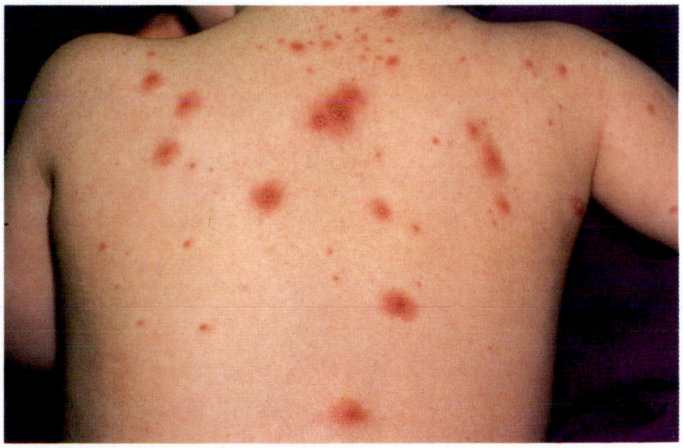

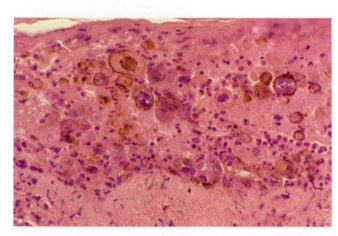

Plate 7-2-7 VARICELLA: A crop of vesicles on an erythematous base on the trunk of a nine-year-old boy.

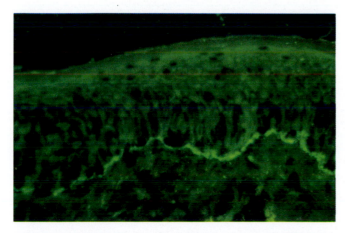

Plate 7-2-8 HERPES ZOSTER: Groups of vesicles with crusting on a hemorrhagic base, localized to the buttock and thigh.

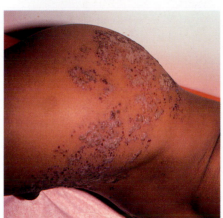

Plate 7-2-9 VARICELLA ZOSTER: Higher magnification of Figure 7-2-12 shows epidermal cell necrosis with epidermal viral giant cells and associated mixed inflammatory infiltrate. (400×)

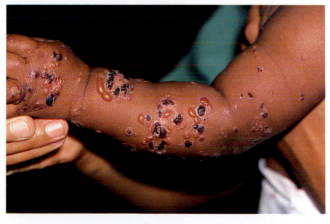

Plate 7-3-1 EBA: Direct immunofluorescence showing IgG in a linear arrangement at the dermal-epidermal junction. (400×)

Plate 7-3-2 CHRONIC BULLOUS DISEASE OF CHILDHOOD: Annular arrangement of sausage-shaped bullae around crusted lesions.

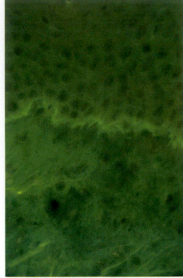

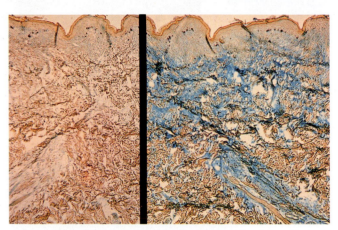

Plate 7-3-3 CHRONIC BULLOUS DISEASE OF CHILDHOOD: Direct immunofluorescence shows linear deposition of IgA at the dermal-epidermal junction. (200×)

Plate 7-3-4 DERMATITIS HERPETIFORMIS: Direct immuno-fluoresence shows papillary dermal collections of granular IgA.

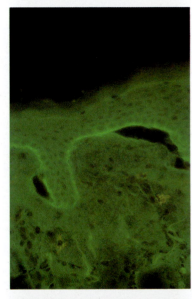

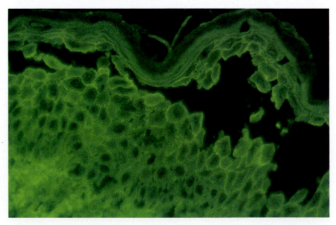

Plate 7-3-5 JUVENILE BULLOUS PEMPHIGOID: Direct immunofluorescence of bullous pemphigoid, showing IgG at the dermal-epidermal junction. (200×)

Plate 7-3-6 LUPUS ERYTHEMATOSUS: Paired section, showing dermal mucin as demonstrated by the colloidal iron technique. The section on the left was predigested with hyaluronidase to remove the hyaluronic acid. The section on the right stains positively. These paired sections demonstrate that the mucin or edematous changes seen within the dermis in lupus erythematosus is that of hyaluronic acid. (40×)

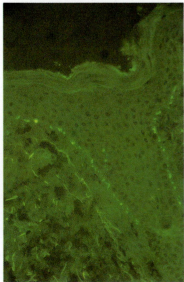

Plate 7-3-7 LUPUS ERYTHEMATOSUS: Direct immunofluorescence demonstrates granular immunoreactants (IgG, C3, IgM, and IgA) at the dermal-epidermal-follicular junction. (400×)

Plate 7-3-8 PEMPHIGUS: Direct immunofluorescent staining with IgG shows positive staining with IgG in the intercellular spaces (pemphigus foliaceous pattern). (400×)

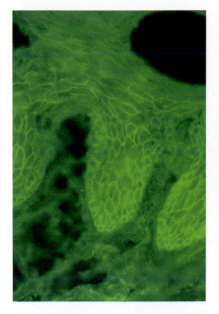

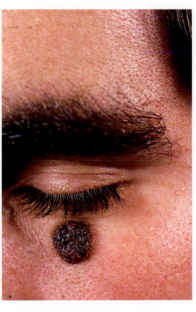

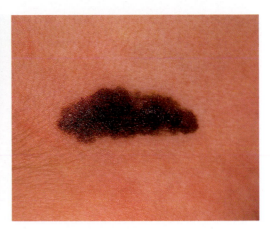

Plate 8-1-2 CONGENITAL NEVUS: Velvety brown plaque with slightly fuzzy borders on the abdomen.

Plate 7-3-9 PEMPHIGUS VULGARIS: Indirect immunofluorescence shows positive intercellular staining with IgG, which indicates circulating antibodies to intercellular substance. (400×)

Plate 8-1-1 COMPOUND NEVUS: Exophitic papillomatous dark brown nodule. Note the similarity to dermal (Plate 8-1-2) nevus, but with darker pigmentation.

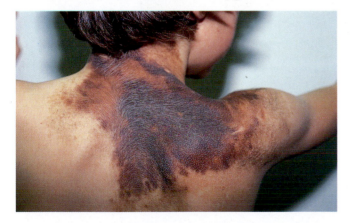

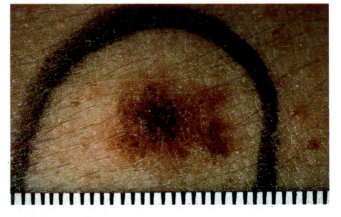

Plate 8-1-3 CONGENITAL HAIRY NEVUS: Extensive brown-black mottled pigmentation on the upper back, extending to the neck and shoulders, associated with increased terminal hair growth. (Courtesy of L. Robert Smith, M.D.)

Plate 8-2-1 DYSPLASTIC ("ATYPICAL") NEVUS: Note the irregular pigmentation and margins.

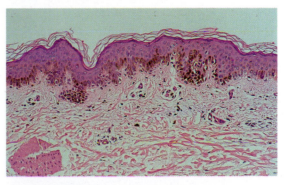

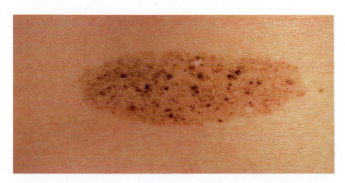

Plate 8-3-2 NEVUS SPILUS: Lentigenous epidermal hyperplasia and basilar pigmentation. Prominent clear cells are seen primarily as single cells at the dermal-epidermal interface. There is one suggestion of a nevus cell nest in the mid-portion of the specimen. Melanophage pigmentation is present in the dermis. (200×)

Plate 8-3-1 NEVUS SPILUS: Smaller islands of pigmentation on a tan background.

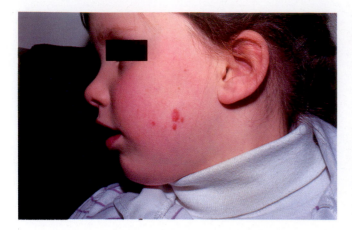

Plate 8-4-1 SPINDLE AND EPITHELIOD CELL NEVUS: Multiple red papules on the cheek, representing Spitz nevi.

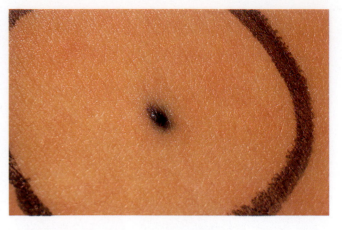

Plate 8-6-1 BLUE NEVUS: A sharply demarcated blue-black nodule on the abdomen.

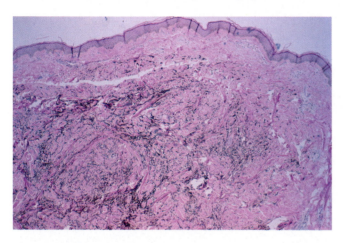

Plate 8-6-2 BLUE NEVUS: Low-power photomicrograph, showing a nodular dermal tumor with pigmentation. (40×)

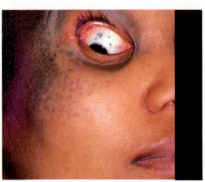

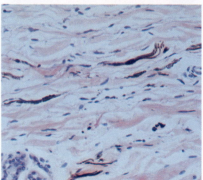

Plate 8-8-1 NEVUS OTA'S/ITO'S: A (top) Scleral and periocular macular slate gray pigmentation in an eight-year-old patient. **B** (bottom) Pigmented bipolar melanocytes in the dermis. (100×)

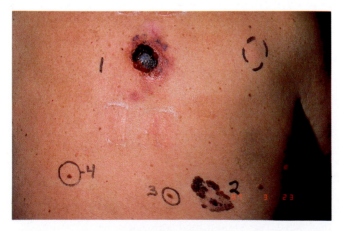

Plate 8-9-1 MALIGNANT MELANOMA: A large exophytic partially ulcerated nodule surrounded by a mottled blue-black macular component. The lesion labeled 2 shows zones of regression within a mottled brown-black plaque.

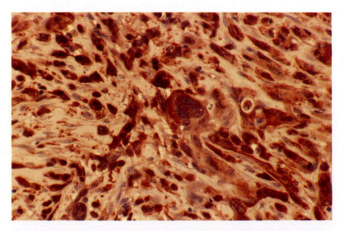

Plate 8-9-2 NODULAR MELANOMA: S-100 protein stain, showing marked S-100 positivity. (400×)

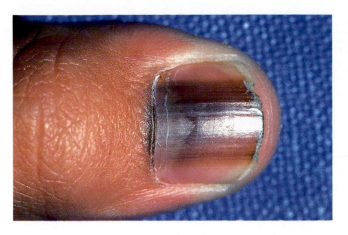

Plate 8-10-1 MELANONYCHIA STRIATA: A pigmented band as seen within the nailplate. Pigmentation is also noted on the posterior nailfold, where the pigment is greatest in intensity.

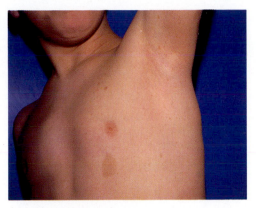

Plate 8-13-1 NEUROFIBROMATOSIS: A child with axillary freckling and a café-au-lait macule beneath the left breast.

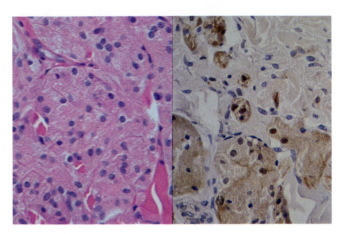

Plate 8-15-1 GRANULAR CELL TUMOR: **A** (left) Higher-power photomicrograph, showing the granular cells, which have a vesicular nucleus with eosinophilic cytoplasm filled with granules. (200×) **B** (right) S-100 stain demonstrates cellular positivity. (200×)

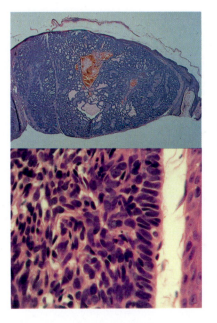

Plate 9-3-1 BASAL CELL CARCINOMA: **A** (top) Low-power magnification, showing islands of basaloid tumor extending into the dermis. (20×) **B** (bottom) Higher-power magnification, showing a basaloid island with distinct peripheral palisading. (400×)

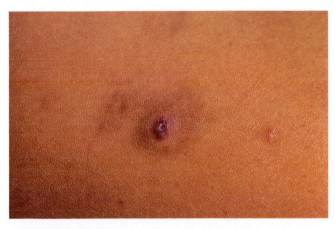

Plate 9-10-1 OSTEOMA CUTIS: Indurated area on the thigh with surrounding inflammation. Suggestion of early extrusion of bony spicule.

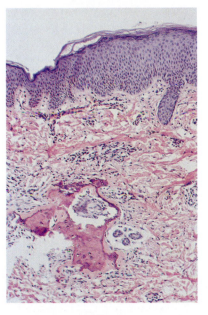

Plate 9-10-2 OSTEOMA CUTIS: Low magnification shows basophilic amorphous material within the dermis. This material represents osteoid or early bone formation. (40×)

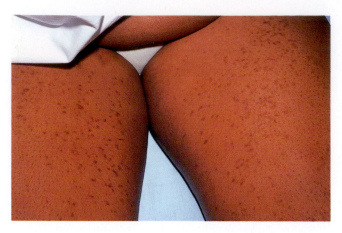

Plate 9-14-1 SYRINGOMA: Numerous firm hyperpigmented papules on both thighs. (Courtesy of Allen Gaisin, M.D.)

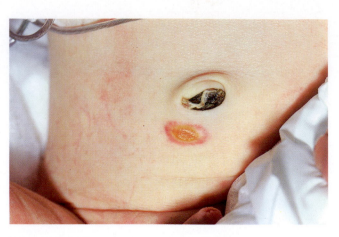

Plate 10-2-1 CONGENITAL FIBROMATOSIS: A reddish brown, somewhat translucent plaque on the abdomen adjacent to the umbilicus of a neonate.

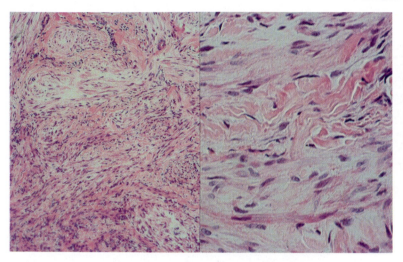

Plate 10-2-2 CONGENITAL FIBROMATOSIS: (left) Variable arrays of basaloid cells in tight fascicles (100×) and (right) in a looser stroma, which contrasts with adjacent normal dermis. (200×) (Courtesy of Jane Chatten, M.D., Department of Pathology of Children's Hospital of Philadelphia.)

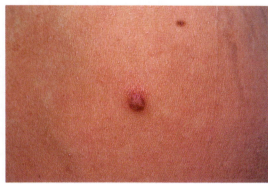

Plate 10-3-1 DERMATOFIBROMA: Elevated firm nodule with a collarette of hyperpigmentation on an adolescent's leg.

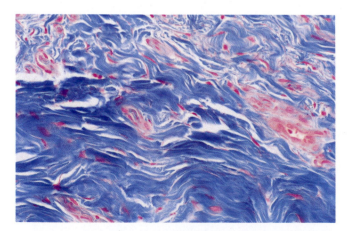

Plate 10-4-1 DESMOID TUMOR: Trichrome stains stain the collagen in this proliferation in blue. (100×) (Courtesy of Jane Chatten, M.D., Department of Pathology of Children's Hospital of Philadelphia.)

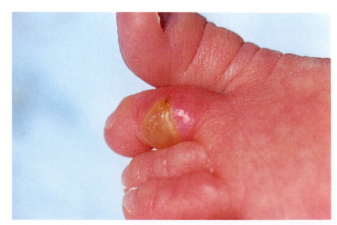

Plate 10-10-1 RECURRENT INFANTILE DIGITAL FIBROMA: A shiny, red nodule on the second toe of a child with a recurrent digital fibroma.

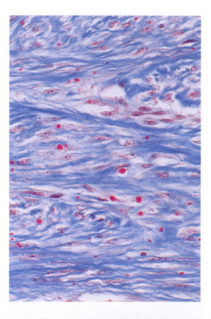

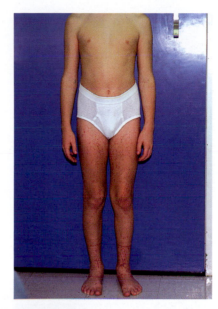

Plate 10-10-2
RECURRENT
INFANTILE DIGITAL
FIBROMA: The
eosinophilic inclusions
shown in Figure
10-10-2 are easily
discerned with tri-
chrome stains. (200×)
(Courtesy of Jane
Chatten, M.D., De-
partment of Pathology
of Children's Hospital
of Philadelphia.)

Plate 11-2-1
HENOCH-
SCHOENLEIN
PURPURA: Typical
distribution. Note
sparing of the trunk.

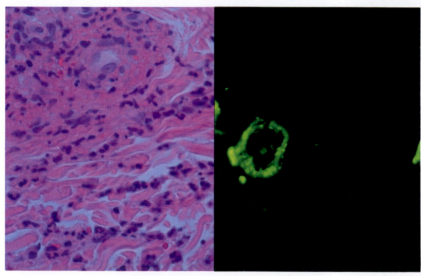

Plate 11-2-2 **HENOCH-SCHOENLEIN**
PURPURA: (left) Leukocytoclastic vasculitis:
vessel wall damage, perivenular fibrin deposition, and fragmented neutrophils. (100×)
(right) Direct immunofluorescence of such
lesion biopsied before forty-eight hours shows
deposition of IgA in a granular pattern in vessel
walls. (100×)

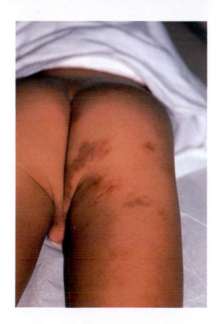

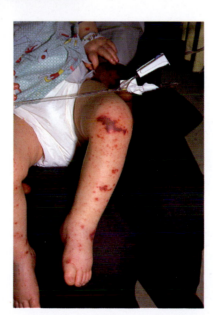

Plate 11-3-1
CHRONIC
PIGMENTED
PURPURA:
Erythematous and
nonerythematous
hyperpigmented
patches on a child's
posterior thigh.

Plate 11-4-1
PURPURA
FULMINANS:
Necrotic lesions in a
patient with meningo-
coccemia.

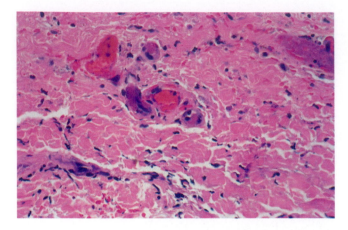

Plate 11-4-2 PURPURA FULMINANS: Occlusion of small dermal vessels by platelets and fibrin thrombi in purpura fulminans. (400×)

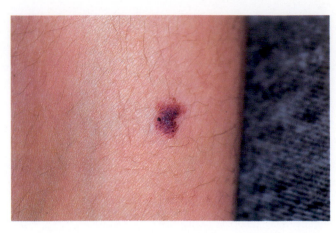

Plate 11-5-1 ANGIOKERATOMA: Sharply circumscribed erythematous and violaceous papule with a verrucous surface.

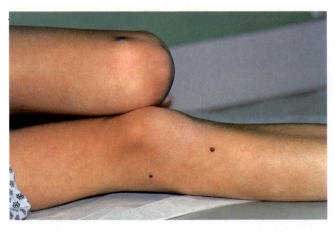

Plate 11-8-1 BLUE RUBBER BLEB NEVUS: Discrete blueblack papules on a child's leg.

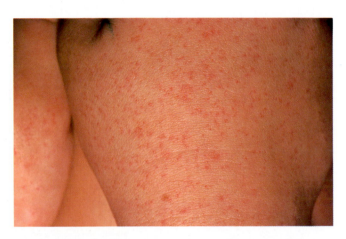

Plate 11-9-1 GENERALIZED ESSENTIAL TELANGIECTASIA: Massive numbers of erythematous blanchable macules.

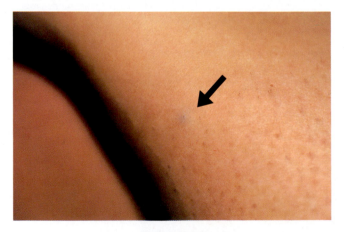

Plate 11-10-1 GLOMUS TUMOR: Deep-seated nodule on the posterior aspect of the lower leg of a ten-year-old.

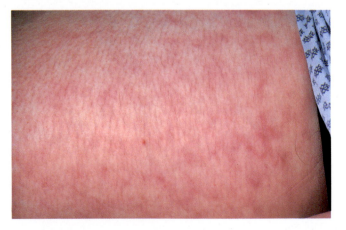

Plate 11-13-1 LIVEDO RETICULARIS: Erythema with a lacelike pattern on a child's back.

REFERENCES

Psoriasis

Farber EM, Carlson RA: Psoriasis in childhood. Calif Med 1966; 105:415.

Farber EM, Mullen RH, Jacobs AH, et al.: Infantile psoriasis: A follow-up study. Pediatr Dermatol 1986; 3:237.

Rasmussen JE: Psoriasis in children. Dermatol Clin North Am 1986; 4:99.

Parapsoriasis

Lambert WE, Everett MA: The nosology of parapsoriasis (review). J Am Acad Dermatol 1981; 5:373.

Pityriasis Rosea

Bjornberg A, Hellgrin L: Pityriasis rosea: A statistical, clinical and laboratory investigation of 826 patients and matched health controls. Acta Derm Venorol 1972; 42 (suppl 50):1.

Parsons JM: Pityriasis rosea update. J Am Acad Dermatol 1986; 15:159.

Pityriasis Rubra Pilaris

Brice SL, Barr RJ, Rattet JP: Childhood lichen planus: A question of therapy. J Am Acad Dermatol 1980; 3:370.

Gelmetti C, Shiuma AA, Cerri D, et al.: Pityriasis rubra pilaris in childhood: A long-term study of 29 cases. Pediatr Dermatol 1986; 3:446.

Lichen Planus

Ellis FA: Histopathology of lichen planus based on analysis of one hundred biopsies. J Invest Dermatol 1967; 48:143.

Lichen Nitidus

Lapius NA, Willoushbis C, Helwis EB: Lichen nitidus: A study of 43 cases. Cutis 1978; 21:634.

Pinkus H: Lichenoid tissue eruptions. Arch Dermatol 1973; 197:840.

Lichen Striatus

Charles CR, Johnson BL, Robinson TA: Lichen striatus. J Cutan Pathol 1974; 1:256.

Reed RJ, Meek T, Ichinose H: Lichen striatus: A mode for the histologic spectrum of lichenoid reactions. J Cutan Pathol 1975; 2:1.

Linear Inflammatory Epidermal Nevus

Hodge SJ, Barr JM, Owen LG: Inflammatory linear verrucous epidermal nevus. Arch Dermatol 1978; 114:436.

Kaidbey KH, Kurban AK: Dermatitic epidermal nevus. Arch Dermatol 1971; 104:166.

Acropustulosis of Infancy

Jarratt M, Ramsdell W: Infantile acropustulosis. Arch Dermatol 1979; 115:834.

Kahn G, Rywlin A: Acropustulosis of infancy. Arch Dermatol 1979; 115:831.

Papular Acrodermatitis of Childhood

Gianotti F: Papular acrodermatitis of childhood and other papulovesicular acro-located syndromes (review). Br J Dermatol 1979; 100:49.

Petrizi A, DiLerna V, Giampaolo G, et al.: Papular and papulovesicular acrolocated eruptions and viral infections. Pediatr Dermatol 1980; 7:22.

Lowe L, Herbert AA, Dovil M: Gianotti-Crosti syndrome associated with Epstein-Barr virus infection. J Am Acad Dermatol 1989; 20:336.

Mucha-Habermann Disease

Hood AF, Mark EJ: Histopathologic diagnosis of pityriasis lichenoides et varioliformis acuta and its clinical correlation. Arch Dermatol 1982; 118:478.

Willemze R, Scheffer E: Clinical and histologic differentiation between lymphomatoid papulosis and pityriasis lichenoides. J Am Acad Dermatol 1985; 13:418.

Mucocutaneous Lymph Node Syndrome

Bierman FZ, Gersony WM: Kawasaki disease: Clinical perspective. Pediatr 1978; 111:789.

Friter BS, Lucky AW: The perineal eruption of Kawasaki syndrome. Arch Dermatol 1988; 124:1805.

Kawasaki T, Kosari F, Owaka S, et al.: A new infantile mucocutaneous lymph node syndrome (MLNS) prevailing in Japan. Pediatrics 1974; 54:271.

7

Bullous Disorders

Contents

7-1 PHYSIOLOGIC BULLOUS DISORDERS

Children with blistering dermatosis are an enjoyable challenge, because the physician can almost always arrive at a specific diagnosis. This requires the use of every available tool: history, physical examination (morphology and distribution of blisters), cultures, Tzank preps, histology, and both direct and indirect immunofluorescence.

     Since many of the blistering disorders look very much alike, a differential diagnosis is not given for each entity. The reader is advised to use the table of contents of this chapter for a differential diagnosis.

     Many of the topics listed are discussed in other chapters. Please refer to those chapters for more information.

ERYTHEMA TOXICUM NEONATORUM

CLINICAL DESCRIPTION

Etiology and Incidence

Erythema toxicum neonatorum occurs in the full-term, normal-weight newborn during the first forty-eight hours of life. Lesions may occur up to two weeks of age. It is rarely seen in infants born before thirty weeks gestation and weighing less than 1,500 g. The incidence ranges between 30% and 70% in children greater than forty weeks gestation and weighing more than 2,500 g. The etiology is unknown.

Clinical Features

Any body area except the palms and soles can be involved. Lesions are 1 to 3 mm, flesh-colored papules to pustules on an erythematous base (Plate 7-1-1). Many are isolated, but clustering is not uncommon. These skin changes do not last long: lesions disappear within hours to days.

Differential Diagnosis

Miliaria
Transient neonatal pustular melanosis
Bullous impetigo
Congenital syphilis
Herpes simplex/varicella zoster
Incontinentia pigmenti
Urticaria pigmentosa
Acropustulosis of infancy
Scabies

HISTOLOGICAL DESCRIPTION

The histological features vary depending on the clinical lesion biopsied. Macular lesions have eosinophils and neutrophils in the outer root sheath of rudimentary follicles (Figure 7-1-1). Papular and pustular lesions show a greater accumulation of

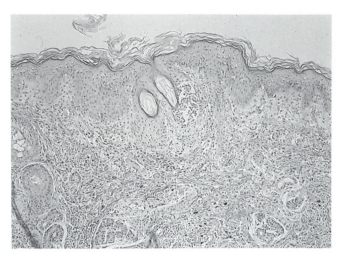

7-1-1 ERYTHEMA TOXICUM NEONATORUM: Low magnification shows hyperkeratosis, follicular plugging, and an infiltrate of cells in the follicular epithelium. (40×)

eosinophils, fewer neutrophils, and a pustule of eosinophils in a subcorneal location at the follicular orifice (Figure 7-1-2). Eosinophils and polymorphonuclear leukocytes may be seen also in the dermis, with associated edema.

Differential Diagnosis

Transient neonatal pustular melanosis
Acropustulosis of infancy
Scabies
Eosinophilic pustular folliculitis
Incontinentia pigmenti

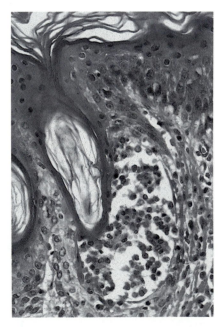

7-1-2 ERYTHEMA TOXICUM NEONATORUM: High magnification shows follicular epithelium filled with a collection of eosinophils. (400×)

MILIARIA

CLINICAL DESCRIPTION

Etiology and Incidence
Obstruction of the eccrine gland ducts produces miliaria.

Clinical Features
These lesions are most commonly found on the head, face, and intertriginous regions. When the sweat is trapped immediately below the stratum corneum, vesicles occur. Erythematous papules are produced, with dermal obstruction and rupture. If polymorphonuclear cells enter, a pustule may be seen. Rapid resolution occurs when the child is kept in a cool environment.

Differential Diagnosis
See Erythema Toxicum Neonatorum

HISTOLOGICAL DESCRIPTION

The distinctive features are an intra- or subcorneal vesicle without inflammatory cells. Vesicles communicate directly with the sweat ducts. The dermis is essentially uninvolved.

There is more epidermal participation in this process, spongiosis, exocytosis of mononuclear cells, and a lymphocytic infiltrate in the dermis. In addition to periductal spongiosis there is spongiosis of the acrosyringum. Miliaria pustulina evolves from this stage, with infiltration of polymorphonuclear leukocytes into the epidermis and sweat duct. There is subsequent formation of subcorneal and intraductal pustules. *Staphylococcus aureus* can be identified in miliaria rubra and miliaria pustulina.

Differential Diagnosis
Bullous impetigo

TRANSIENT NEONATAL PUSTULAR MELANOSIS

CLINICAL DESCRIPTION

Etiology and Incidence
This disorder of the newborn is seen mainly in blacks (4.4%). The cause is unknown.

Clinical Features
Any body surface may be involved. Vesicopustules are found at birth (occasionally only hyperpigmented macules) and disappear within twenty-four to forty-eight hours, leaving behind a hyperpigmented macule (Plate 7-1-2) frequently surrounded by a collarette of fine scales (Plate 7-1-3). All findings disappear within three weeks to three months. All cultures are negative. No associated disorders have been identified.

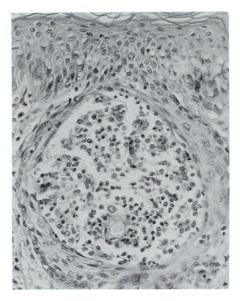

7-1-3 TRANSIENT NEONATAL PUSTULAR MELANOSIS: Dilated follicle filled with neutrophils. (200×)

Differential Diagnosis
See Erythema Toxicum Neonatorum

HISTOLOGICAL DESCRIPTION

The histological features are a subcorneal and intracorneal pustule filled with neutrophils and admixed with a few eosinophils (Figure 7-1-3). This is in contrast to erythema toxicum, which is almost a pure eosinophilic infiltrate. The dermal reaction is mixed with lymphocytes, histiocytes, eosinophils, and neutrophils. The macular hyperpigmented lesions show only basal cell melanocytic hyperpigmentation.

Differential Diagnosis
Erythema toxicum neonatorum
Bullous impetigo

7-2 BULLAE SECONDARY TO INFECTION

BULLOUS IMPETIGO

CLINICAL DESCRIPTION

Etiology and Incidence
Bullous impetigo occurs at most ages, but especially in children less than six years old. *Staphylococcus aureus* releases toxins that produce the clinical skin changes.

Clinical Features
Lesions usually occur on the face, trunk, and extremities (Figure 7-2-1). Erythematous macules go on to form superficial vesicles or bullae that easily rupture, leaving red weeping

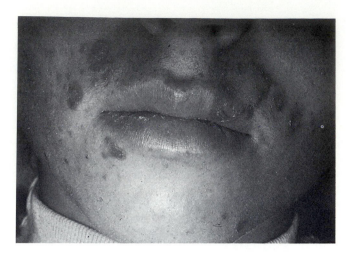

7-2-1 BULLOUS IMPETIGO: Multiple perioral lesions with typical honey-colored crust.

surfaces similar to those seen in staphylococcal scalded skin syndrome. The serous fluid forms typical honeycomb crusts. Surrounding erythema is minimal.

Differential Diagnosis
See Erythema Toxicum Neonatorum

HISTOLOGICAL DESCRIPTION

Although impetigo is not usually grouped with bullous diseases, it is frequently bullous in children. The usual form of impetigo contagiosa can produce blisters in children, and separation occurs within the superficial portion of the epidermis, either subcorneal-intragranular or subgranular-superficial epidermis. Acute inflammatory and acantholytic epidermal cells may be found as well as organisms within the crust and in the superficial portion of the epidermis (Figure 7-2-2). The inflammatory infiltrate in the dermis is mixed and contains acute as well as chronic inflammatory cells and may be severe.

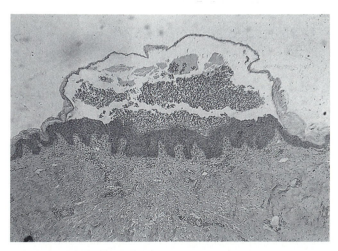

7-2-2 BULLOUS IMPETIGO: Large subcorneal pustule filled with neutrophilic acute inflammatory cells. (40 ×)

Differential Diagnosis
Staphylococcal scalded skin syndrome

CONGENITAL SYPHILIS
CLINICAL DESCRIPTION

Etiology and Incidence
Up to one-half of infants with congenital syphilis have cutaneous findings. *Treponema pallidum* is found in these newborns and produces these changes.

Clinical Features
This condition usually presents the same clinical picture as other intrauterine infections. Vesicular lesions on the palms and soles in the newborn are rare but highly diagnostic (Figure 7-2-3). Other skin changes may appear on any body surface but seem to favor the face, abdomen, diaper area, legs, palms, and soles. Ham-colored, oval or round maculopapular or papulosquamous lesions are common. The palms and soles may show ham-colored macules, desquamation, or a very shiny erythematous skin surface. Mucous membrane lesions include white patches (seen in one-third of infants), fissures radiating from the mouth that eventually scar (rhagades), and condylomata lata (raised, flat, moist, warty lesions). Many of the transient lesions disappear within one to three months.

Differential Diagnosis
See Erythema Toxicum Neonatorum

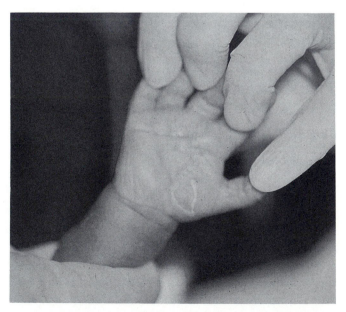

7-2-3 CONGENITAL SYPHILIS: Neonate with findings highly diagnostic of bullae on the palms and remnants of a ruptured blister.

HISTOLOGICAL DESCRIPTION

Bullae occur two weeks to six months after birth, on any cutaneous surfaces. On the mucosal surface only erosions are seen, due to the fragility of the blister roof. There is a dermal-epidermal interface inflammatory response in addition to a perivascular reaction (Figure 7-2-4). These severe inflammatory changes produce the bullae. Children develop bullae with a greater frequency than do adults because of less well developed anchoring fibrils and immaturity of the dermal-epidermal attachment.

The inflammation contains a varying number of plasma cells and lymphocytes. Plasma cells may not be the predominant cell in this infiltrate (Figure 7-2-5). The vessels exhibit endothelial swelling without vascular occlusion.

Spirochetes can be demonstrated, especially on mucosal lesions, and are best visualized with silver stains, such as the Warthin-Starry or Dieterle. Spirochetes are found in the epidermis, about vessels and in the epithelium of the follicles (Plate 7-2-2). The identification of spirochetes in the dermis is not without hazard since the dermal fibers can easily be confused with organisms.

Differential Diagnosis

Pityriasis lichenoides et varioliformis acuta (PLEVA)
Lichen planus

HERPES SIMPLEX

CLINICAL DESCRIPTION

Etiology and Incidence

More than 50% of neonates infected with herpes simplex virus (HSV) will have cutaneous manifestations two to thirty

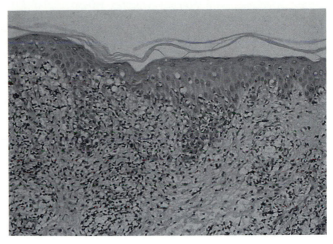

7-2-5 CONGENITAL SYPHILIS: Higher magnification of Figure 7-2-4 shows interface dermatitis as well as a perivascular infiltrate of lymphocytes, plasma cells, and histiocytes. Bullae develop at the dermal-epidermal interface secondary to the inflammatory response. (200×)

days following exposure. The etiologic agent, HSV, is cultured best from vesicular fluid.

Clinical Features

Lesions occur on the presenting part (i.e., the scalp in vertex deliveries, the buttocks in breech births) (Plate 7-2-3). The lesions are usually grouped vesicles on an erythematous base. However, the infection may present as individual vesicles, pustules, bullae, or denuded skin (Plate 7-2-4). On occasion a zosteriform distribution is seen. Recurrences, as with cold sores, are common.

Other Infections with Herpes Simplex Virus

The initial infection with HSV in young children is usually herpetic gingivostomatitis. Vesicles involve the lips and the rest of the mouth. The gingiva becomes inflamed, eroded, ulcerated, and edematous and bleeds easily. This primary infection, as well as any other primary infection with HSV, is usually associated with fever and regional lymphadenopathy.

Herpes progenitalis may produce fever and local lymphadenopathy as well as characteristic clusters of vesicles on an erythematous base. Frequently erosions or ulcerations evolve on the vulva or penis. Pain and dysuria are present. Herpes labialis, herpetic whitlow, Kaposi's varicelliform eruption, and keratoconjunctivitis are other manifestations of infection with this virus.

Differential Diagnosis
Herpes Simplex Virus
Vesicopustules of any of the congenital infections

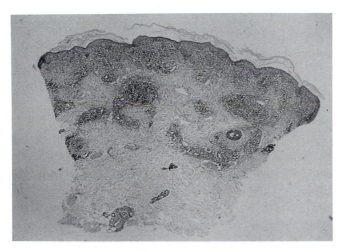

7-2-4 CONGENITAL SYPHILIS: Low power shows a dense perivascular inflammatory infiltrate that extends from the dermal-epidermal interface to the lower reticular dermis. (40×)

Other Infections with Herpes Simplex Virus
Vincent's infection
Hand-foot-mouth disease
Aphthous stomatitis
Erythema multiforme
Behçet syndrome

HISTOLOGICAL DESCRIPTION

Herpes simplex in children involves greater cutaneous areas than the localized variety in adults. Children have herpetic gingivostomatitis, ulcerative herpes, and often systemic herpes simplex.

The histological features are similar in all of the cutaneous forms and can be diagnostic of viral disease when the appropriate site is biopsied. The distinguishing factors are: (1) intraepidermal vesicles, produced because of severe intracellular and intercellular edema (ballooning and reticular degeneration); (2) multinucleated epidermal cells; (3) epidermal giant cells, either multinucleated or cells with a large single nucleus; and (4) acantholytic epidermal cells with eosinophilic intranuclear inclusions. These changes are best seen in early vesicles or bullae or at the margin of a later lesion (Figures 7-2-6 and 7-2-7).

As the process progresses, acute inflammatory cells appear and ulceration occurs. In chronic ulcerative herpes simplex, distinctive changes may not be found because of the ulceration, but a careful study of the crusted margins often shows typical viral giant cells, which stain almost entirely eosinophilic but are distinct enough to be diagnostic. Biopsy of the lesion margins may be more rewarding. The dermal reaction may be severe enough to include vascular necrosis. The inflammatory infiltrate is mixed. Diagnostic epithelial viral giant cells can be demonstrated on smears from scraped blister bases and roofs (Tzanck smears) (Plate 7-2-5).

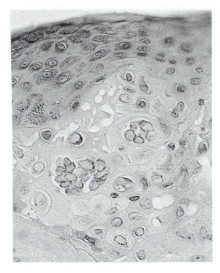

7-2-7 HERPES SIMPLEX: Ballooning and reticular degeneration have resulted in the formation of intraepidermal blister. (100×)

Differential Diagnosis
Acantholytic dermatoses

STAPHYLOCOCCAL SCALDED SKIN SYNDROME

CLINICAL DESCRIPTION

Etiology and Incidence
This syndrome is usually seen in children younger than six years of age; only rarely is it seen in adolescents and adults. Included under the heading of staphylococcal scalded skin syndrome are bullous impetigo (see above), staphylococcal pustulosis in the newborn, staphylococcal scarlatina, Ritter's disease (newborn), and Lyell's disease (children). This process occurs via an epidermolytic toxin produced by the staphylococcal organism (Table 7-2-1).

Clinical Features
The skin changes are distributed on the neck, intertriginous areas, and periorificially (especially the eyes and mouth) (Plate 7-2-6). The illness begins with malaise, fever, and irritability (due to marked tenderness of the skin). A "sunburn" erythema and edema soon appear in the areas described and then may spread to involve varying portions of the rest of the skin surface. With severe involvement, large sheets of skin come off, leaving a denuded, oozing surface (Figure 7-2-8). Vesicles, bullae, and pustules can also be seen during the exfoliative phase. Mild involvement produces flaking of the skin much like after a sunburn. Clearing occurs in twelve to fourteen days without scarring.

Differential Diagnosis
Drug-induced toxic epidermal necrolysis

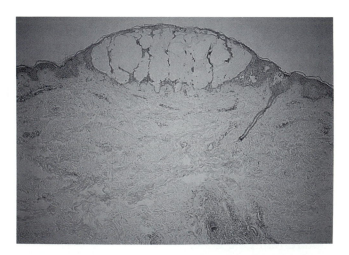

7-2-6 HERPES SIMPLEX: Intraepidermal multilocular bulla containing erythematous amorphous material. (20×)

7-2-1 Differential Features of Superficial Epidermal Necrotic Processes

	Impetigo	*Staphylococcal Scalded Skin Syndrome*	*Erythema Multiforme (TEN)*
Pathology	Vesicopustule above, within, or below granular cell layer containing numerous polys: possibly some acantholytic cells in the blister; occasional Gram-positive cocci	Cleavage plane in upper epidermis, within or below granular cell layer; possibly 1–2 acantholytic cells; little inflammatory cell infiltrate	Vacuolar change to subepidermal split; may be changes of erythema multiforme elsewhere on the slide (vacuolar change, dyskeratotic cells); in TEN full-thickness necrosis
Etiology	Organisms may be seen in the lesion; caused by group A streptococcus (impetigo contagiosum) or *S. aureus* (bullous impetigo)	No organisms in the lesion; blisters caused by exfoliative toxin produced by *S. aureus* (phage group II, type 3A, 3B, 3C, 55, or 71)	Associated with drugs, herpes, severe GVH, etc.
Diagnosis	Gram stain; culture; biopsy	Biopsy; frozen section; clinical appearance	Biopsy (frozen section; jellyroll); clinical appearance
Differential Diagnosis	1. Pustular psoriasis (spongiform pustule of Kogoj and thinned suprapapillary plate) 2. Superficial pemphigus (more acantholytic cells, fewer polys, no bacteria) 3. Subcorneal pustular dermatosis of Sneddon-Wilkinson 4. *Candida* (do PAS)	1. Superficial pemphigus 2. Bullous impetigo (more inflammatory cells; occasional Gram-positive cocci)	Erythema multiforme: 1. Graft vs. host disease 2. Fixed drug reaction 3. Subacute lupus TEN: 1. Necrosis due to ischemia (coma blisters; involves eccrine ducts, vasculitis emboli, etc.)

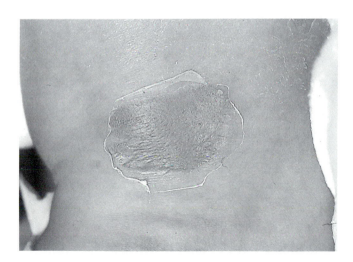

7-2-8 STAPHYLOCOCCAL SCALDED SKIN SYNDROME: A sharply circumscribed zone of erythema delineates the blister base. The peripheral collarette is the remnant of the blister roof.

HISTOLOGICAL DESCRIPTION

There is superficial epidermal necrosis, with a mixed inflammatory infiltrate that is exocytotic to the overlying epidermis (Figure 7-2-9). There is separation in the stratum corneum or the granular layer. Lack of full thickness epidermal necrosis distinguishes staphylococcal scalded skin syndrome from toxic epidermal necrolysis. The latter disorder is usually drug-induced and occurs in older children and adults.

The dermis may show edema and a rather dense infiltrate of mononuclear cells as well as a few polymorphonuclear cells. Frozen sections of intact bullae can be used to differentiate staphylococcal scalded skin from toxic epidermal necrolysis (Figures 7-2-10 and 7-2-11).

Differential Diagnosis

Superficial pemphigus
Bullous impetigo

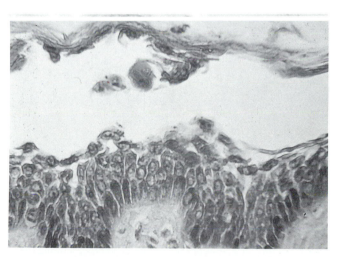

7-2-9 STAPHYLOCOCCAL SCALDED SKIN SYNDROME: Superficial epidermal necrosis with epidermal separation without a significant inflammatory response in the papillary dermis. (200×)

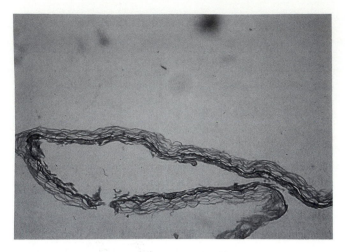

7-2-10 STAPHYLOCOCCAL SCALDED SKIN SYNDROME: Frozen section whole mount of a blister roof shows only a portion of the epidermis. (40×)

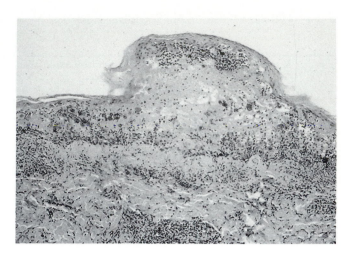

7-2-12 VARICELLA ZOSTER: Low-power photomicrograph, showing a necrotic intraepidermal blister. The dermis shows a mixed chronic inflammatory infiltrate. (40×)

VARICELLA ZOSTER

CLINICAL DESCRIPTION

Etiology and Incidence

Varicella occurs mainly during childhood (50% by five years of age, 90% by fifteen years), however nonimmune adolescents and adults are susceptible. Herpes zoster also occurs in the pediatric population, especially if varicella is contracted prior to one to two years of age. Herpes zoster in the first year of life indicates fetal exposure to varicella.

Clinical Features

A delicate teardrop vesicle is characteristic. Lesions usually begin on the trunk and rapidly progress (within six to twenty-four hours) from papules to vesicles to crusts (Plate 7-2-7). All stages are present in one area. Mucous membranes are usually involved. Children are contagious until all lesions have crusted (generally 7 days).

Herpes zoster in childhood is somewhat different than the infection in adults (Plate 7-2-8). Children rarely have postinfectious neuralgia or associated malignancies. Papules and vesicles are distributed over a dermatome innervated by the affected sensory nerve. Frequently, scattered, distant, isolated lesions resembling varicella are seen. Involvement of the tip of the nose indicates corneal involvement. Lesions continue to erupt for seven days and resolve in seven to fourteen days.

HISTOLOGICAL DESCRIPTION

On histological study, varicella zoster and herpes simplex appear to be the same. The intensity of the dermal reaction in early varicella zoster is helpful in the diagnosis. This can be and usually is more severe than in herpes simplex. The vascular reaction is also more intense, with endothelial swelling and necrosis. Giant cells, multinucleated and uninucleated, are prominent in varicella zoster. The features of reticular degeneration, spongiosis, and acantholysis are also present (Figure 7-2-12; Plate 7-2-9).

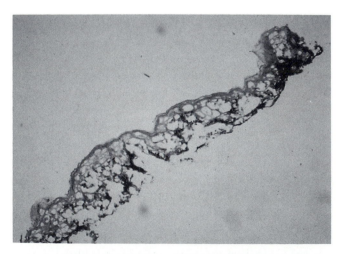

7-2-11 TOXIC EPIDERMAL NECROLYSIS: Blister roof from toxic epidermal necrolysis of the drug-induced type, showing the entire thickness of the epidermis on a frozen section whole mount. This technique is useful in rapid differentiation of staphylococcal scalded skin syndrome from toxic epidermal necrolysis. (40×)

Differential Diagnosis

See Herpes Simplex

7-3 IMMUNOLOGICALLY MEDIATED DISORDERS

EPIDERMOLYSIS BULLOSA ACQUISITA

CLINICAL DESCRIPTION

Etiology and Incidence

Epidermolysis bullosa acquisita (EBA) is a rare acquired bullous disorder. Very few cases have been described in children. Although it may occur at any age, the youngest child described thus far in the literature has been three months old. This disorder seems to be an autoimmune disease in which patients have autoantibodies directed against type VII collagen (the EBA antigen).

Clinical Features

Classically, EBA resembles the hereditary forms of scarring epidermolysis bullosa. Diagnosis is based on the criteria outlined in Table 7-3-1. Children present with a trauma-induced bullous eruption that involves the skin and mucous membranes (Figure 7-3-1). The changes include skin fragility, atrophic scarring, and milia in an acral and extensor distribution. Patients may demonstrate alopecia and nail dystrophy.

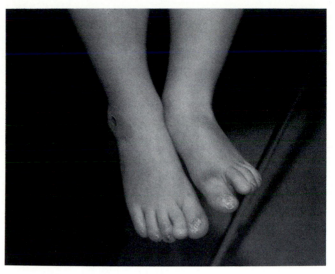

7-3-1 EBA: Acral blisters are especially notable over bony prominences and areas prone to trauma.

An inflammatory presentation may also occur and resemble changes seen in erythema multiforme, cicatricial pemphigoid, and bullous pemphigoid.

Differential Diagnosis

Dominant dystrophic epidermolysis bullosa
Recessive dystrophic epidermolysis bullosa
Porphyria cutanea tarda
Erythema multiforme
Bullous pemphigoid
Cicatricial pemphigoid
Bullous systemic lupus erythematosus

HISTOLOGICAL DESCRIPTION

A subepidermal blister is seen and is indistinguishable on hematoxylin and eosin-stained sections from other varieties of epidermolysis bullosa , or cicatricial pemphigoid if it occurs on the mucosal surface (Figure 7-3-2).

    Immunodiagnostic studies, including immunoelectronmicroscopy, are necessary to differentiate this type of epidermolysis bullosa from other types. Direct immunofluorescence studies usually show IgG, C3, IgM, IgE, and fibrin in a linear arrangement at the dermal-epidermal interface (Plate 7-3-1). Indirect immunofluorescence study is usually negative. On immunoelectronmicroscopy, tissue-bound immunoreactants, which may include IgG and C3, are found within the lamina densa and/or sublamina densa region.

Differential Diagnosis

Other subepidermal blistering dermatoses

7-3-1   Diagnostic Criteria for Epidermolysis Bullosa Acquisita

Diagnostic Criteria
Variable age of onset (not congenital)
Negative family history of epidermolysis bullosa
Exclusion of other bullous diseases: hereditary EB, porphyria, pseudoporphyria, bullous drug eruption, bullous erythema multiforme, bullous pemphigoid, cicatricial pemphigoid, pemphigus vulgaris, bullous systemic lupus erythematosus
Relatively recalcitrant to therapy
Inflammatory or noninflammatory mucocutaneous bullae
Light microscopic findings: subepidermal bulla and/or inflammation
Direct immunofluorescence of perilesional skin: linear deposits at Dermal epidermic junction of IgG and/or IgM, IgA, C3, fibrinogen
Direct immunoelectron microscopic examination of perilesional skin: immune deposits in sublamina densa zone
Indirect immunofluorescence using sample of patient's serum: normal epithelium—IgG in linear deposit at DEJ; saline-split human skin—IgG on dermal side of split
Western immunoblot: serum antibodies to specific major 290-kd and minor 145-kd proteins (the EBA antigen)

From McGuaig CC, et al.: EBA in childhood. Arch Dermatol 1989; 125:949–999.

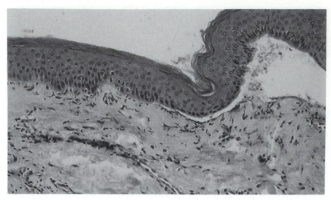

7-3-2 EBA: Subepidermal blister with hemorrhage and epithelial regrowth. This biopsy demonstrates the diagnostic difficulty when later lesions are biopsied. The inflammatory infiltrate is lymphocytic about superficial dermal vessels. (40×)

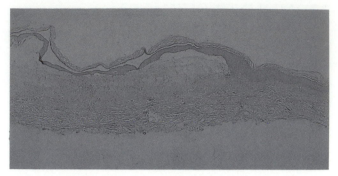

7-3-3 CHRONIC BULLOUS DISEASE OF CHILDHOOD: A broad-based subepidermal blister. (20×)

HISTOLOGICAL DESCRIPTION

Chronic bullous disease of childhood is a bullous disorder that can now be separated from other bullous diseases on the basis of clinical and histological findings. The characteristic findings are those of IgA in a linear pattern at the epidermal-dermal interface. On routine histology, differentiation may not be as clear. There is a subepidermal bulla (Figure 7-3-3) and an infiltrate that varies in predominant cells. When neutrophiles predominate the changes resemble linear IgA disease (Figure 7-3-4), or dermatitis herpetiformis. When eosinophiles predominate, the features resemble bullous pemphigoid. Immunofluorescence study helps differentiate these conditions: dermatitis herpetiformis has granular deposits of IgA at the papillae tips; bullous pemphigoid has linear (tubular) IgG at the dermal-epidermal interface; and chronic bullous disease of childhood has linear IgA of the dermal-epidermal interface (Plate 7-3-3).

Differential Diagnosis
Bullous pemphigoid
Dermatitis herpetiformis

CHRONIC BULLOUS DERMATOSIS OF CHILDHOOD

CLINICAL DESCRIPTION

Etiology and Incidence
This bullous disorder occurs mainly in the preschool age group. It is the most common chronic bullous dermatosis in the first ten years of life. An immunologic etiology is suggested by the deposits of IgA (in a linear pattern) on the basement membrane, as well as circulating IgA basement membrane zone antibodies.

Chronic bullous dermatosis of childhood (CBDC) differs from childhood dermatitis herpetiformis and bullous pemphigoid, in that the latter two are much like the adult form of the disease (Table 3-3-1).

Clinical Features
The lesions commonly involve the perioral skin, lower trunk, inner thighs, genitalia, and perineum. The mucous membranes may be affected. Bullae are the major finding, and their appearance is characteristic. An annular arrangement of sausage-shaped bullae is seen around resolving crusted lesions (Plate 7-3-2). Pruritus is mild to severe. The disorder is self-limiting, clearing within several months to three years. It is not associated with celiac disease.

Differential Diagnosis
Erythema multiforme
Dermatitis herpetiformis
Bullous impetigo
Epidermolysis bullosa acquisita (EBA)
Bullous pemphigoid

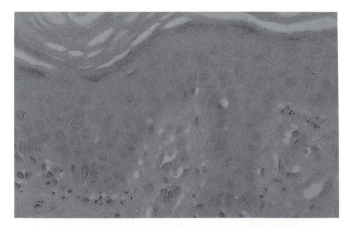

7-3-4 CHRONIC BULLOUS DISEASE OF CHILDHOOD: Characteristic alignment of neutrophils along the dermal-epidermal junction at intact blister edges. (400×)

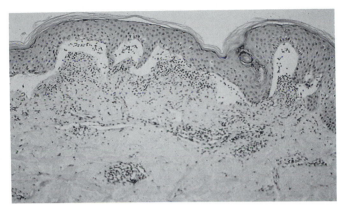

7-3-5 DERMATITIS HERPETIFORMIS: A subepidermal blister, showing distinct separation over the tips of the papillae. Inflammatory cells can be seen within the papillae tips. (40×)

DERMATITIS HERPETIFORMIS

HISTOLOGICAL DESCRIPTION

The histological features seen in this condition are discrete areas of subepidermal blister formation that may involve only one or two papillae (Figure 7-3-5). In papillae adjacent to the blister collections of polymorphonuclear leukocytes at the tips of the dermal papillae are seen (Figure 7-3-6). The other change in the dermis is chronic inflammation about the dermal vessels, with lymphocytes, histiocytes, and an occasional eosinophil. Immunofluorescence study reveals granular IgA at the tips of the dermal papillae (Plate 7-3-4).

Differential Diagnosis
Bullous pemphigoid
Linear IgA bullous dermatosis

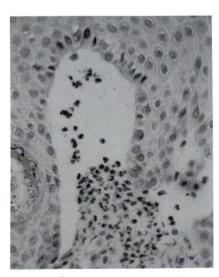

7-3-6 DERMATITIS HERPETIFORMIS: Higher-power magnification of Figure 7-3-5, showing distinct dermal-epidermal separation with collections of polymorphonuclear leukocytes within the papillae tips. (400×)

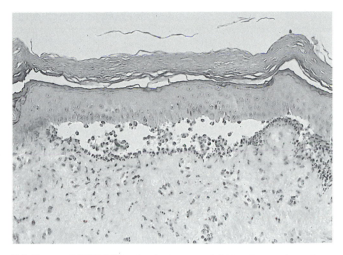

7-3-7 JUVENILE BULLOUS PEMPHIGOID: Extremity skin, showing a subepidermal blister with inflammatory cells, many of them eosinophils within the blister space. (40×)

JUVENILE BULLOUS PEMPHIGOID

HISTOLOGICAL DESCRIPTION

The histological features in this condition are usually large subepidermal blisters with an inflammatory infiltrate in the dermis of lymphocytes, histiocytes, and numerous eosinophils, the latter of which may also be seen filling the blister space (Figure 7-3-7). Adjacent dermal papillae may show edema and small areas of dermal-epidermal separation with the presence of eosinophils in the small cleftlike spaces where the epidermis is separating from the dermis (Figure 7-3-8).

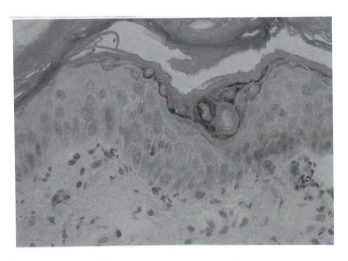

7-3-8 JUVENILE BULLOUS PEMPHIGOID: Higher-power magnification of Figure 7-3-7 at the edge of the blister, showing eosinophils within the dermal papillae and early dermal-epidermal separation. (400×)

7-3-2   Dermatitis Herpetiformis and Bullous Pemphigoid

	Dermatitis Herpetiformis	*Bullous Pemphigoid*
Usual age at onset	Greater than 8 y; rarely younger	Greater than 8–10 y; rarely younger
Type of lesions	Grouped papulovesicles, bullae, or urticarial lesions	Large, tense bullae
Distribution	Back, buttocks, scalp, extensors of extremities; often symmetric	Trunk and flexor surfaces of extremities
Pruritus	Intense	Mild
Mucous membrane involvement	No	Yes
Duration	5–10	2–3

Eosinophilic spongiosis may also be seen in bullous pemphigoid in areas away from the blister. In addition to lymphocytes, histiocytes, and eosinophils, the dermis often shows rather marked reticular dermal edema. Immunofluoresence in this condition shows IgG and C_3 in a linear band at the dermal-epidermal interface (Plate 7-3-5; Tables 7-3-2 and 7-3-3).

Differential Diagnosis
Dermatitis herpetiformis
Epidermolysis bullosa
Porphyrias

ERYTHEMA MULTIFORME

CLINICAL DESCRIPTION

Erythema multiforme ranges in severity from macular-urticarial lesions to vesiculobullous lesions with (Stevens-Johnson syndrome) or without mucous membrane involvement. The most severe form is toxic epidermal necrolysis (TEN).

Etiology and Incidence
The disorder is an acute and frequently recurrent inflammatory hypersensitivity syndrome. Drug-induced TEN must be differentiated from an illness caused by a circulating staphylococcal exotoxin. The drug-related disorder is usually seen after six years of age. Herpes simplex virus has now been identified as a precipitating factor in many "idiopathic" cases. Death occurs in 3% to 15% of patients.

Clinical Features
Any body surface may be involved, as well as the mucous membranes, gastrointestinal tract, and tracheobronchial tree. There is a predilection for the backs of the hands, palms, soles, and extensor surfaces of the limbs. Twenty-five percent of patients have mucous membrane involvement. Simple conjunctivitis or severe panophthalmitis leading to blindness may occur (3% to 10%). Lesions may continue to erupt for two to three weeks.

Lesions are macules, papules, or blisters, some of which form into the characteristic "iris" or "target" lesion (Figure 7-3-9). Large sheets of skin are lost in TEN, producing the potential for fluid and electrolyte disturbances and bacterial invasion (Figure 7-3-10).

Differential Diagnosis
See Chronic Bullous Disease of Childhood

HISTOLOGICAL DESCRIPTION

Subepidermal blisters occur in erythema multiforme on the basis of two mechanisms. In one there is disruption of the dermal-epidermal interface with separation of the epidermis from the dermis. In the other mechanism, marked dermal edema pushes the epidermis off the dermis, leaving strands of

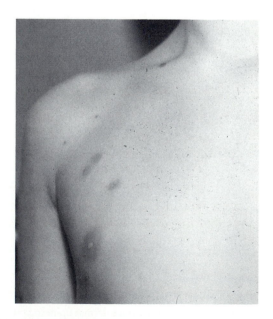

7-3-9 ERYTHEMA MULTIFORME: Target lesion on child's chest.

7-3-3   Chronic Bullous Diseases of Childhood

	Dermatitis Herpetiformis	Bullous Pemphigoid	Linear IgA Disease	Bullous Lupus Erythematosus	Epidermolysis Bullosa Acquisita	Erythema Multiforme
Histopathology						
Vesicle	Subepidermal	Subepidermal	Subepidermal	Subepidermal	Subepidermal	Subepidermal
Inflammation	Neutrophilic	Eosinophilic	Neutrophilic	Neutrophilic	None or mononuclear	Mononuclear
Immunopathology (DE junction)	Granular IgA (dermal papilla)	Linear IgG and C_3	Linear IgA	Granular IgG and C_3	Linear IgG	None
Circulating antibodies	None	50–60% IgG	50% IgA	None	Most patients IgG	None
Immunoelectron- microscopic deposits	Granular sublamina densa	Lamina lucida	Linear lamina lucida or sublamina densa	Sublamina densa	Sublamina densa	None
Treatment	Sulfapyridine or dapsone	Steroids	Self-limited sulfapyridine or steroid/ sulfa	Steroids/ immuno- suppressives or dapsone	Resistant to steroids; dapsone	Steroids
Clinical features						
Age	8–10 y	8–10 y	6 mo–9 y		Rare in childhood	
Blisters	Tense	Tense	Tense	Tense	Tense	Tense
Base	Normal/ inflamed	Normal/ inflamed	Normal/inflamed	Normal/ inflamed	Normal/ inflamed	Inflamed
Skin fragility	—	—	—	—	—	—
Distribution	Generalized, flexural	Generalized, flexural	Generalized, flexural, "cluster of jewels"	Generalized	Extensor	Generalized
Mucous membranes	±	±	±	–	–	+ +
Palms and soles	±	±	±	–	–	+ +
Pruritus	+	+	+	+	–	–
Atrophy and scarring	–	–	–	+	+ +	±
Milia	–	–	–	–	+	–

collagen in the intervening blister space (Figure 7-3-11). In both conditions there is usually a dense inflammatory infiltrate of lymphocytes and histiocytes about the dermal vessels. In the dermal-epidermal variety, there is an interface dermatitis of mononuclear cells at the dermal-epidermal junction with exocytosis of lymphocytes and the production of necrotic keratinocytes (satellite cell necrosis) within the epidermis (Figures 7-3-12 and 7-3-13). Colloid bodies are also seen.

Eosinophils may be seen in this condition, although they may not be prominent. In the epidermal variety necrotic keratinocytes and satellite cell necrosis are seen. In TEN there is full-thickness epidermal necrosis (Figure 7-3-14). This is in contrast to staphylococcal scalded syndrome skin, in which there is only superficial epidermal necrosis. The inflammatory response in the dermis is mainly lymphocytic, although eosinophils and neutrophils can be seen in some vesicles of erythema multiforme.

Differential Diagnosis
Mucha-Habermann disease
Staphylococcal scalded skin syndrome
Graft versus host disease
Secondary syphilis

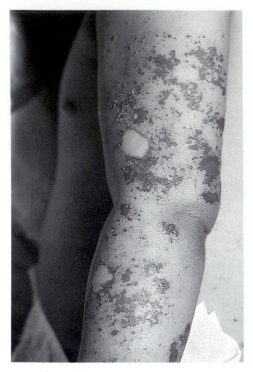

7-3-10 ERYTHEMA MULTIFORME: Denuded skin in patient with TEN.

LUPUS ERYTHEMATOSUS (BULLOUS)

CLINICAL DESCRIPTION

Etiology and Incidence

Besides the usual skin manifestations of lupus erythematosus, a small number of patients develop a severe, generalized vesicobullous eruption. Although the bullae may suggest the presence of bullous pemphigoid or dermatitis herpetiformis,

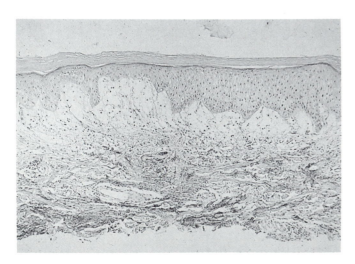

7-3-11 ERYTHEMA MULTIFORME: Low-power photomicrograph, showing a subepidermal blister. In the blister space there are strands of collagen that are still attached to the epidermis. (40×)

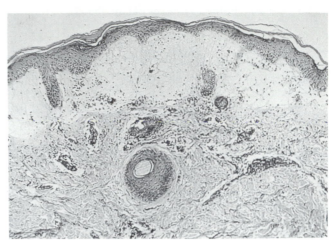

7-3-12 ERYTHEMA MULTIFORME: High-power photomicrograph, showing a subepidermal blister and erythema multiforme on the basis of severe edema. (200×)

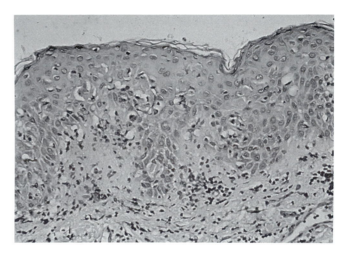

7-3-13 ERYTHEMA MULTIFORME: Individual necrosis of keratinocytes at various levels of the epidermis. (400×)

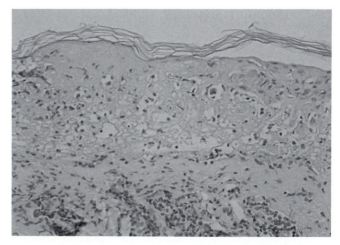

7-3-14 ERYTHEMA MULTIFORME: Full-thickness necrosis of the epidermis, characteristic of toxic epidermal necrolysis. (400×)

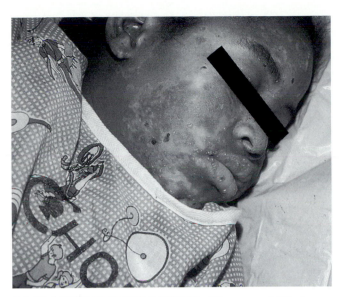

7-3-15 LUPUS ERYTHEMATOSUS: Blister on a child's face.

the histologic and immunofluorescence findings are atypical. At times the bullous lesions indicate the presence of epidermolysis bullosa acquisita in association with systemic lupus erythematosus.

Clinical Features

The skin changes are those usually found in systemic lupus erythematosus, plus the blisters (Figure 7-3-15). Response to dapsone rather than systemic steroids is common in these patients.

Differential Diagnosis

Bullous pemphigoid
Dermatitis herpetiformis
Epidermolysis bullosa aquisita

HISTOLOGICAL DESCRIPTION

Lupus erythematosus, like lichen planus, is not usually a blistering disease but may present as blisters in the skin of young children. When blisters occur in this condition, they are subepidermal in location and are on the basis of dermalepidermal interface dissolution because of the inflammatory infiltrate (Figure 7-3-16). In sites adjacent to the blister, there are more typical changes of lupus erythematosus: basal layer vacuolar degeneration with a lymphocytic inflammatory infiltrate. The epidermis shows hyperkeratosis and follicular hyperkeratosis and may also show atrophy. In the dermis there is an increase in ground substance (mucin-hyaluronic acid) as well as periadnexal inflammation of lymphocytes (Plate 7-3-6). Immunofluorescence studies in this condition will show granular IgG, C_3, IgA, or IgM in a linear formation at the dermal-epidermal interface (Plate 7-3-7).

Differential Diagnosis

Lichen planus
Dermatitis herpetiformis (bullous lupus)
Lichenoid dermatoses

PEMPHIGUS

CLINICAL DESCRIPTION

Etiology and Incidence

Pemphigus is an extremely rare disorder in childhood. One review (Smitt) in 1985 cited thirty-one published reports of this disorder. Of the varieties of pemphigus seen in children, pemphigus foliaceus is more common than pemphigus vulgaris.

Pemphigus vulgaris is thought to be due to the effects of intercellular antibodies. The stimulus for the production of those antibodies is unknown.

Clinical Features

The distribution of lesions in pemphigus favors the seborrheic regions. Vesicles or flaccid bullae arise in these areas on normal or inflamed skin (Figure 7-3-17). The mucous membranes are involved in more than 90% of patients and may be the presenting sign. Nikolsky's sign is present. The bullae break and leave slowly healing painful erosions. The disorder is a chronic one.

Erosions that become vegetative, especially in the intertriginous regions and face, indicate pemphigus vegetans.

Pemphigus foliaceus is more superficial and, therefore, milder. The mucous membranes are infrequently involved. Though symptomatic (pruritus, pain, and burning), patients with this disorder are not very ill.

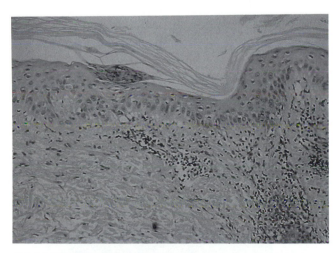

7-3-16 LUPUS ERYTHEMATOSUS: Low-power photomicrograph, showing interface reaction as well as periadnexal inflammatory reaction of lymphocytes about a rudimentary follicular structure. The adjacent dermis shows increased ground substance. (200×)

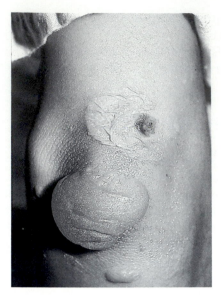

7-3-17 PEMPHIGUS VULGARIS: Flaccid bulla on patient's knee.

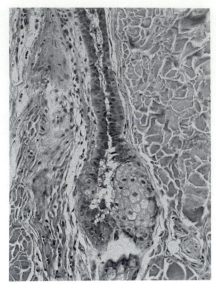

7-3-19 PEMPHIGUS VULGARIS: Acantholysis in a follicular structure, a classic and typical finding. (400×)

Differential Diagnosis
Bullous impetigo

HISTOLOGICAL DESCRIPTION

Pemphigus Vulgaris
The histological features in pemphigus vulgaris are suprabasalar acantholysis with the formation of an intraepidermal blister (Figure 7-3-18). The acantholytic process extends down the sides of follicular structures (Figure 7-3-19), a feature that helps to distinguish pemphigus vulgaris from other intraepidermal acantholytic processes. The inflammatory in-

filtrate in the dermis is usually perivascular in location and not intense, unless there has been erosion, ulceration, and secondary infection.

Pemphigus Foliaceus
The histological features in pemphigus foliaceus are superficial acantholysis, either in or just below the granular cell layer (Figure 7-3-20). A cleftlike space develops and may give rise to a bulla (although not common). Dyskeratotic cells can be seen within the granular layer; they resemble grains of Darier's disease. Dyskeratotic cells are not seen in pemphigus vulgaris. Eosinophilic spongiosis can be seen in both varieties of pemphigus. Immunofluorescence findings in pemphigus

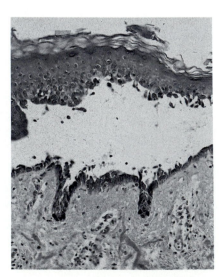

7-3-18 PEMPHIGUS VULGARIS: Suprabasilar acantholysis with the production of an intraepidermal blister. Acantholytic cells can be seen on the roof of the blister (200×)

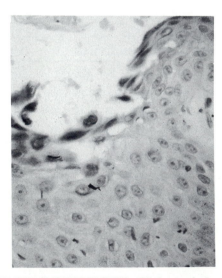

7-3-20 PEMPHIGUS FOLIACEUS: High-power photomicrograph, showing acantholytic cells in the superficial epidermis and absence of the stratum corneum and stratum granulosum. (200×)

are IgG and complement in the intercellular spaces of the epidermis. Immunofluorescence findings are positive on direct or indirect immunofluorescence (Plates 7-3-8 and 7-3-9).

Differential Diagnosis
Hailey and Hailey disease
Pemphigus foliaceus
Erythematoides and erythematosus

7-4 OTHERS

FLEA BITES

CLINICAL DESCRIPTION

Etiology and Incidence
Flea bites occur less frequently than mosquito bites in childhood. Because of the close relationship between humans and pets, dog and cat flea bites are most common. Individuals become sensitized to injected toxins and allergens contained in the saliva of fleas.

Clinical Features
The distribution and grouping of lesions is valuable in making the diagnosis of flea bites. Exposed skin surfaces (head, face, and extremities) are usually involved. Lesions are usually grouped because fleas feed at various sites during one meal (Figure 7-4-1). Usually urticarial papules occur after sensitization. Extreme sensitivity frequently leads to the development of bullous lesions. Flea bites induce vesicular, pustular, or bullous reactions more often than any other insect bite. Severe pruritus is experienced by the patient.

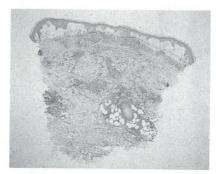

7-4-2 FLEA BITES: Low-power photomicrograph shows a subepidermal blister with dense inflammatory infiltrate, somewhat nodular, about dermal vessels. (20×)

Differential Diagnosis
Bullous impetigo
Varicella
Rickettsialpox
Bullous pemphigoid

HISTOLOGICAL DESCRIPTION

The histological features are interface dermatitis and superficial and deep perivascular infiltrate. The infiltrate consists of lymphocytes, histiocytes, and many eosinophils. There is also exocytosis of inflammatory cells into the epidermis associated with spongiosis and sometimes epidermal cell necrosis. Bullae are due to papillary dermal edema or the interface inflammatory response (Figures 7-4-2 and 7-4-3).

Differential Diagnosis
Erythema multiforme
Drug eruptions

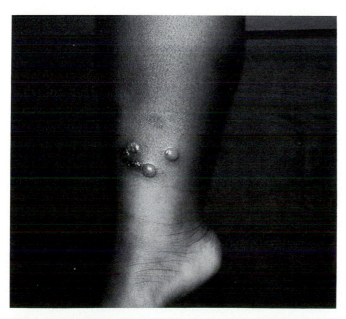

7-4-1 FLEA BITES: Three bullous lesions on a child's leg.

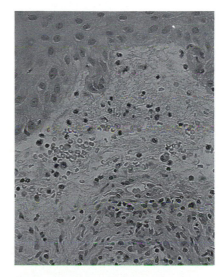

7-4-3 FLEA BITES: High-power photomicrograph, showing a subepidermal blister. In the blister space there is hemorrhage and an inflammatory infiltrate of lymphocytes in many eosinophils. (100×)

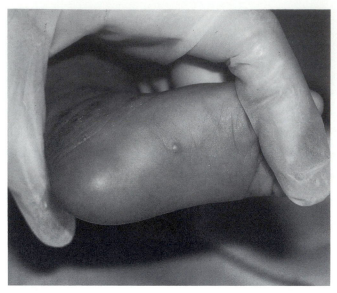

7-4-4 SCABIES: Toddler with scabies. Note blistering on the sole.

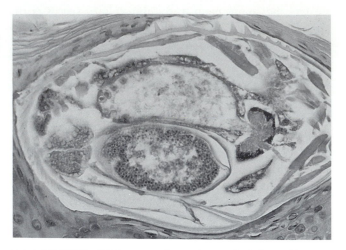

7-4-6 SCABIES: High-power photomicrograph of the scabies mite within the burrow, showing overlying parakeratosis. Blisters, when they develop, are subepidermal. (400×)

SCABIES

CLINICAL DESCRIPTION

Etiology and Incidence
The mite that produces scabies affects any age group.

Clinical Features
Diagnosis is based on the distribution of skin lesions and involvement of significant contacts (parents or other caretakers). Lesions are concentrated on the hands, feet (palms and soles), and folds of the body. Infants, unlike older children, will have involvement of the skin of their face and head. The skin lesions include papules, pustules, and vesicles. Infants are more likely to develop blisters (Figure 7-4-4). Ten percent of patients will have the pathognomonic linear burrow.

Unfortunately, burrows are difficult to identify because of distortion by scratching; severe pruritus is the major symptom. The eruption will persist indefinitely unless the individual is treated. The signs and symptoms are secondary to sensitization, therefore one month will elapse following infestation before pruritus and skin changes are noted.

Differential Diagnosis
Atopic eczema
Insect bite reaction
Bullous impetigo
Dyshidrotic eczema
Contact dermatitis
Histiocytosis X (Letterer-Siwe disease)

HISTOLOGICAL DESCRIPTION

Scabies may be vesicular or bullous in infants and very young children. The features seen are an intraepidermal spongiotic vesicle filled with lymphocytes and eosinophils. The organism may sometimes be found in sections associated with the spongiosis (Figures 7-4-5 and 7-4-6). The organism is subcorneal in location and is seen on cross section. Sections may only show fecal deposits (scybala) in the subcorneal location. A subepidermal blister may develop when there is marked edema of the papillary dermis. The infiltrate in the dermis is composed of lymphocytes, histiocytes, and eosinophils. There is associated dermal edema.

Differential Diagnosis
Other bite reactions (tick, flea)
Drug eruptions

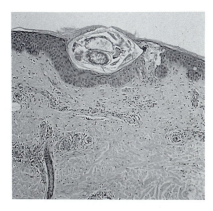

7-4-5 SCABIES: A scabetic burrow containing the organism as seen in a substratum corneum location. There is an inflammatory infiltrate about dermal vessels. (40×)

REFERENCES

Erythema Toxicum Neonatorum

Luder D: Histologic observations in erythema toxicum neonatorum. Pediatrics 1960; 26:219.

Schachner L, Press S: Vesicular, bullous and pustular disorders in infancy and childhood. Pediatr Clin North Am 1983; 30:609.

Miliaria

Holzle E, Kligman A: The pathogenesis of miliaria rubra: Role of the resident microflora. Br J Dermatol 1978; 99:117.

Transient Neonatal Pustular Melanosis

Barr RJ, Globeman LM, Weber FA: Transient neonatal pustular melanosis. Int J Dermatol 1979; 18:636.

Ramamurthy RS, Reveri M, Esterly NB, et al.: Transient neonatal pustular melanosis. J Pediatr 1976; 88:830.

Bullous Impetigo

Elias PM, Levy SW: Bullous impetigo: Occurrence of localized scalded skin syndrome in an adult. Arch Dermatol 1976; 112:856.

Kouskoukis CE, Ackerman AB: What histological finding distinguishes superficial pemphigus and bullous impetigo. Am J Dermatopathol 1984; 66:179.

Schachner L, Taplin D, Scott GB, et al.: A therapeutic update of superficial skin infections. Pediatr Clin North Am 1983; 30:397.

Congenital Syphilis

Jeerapaet P, Ackerman AB: Histologic patterns of secondary syphilis. Arch Dermatol 1973; 107:373.

Masciola L, Pelosi R, Blount JH, et al.: Congenital syphilis revisited. Am J Dis Child 1985; 139:575.

Noppakun N, Dinehart SM, Soloman AR: Pustular secondary syphilis. Int J Dermatol 1987; 26:112.

Herpes Simplex

Catalano LW Jr, Satley GH, Muceles M, et al.: Disseminated herpes virus infection in a newborn infant: Virologic, serologic, coagulation and interferon studies. J Pediatr 1971; 79:313.

Corey L, Spear PG: Infections with herpes simplex viruses. N Engl J Med 1986; 314:686.

Komorous JM, Wheeler CE, Briggaman RA, et al.: Intrauterine herpes simplex infections. Arch Dermatol 1977; 113:918.

Prober LG, Hensleigh PA, Boucher FD, et al.: Use of routine viral cultures at delivery to identify neonates exposed to HSV. N Engl J Med 1988; 318:887.

Staphylococcal Scalded Skin Syndrome

Elias PM, Fritsch P, Epstein EH Jr: Staphylococcal scalded skin syndrome (review). Arch Dermatol 1977; 113:207.

Lillibridge CB, Melish ME, Glasgow LA: Site of action of exfoliative toxins in the staphylococcal scalded skin syndrome. Pediatrics 1972; 50:723.

Varicella Zoster

Rogers RS III, Tindall JP: Herpes zoster in children. Arch Dermatol 1972; 106:204.

Wurzel CL, Kahan J, Heitler M, et al.: Prognosis of herpes zoster in healthy children. Am J Dis Child 1986; 140:477.

Epidermolysis Bullosa

Barthelemy H, Kantankis J, Cambazaro F, et al.: Epidermolysis bullosa acquisita: Mapping of antigen determinants by an immunofluorescence technique. Clin Exp Dermatol 1986; 11:378.

McCuaig CC, Chau LS, Woodley DT, et al.: Epidermolysis bullosa acquisita in childhood: Differentiation from hereditary epidermolysis bullosa. Arch Dermatol 1989; 125:944.

Bullous Disease of Childhood

Blenkinsoff WK, Tury L, Haffenden GP, et al.: Histology of linear IgA disease, dermatitis herpetiformis, and bullous pemphigoid. Am J Dermatopathol 1983; 5:547.

Chorzelski TP, Beutner EH, Jablonska S, et al.: Immunofluorescence studies in the diagnosis of dermatitis herpetiformis and its differentiation from bullous pemphigoid. J Invest Dermatol 1971; 56:373.

Wojnarowska F, Marsden RA, Bhogal B, et al.: Chronic bullous disease of childhood, childhood cicatricial pemphigoid, and linear IgA disease of adults: A comparative study demonstrating clinical and immunopathologic overlap. J Am Acad Dermatol 1988; 19:792.

Erythema Multiforme

Corticosteroids for erythema multiforme (Symposium). Pediatr Dermatol 1989; 6:229.

Howland WW, Galetz LE, Weston WL: Erythema multiforme: Clinical, histopathologic and immunologic study. J Am Acad Dermatol 1984; 10:438.

Lupus Erythematosus

Boh E, Roberts LJ, Lien TS, et al.: Epidermolysis bullosa acquisita preceding the development of systemic lupus erythematosus J Am Acad Dermatol 1990; 22:587.

Camisa C: Vesicobullous systemic lupus erythematosus. J Am Acad Dermatol 1988; 18:93.

Camisa C, Sharma HM: Vesicobullous systemic lupus erythematosus. J Am Acad Dermatol 1983; 9:924.

Olawsky AJ, Briggaman RA, Gamman WR, et al.: Bullous systemic lupus erythematosus. J Am Acad Dermatol 1982; 7:511.

Pemphigus

Furtaoo TA: Histopathology of pemphigus foliaceous. Arch Dermatol 1959; 80:66.

Merlog P, Metzker A, Aazar B, et al.: Neonatal pemphigus vulgaris. Pediatrics 1986; 78:1102.

Smitt JHS: Pemphigus vulgaris in childhood: Clinical features, treatment and prognosis. Pediatr Dermatol 1985; 2:185.

Storer JS, Galen WK, Nesbitt LT, et al.: Neonatal pemphigus vulgaris. J Am Acad Dermatol 1982; 6:929.

Bite Reactions

Fernandez N, Torres A, Ackerman AB: Pathological findings in human scabies. Arch Dermatol 1977; 113:320.

Honig PJ: Arthropod bites, stings, and infestations: Their prevention and treatment. Pediatr Dermatol 1986; 3:189.

Honig PJ: Bites and parasites. Pediatr Clin North Am 1983; 30:563.

Schaffer B, Jacobson C, Beerman H: Histopathologic correlation of lesions of papular urticaria and positive skin test reactions to insect antigens. Arch Dermatol 1954; 70:437.

Dermatitis Herpetiformis

Ackerman AB, Tolman MM: Papular dermatitis herpetiforonis in childhood. Arch Dermatol 1969; 100:286.

Ermacora E, Prampolini L, Tribbia G, et al.: Longterm follow up of dermatitis herpetiformis in children. J Am Acad Dermatol 1986; 15:24.

8

Nevi, Melanoma, and Neural Tumors

Contents

8-1 JUNCTION, COMPOUND, DERMAL, AND CONGENITAL NEVI

CLINICAL DESCRIPTION

Etiology and Incidence

Nevi can be found in newborns, although most arise during childhood and adolescence. Peak incidence occurs around the midtwenties, after which nevi diminish. Approximately 1% of newborn infants have true melanocytic nevi. This is the most common tumor in humans; its incidence increases sharply at puberty and is associated with pigment darkening at the same time. Nevi are tumors of melanocytic cells in the epidermis or dermis or both.

The importance of congenital nevi other than cosmetic concerns is the potential for development of malignant melanoma. The incidence of the development of melanoma varies in many series from a low of 5% to 6% to a high of 11% to 12%. In congenital nevi the predicted incidence for melanoma is approximately 0.9% to 1%, versus 0.3% to 0.4% in the general nonpigmented population. The predicted development of melanoma in these tumors is the factor that drives treatment and causes so much frustration on the part of the patient, family, and clinician.

Clinical Features

All nevi have similar color and substance. Differentiation of dermal, junctional, and compound nevi on a clinical basis is difficult if not impossible, but there are some features that

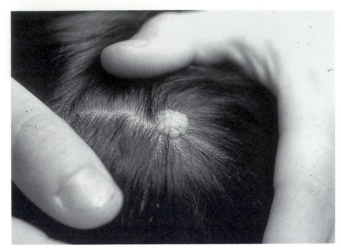

8-1-2 DERMAL NEVUS: Exophytic papillomatous flesh-colored nodule on a young child's scalp.

suggest one type of nevus over another. Junctional nevi are usually flat and well-circumscribed and have diffuse brown-black pigmentation or may have a centrally placed darker pigmented area with peripheral lightening (Figure 8-1-1). Most nevi in prepubertal children are junctional. Dermal nevi are raised, approximately 0.5 cm in diameter, and the color of the patient's skin or slightly browner (Figure 8-1-2). Compound nevi are raised and about the same size as dermal nevi but are darker in color, their color being most closely akin to that of junctional nevi (Plate 8-1-1).

Congenital nevi all show pigmentation of the skin and are larger than 1 cm in diameter. Some, in addition, show prominent hair growth within the pigmented areas. Congenital nevi vary in size and cover areas that include an entire arm (coat sleeve), a hand (glove), or leg (pants leg), or the trunk (bathing suit). The pigmentation within congenital nevi varies from brown to black. As with other nevi, the color increases in intensity at puberty. Almost all congenital nevi show some surface irregularities from papulation to nodule formation (Plate 8-1-2). Congenital nevi of the giant hairy type that overlie the scalp or spine may be associated with neurologic disorders, which are related to nevoid melanocytic changes in the central nervous system (Plate 8-1-3). The significance of the large garment type congenital nevi is the propensity for the development of melanoma. It is thought that this type of congenital nevus gives rise to melanoma with a greater frequency than do the smaller congenital nevi. All congenital nevi should be followed carefully.

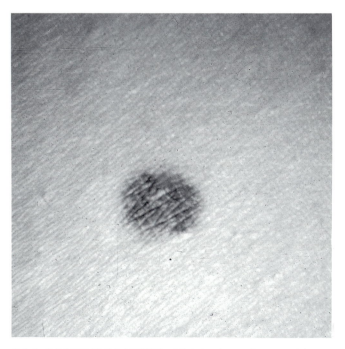

8-1-1 JUNCTIONAL NEVUS: Slightly elevated nevus with an irregular border and mottled brown pigmentation.

Differential Diagnosis

Blue nevus
Café-au-lait spot
Pigmented Spitz nevus
Urticaria pigmentosa

Pigmented basal cell epithelioma
Becker's nevus
Nevoid hyperpigmentation
Linear epidermal nevus

HISTOLOGICAL DESCRIPTION

Nevus cells vary in their cytological appearance, often depending on location in the skin. Epidermal nevus cells are usually round to oval with a large, pale-staining nucleus; they may or may not have a well-defined nucleolus. Nevus cells in the epidermis often have cytoplasmic melanin pigment granules. Nevus cells are recognized not only by their cytological characteristics, but, most often, by their arrangement in nests or theques in the epidermis and dermis.

Dermal nevus cells may vary in their cytological appearance depending on their location in the dermis. Nevus cells in the papillary and upper reticular dermis tend to be more cuboidal and have more pigment. Midreticular dermal nevus cells have less cytoplasm and begin to resemble lymphocytes. These are almost never pigmented. Nevus cells in the lower dermis may resemble the midlevel cells or be more bipolar or spindle-shaped, resembling fibroblasts. Pigment within these cells is rare. Mast cells cytologically resemble nevus cells but do not form nests.

Nevus cells stain with silver stains and with the immunoperoxidase technique, S-100 protein, and some nevus cells stain with HMB 45.

Nevi in children show more cellularity at the epidermal-dermal interface and within the epidermis, a change that when seen in adults may be considered alarming. Nevi in children often have junctional activity that extends laterally well beyond the dermal component, giving an asymmetrical appearance. Nevi in children may show pagetoid growth and have nests of cells in parakeratotic scales. These are still considered benign, though in adults they would be cause for concern. Nevi in children under ten years of age rarely, if ever, show neurotization, a frequent finding in adults. Nevus cell nests in the epidermis in children are large, with large nevus cells that have abundant cytoplasm and dusty cytoplasmic pigment. Mitoses may be present at the epidermal-dermal interface.

Junctional Nevi

The striking feature in junctional nevi is large succulent nevus cell nests in the epidermis at the epidermal-dermal interface (Figure 8-1-3). There may be pigmented parakeratosis overlying the epidermal changes. There are no dermal nevus cells. The inflammatory infiltrate varies from sparse to moderate and is lymphocytic in character and mainly perivascular in location. Dermal melanophage pigmentation may be present. Nevus cell nests in children over twelve years of age become smaller, due to the decrease in cell cytoplasm and nuclear shrinkage.

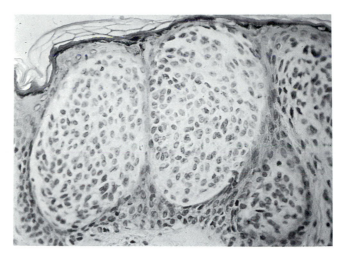

8-1-3 JUNCTIONAL NEVUS: High magnification shows large nevus cell nests within an expanded epidermis. Note the size and shape of the intraepidermal nests, a characteristic feature. (400×)

Compound Nevi

Compound nevi show, in addition to the epidermal component, dermal nests and groups of mature plump nevus cells (Figure 8-1-4). An inflammatory component may be seen that is perivascular and lymphocytic. Lymphocytes may also be seen in the dermis, about the nevus cell nests. The epidermal component may extend well beyond the dermal component.

Dermal Nevi

Dermal nevi have nevus cells in nests and groups in the dermis and are found in older children and teenagers (Figure 8-1-5). Pigmentation is variable; those nevus cells in the papillary dermis usually possess cytoplasmic pigmentation. The inflammatory infiltrate is lymphohistiocytic, perivascular, and sometimes diffuse. Mitoses and cellular atypia are rare.

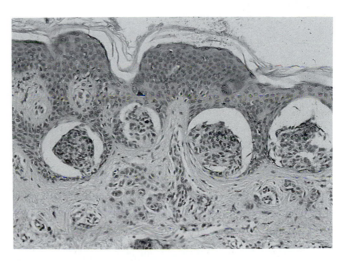

8-1-4 COMPOUND NEVUS: Melanocytic cell nests are present in the dermis and epidermis. (200×)

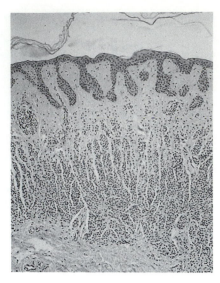

8-1-5 DERMAL NEVUS: Nests of melanocytic cells in the dermis in cords and strands, extending to the midreticular dermis. The epidermis shows adenoid acanthosis with basilar pigmentation. No nests are seen within the epidermis. (40×)

Congenital Nevi

Congenital nevi are usually defined by size: small and large (giant or garment). The large congenital nevi measure greater than 20 cm in diameter.

The striking feature of congenital nevi that most often differentiates them from usual acquired nevi is the volume of cells per unit of tissue (Figure 8-1-6). Congenital nevi may also show only a superficial component. The pattern of a superficial and deep component is often age-related.

The difficult differential diagnosis is superficial congenital nevi and acquired nevi. Congenital nevi have melanocytes in the sweat ducts and about the hair follicles and sebaceous glands. Melanocytic cells can be found extending singly between collagen bundles and in blood vessel walls. Signs of immature skin, young fat cells, cellular collagen, immature sebaceous, and sweat glands are other features that help identify congenital nevi. When there is a deep component the diagnosis is easier. In congenital nevi myriads of cells extend into the subcutaneous fat. These melanocytic cells at the lower border of the tumor resemble lymphocytes in that they are basophilic with scant cytoplasm. Pigmentation within the tumor is variable and can be seen at all levels. It can be quite dense in the mid- and lower portions.

Large or garment congenital nevi may show, in addition, neurotization (neuroid elements and neuroid-appearing melanocytic cells) and dendritic cells (Figure 8-1-7). The dendritic cell component of congenital nevi resembles that of a blue nevus, but these spindle cells represent only a small portion of the overall tumor.

The inflammatory response in all of these tumors is variable, usually lymphocytic, perivascular as well as tumor admixed.

Differential Diagnosis
Dermal Nevi
Mast cell tumor

Congenital Nevi
Neural tumor
Blue nevus

Junctional Nevus
Paget's disease

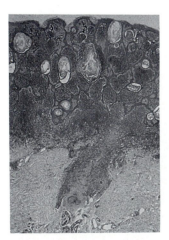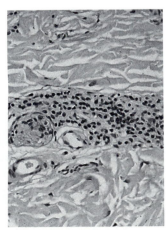

8-1-6 CONGENITAL NEVI: Split photo, showing nevic cells permeating the dermis. Close apposition of melanocytes to the preexisting appendages (right panel) is a characteristic feature. (40×, 200×)

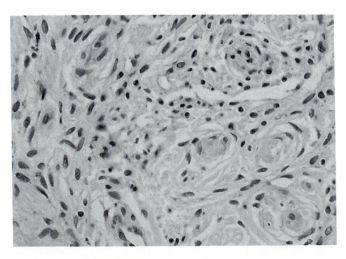

8-1-7 CONGENITAL NEVI: Neuroid differentiation in a congenital hairy nevus. (100×)

8-2 DYSPLASTIC (ATYPICAL) NEVUS

CLINICAL DESCRIPTION

Etiology and Incidence

Dysplastic nevi occur in approximately 5% of the white population in the United States. They occur in a syndromic pattern in certain families but are most often found on a sporadic basis.

Clinical Features

Dysplastic nevi occur most commonly on non-sun-exposed skin (e.g., the scalp and buttocks). Dysplastic nevi have irregular, ill-defined borders. Pigmentation over the surface is irregular and may be speckled (Plate 8-2-1). The surface may be pebbly or somewhat rugose. Dysplastic nevi vary in size and can be up to 0.6 mm in diameter.

Differential Diagnosis

Cockarde nevus
Malignant melanoma
Compound nevus
Junctional nevus

HISTOLOGICAL DESCRIPTION

Dysplastic (atypical) nevi occur as part of a syndrome and were formerly thought to be a constant precursor for melanoma. It is now known that dysplastic nevi occur sporadically in the population, and not all of them portend the development of melanoma. Dysplastic nevi rarely occur below the age of ten years.

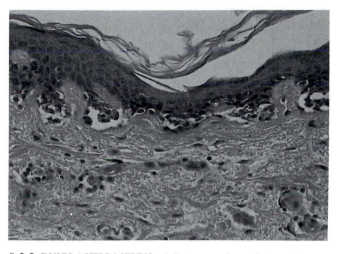

8-2-2 DYSPLASTIC NEVUS: Adjacent sections of the melanocytic process in Figure 8-2-1 shows atypical melanocytic cells in nests at the dermal-epidermal interface. Some nests are oriented parallel to the epidermal surface. This portion of the specimen shows cytologic atypia as well as architectural atypia. (200×)

Histologically there are two patterns: architectural atypia and cytological atypia. In the former there is lentiginous hyperplasia with fusion of some of the rete ridges. The lentiginous rete show an increased number of melanocytes along the sides, and some may appear pleomorphic (Figures 8-2-1 and 8-2-2). Nests of melanocytes can be found in the upper dermis, the cells within them spindle-shaped or epithelioid, with abundant dusky pigmented cytoplasm. Dermal nests appear normal. There is often an associated lymphocytic inflammatory infiltrate. The papillary dermis shows a varying degree of fine lamellar fibroplasia.

The dysplastic nevus has cytologic atypia in addition to the other features noted. There are atypical melanocytes at

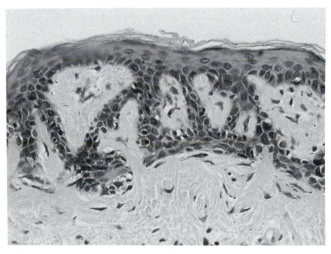

8-2-1 DYSPLASTIC NEVUS: This is architectural atypia with lentiginous hyperplasia of the epidermis and the presence of hyperchromatic melanocytic cells at the dermal-epidermal interface. Associated with this in the dermis there is lamellar fibroplasia. (200×)

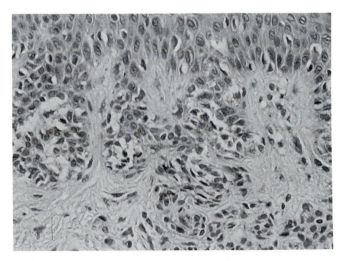

8-2-3 DYSPLASTIC NEVUS: Melanocytes in the dermis and epidermis. The epidermal component shows disorganized nests of pleomorphic melanocytes. The dermal component does not show significant atypia. (400×)

the tips and sides of the elongated rete, occurring singly or in small groups (Figure 8-2-3). Nests of atypical melanocytes are in elongate nests at the dermal-epidermal interface, oriented parallel to the surface. Atypical melanocytic cells, appearing in nests or singly, can be found in the upper epidermis, but there is not distinct pagetoid spread. There is distinct papillary lamellar fibroplasia and an associated, often brisk, lymphocytic infiltrate.

Differential Diagnosis
Compound nevus
Malignant melanoma

8-3 NEVUS SPILUS

CLINICAL PRESENTATION

Etiology and Incidence
Nevi spilus (nevoid lentigo) may occur at any age and is often present at birth.

Clinical Features
These nevi are large, yellow-brown macules that can measure several centimeters in diameter (Plate 8-3-1). The borders are sharply defined. The pigmentation may be speckled with darker spots on a background of yellow-brown.

Differential Diagnosis
Café-au-lait spot
Becker's nevus

HISTOLOGICAL DESCRIPTION

Nevus spilus is essentially a lentigo in which nevus cells are sometimes found. There is acanthosis with increased pigment at the tips and sides of the acanthotic rete ridges (Plate 8-3-2). There may also be dermal or epidermal collections of nevus cells. Giant melanosomes have been seen in the melanocytes of these lesions. The inflammatory response is variable, usually being sparse numbers of perivascular lymphocytes.

Differential Diagnosis
Lentigo
Compound nevus

8-4 SPINDLE CELL AND EPITHELIOID CELL NEVUS (SPITZ NEVUS)

CLINICAL DESCRIPTION

Etiology and Incidence
Spindle cell and epithelioid cell nevi are uncommon forms of melanocytic tumors that occur frequently in children aged

one to thirteen years. Fifteen percent occur on the cheek. As with junction, compound, and dermal nevi, this is a tumor of melanocytic cells.

Clinical Features
Spindle cell and epithelioid cell nevi are usually solitary nodules found in any location, with a greater tendency to occur on the face and extremities. They do not have the usual characteristics of melanocytic tumors in that they are usually not clinically pigmented. Spindle cell and epithelioid cell nevi are reddish to purple to pink in color and are commonly mistaken clinically for vascular tumors or verrucae (Plate 8-4-1). They are larger than the usual nevi of childhood, varying from 1 to 2 cm in diameter.

Differential Diagnosis
Hemangioma
Pyogenic granuloma
Angiofibroma
Dermatofibroma
Verruca

HISTOLOGICAL DESCRIPTION

This tumor has been called a Spitz nevus or tumor, as well as by the unfortunate term *benign juvenile melanoma*. Of all benign nevi, this tumor is most often misdiagnosed as melanoma. Although this lesion is most common in childhood, about 20% occur in adults. In adults, the clinical diagnosis is rarely if ever made and in children it is made infrequently. The most common clinical diagnosis is verruca.

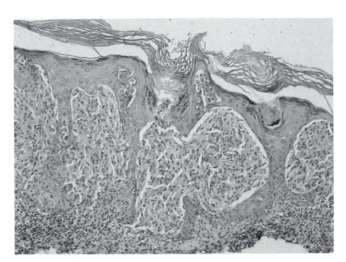

8-4-1 SPINDLE AND EPITHELIOID CELL NEVUS: Low-power photomicrograph, showing nests of spindle and epithelioid cells at the dermal-epidermal interface with the presence of a small crust on the surface. The dermis is filled with nests of epithelioid melanocytes. (20 ×)

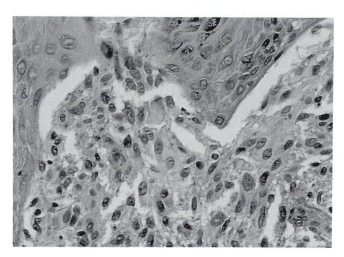

8-4-2 SPINDLE AND EPITHELIOID CELL NEVUS: High-power photomicrograph, showing spindle melanocytic cells within the epidermis. These have abundant amphophilic cytoplasm. Eosinophilic bodies (Kamino bodies) are seen within the epidermis. (400×)

The histological features in this tumor vary depending on the predominant type or admixture of cells seen in the specimen—epithelioid or spindle. Almost all are compound nevi, which most commonly show grouped and single spindle or epithelioid nevus cells at the epidermal-dermal interface (Figure 8-4-1). There may be single-cell upward growth of pigmented cells in the epidermis. Dyskeratotic epidermal cells (Kamino bodies) are almost always found in the epidermis (Figure 8-4-2). In the papillary dermis, mitotic figures are not uncommon. Nevus cells in the reticular dermis tend to nest less and are found as single epithelioid or spindle cells. Approaching the lower reticular dermis, melanocytic cells have less cytoplasm and infiltrate the dermis as single cells. Pigmentation and inflammation are variable in these tumors. When pigment is present it is most often found in the papillary dermis.

Differential Diagnosis
Malignant melanoma

8-5 HALO NEVUS

CLINICAL DESCRIPTION

Etiology and Incidence
Halo nevi are junction, dermal, or compound nevi that undergo an inflammatory or immunologic event. This response causes a loss of pigment around the melanocytic process, giving it its characteristic appearance. This change can occur in

any nevus and at any age but is most common in late adolescence. Halo nevi are often associated with vitiligo, suggesting an immunologic basis for this process.

Clinical Features
Halo nevi present a striking clinical picture. A pigmented nevus is surrounded by a depigmented halo (Figure 8-5-1). There may be an associated flare of erythema about the halo. As the process continues there is complete destruction of the nevus; the area of depigmentation persists from months to years. This reaction (halo formation) can occur in other pigmented lesions, including blue nevi, giant congenital nevi, melanomas, cutaneous metastatic melanomas, and sometimes neuromas. Because of the histologic atypia seen in these lesions and the rare possibility of the development of melanoma, some physicians recommend the unnecessary excision of all halo nevi. Excision should be considered only if the nevus exhibits atypical characteristics suggestive of malignant change.

Differential Diagnosis
Vitiligo
Melanoma
Morphea

HISTOLOGICAL DESCRIPTION
Halo nevi were originally considered benign inflammatory changes in normal nevi. There have been some data to suggest otherwise, because of the presence of atypical melanocytic cells in the inflammatory infiltrate. Despite these data that suggest an aggressive course of action, the majority of data indicate that halo nevi are benign lesions.

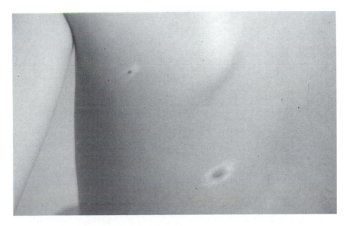

8-5-1 HALO NEVUS: Multiple halo nevi on patient's back show perinevoid vitiligo with a central erythematous papule.

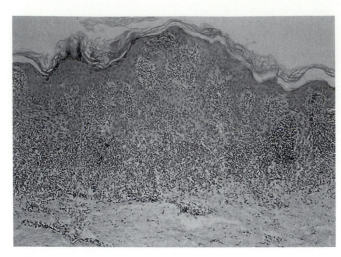

8-5-2 HALO NEVUS: A dense inflammatory infiltrate in the dermis surrounds and obscures dermal nevus cell nests as well as those at the dermal-epidermal interface. The inflammatory infiltrate is composed entirely of lymphocytes. (40×)

The striking histological feature is a dense, plaquelike inflammatory infiltrate that occupies the papillary and upper reticular dermis (Figure 8-5-2). The mainly lymphocytic infiltrate obscures the dermal-epidermal interface, is exocytotic to the epidermis, and obscures nevus cells and nevus cell nests (Figure 8-5-3). The section at the lateral margins may show a well-defined dermal, compound, or junction nevus.

The melanocytic cells in the inflammatory infiltrate may show cytoplasmic and nuclear alteration and appear cytologically atypical. Often it is difficult to decide whether this is a melanocytic lesion. Immunoperoxidase stains with S-100

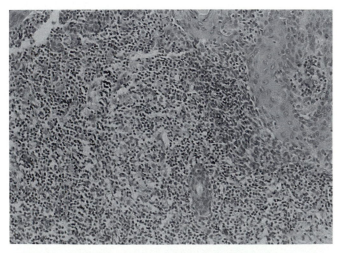

8-5-3 HALO NEVUS: Higher-power photomicrograph, showing the inflammatory infiltrate, within which an occasional pigmented cell can be seen. There is one melanocytic nest underlying the epidermis (at the right). (400×)

protein or HMB45 can be invaluable in identifying melanocytic cells in the infiltrate and at the dermal-epidermal interface.

Differential Diagnosis
Malignant melanoma
Lymphocytic infiltrates

8-6 BLUE NEVUS AND CELLULAR BLUE NEVUS

CLINICAL DESCRIPTION

Etiology and Incidence
Blue nevi may be present at birth or may develop at any age. Females tend to have a greater number of blue nevi than males. Blue nevi develop from dermal dendritic melanocytes that are found in greater numbers than seen in the mongolian spot or Ota's nevus. They can occur as the common pigmented dendritic type or the cellular type, which contains less pigment.

Clinical Features
Blue nevi are distinctive. They are blue-black in color and dome-shaped, with a smooth surface having normal skin markings (Plate 8-6-1). They are usually less than 1 cm in diameter. Blue nevi are stable in size and rarely exhibit growth patterns. The majority of blue nevi are benign; malignant changes occur rarely.

Cellular blue nevi are less pigmented than common blue nevi. They are larger in size, being 1 cm in diameter or greater. Cellular blue nevi are more site-specific than noncellular, often occurring on the buttocks and sacrococcygeal area but also found in other sites. Cellular blue nevi have a greater tendency to develop malignancy than do regular pigmented blue nevi.

Differential Diagnosis
Other types of nevi
Melanoma
Dermatofibroma

HISTOLOGICAL DESCRIPTION

Blue nevi are tumors of dendritic melanocytes in the dermis (Plate 8-6-2). These dendritic cells, usually bipolar, carry their own dense fibrocellular stroma, which is often distinct from the surrounding collagen (Figure 8-6-1). Pigment is common, usually coarse and intracytoplasmic. Inflammation is sparse, usually lymphohistiocytic in type. The pigment-producing cells in blue nevi may aggregate about adnexae or blood vessels.

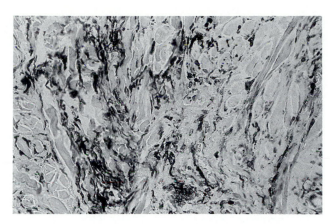

8-6-1 BLUE NEVUS: Higher-power photomicrograph, showing spindle-shaped pigmented melanocytes within a fibrocellular dermis. (400×)

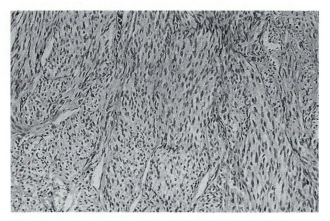

8-6-3 CELLULAR BLUE NEVUS: High-power photomicrograph, showing the fascicles and cords of melanocytic cells separated by compressed collagen. No pigmentation is noted in this field. (400×)

Cellular blue nevi may be biphasic, with superficially placed pigmented spindle cell melanocytes and deeper spindle-shaped cells melanocytes without pigment (Figure 8-6-2). These latter cells occur in patterns resembling the storiform pattern of fibrocellular tumors, in that they consist of intersecting fascicles and streams of cells (Figure 8-6-3). The melanocytic cells of the latter group have more cytoplasm than usual melanocytes in blue nevi and little if any pigment. They are deeply placed, often extending into the subcutaneous fat. When cellular blue nevi are composed of only nonpigmented spindle cell melanocytes the diagnosis can be difficult. The immunoperoxidase technique (S-100 protein and HMB 45) is invaluable in assisting with the diagnosis when there is no cytoplasmic pigment. Cellular blue nevi may show cytologic atypia without being malignant. Giant, bizarre multinucleated cells with or without inflamma-

tion may be seen. The lack of mitoses, cellular necrosis, and the presence of the more characteristic spindle-shaped cells speak for a benign condition.

Differential Diagnosis
Dermatofibrosarcoma protuberans
Pigmented neurofibroma
Dermatofibromas

8-7 MONGOLIAN SPOTS

CLINICAL DESCRIPTION

Etiology and Incidence
Mongolian spots are most commonly seen in the pigmented races. Approximately 85% to 90% occur at birth in African-American children. They are also common in Hispanics, Asians, Native Americans, and, on occasion, Caucasians. These spots are dermal dendritic melanocytic lesions representing a type of blue nevus.

Clinical Features
Mongolian spots are blue-black macular discolorations of the skin commonly located in the sacral-coccygeal area (Figure 8-7-1). They can occur as one large spot, 1 cm or greater in diameter, or multiple small pigmented macular areas. The pigmentation is present at birth and persists into adulthood but does diminish somewhat in intensity in the adult years.

Differential Diagnosis
Blue nevus

HISTOLOGICAL DESCRIPTION
This condition has in common with blue nevus the presence of pigmented dermal dendritic cells. The overlying epidermis

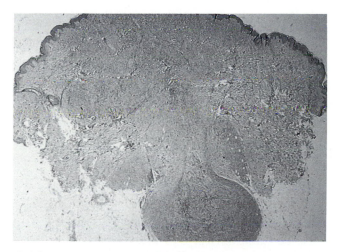

8-6-2 CELLULAR BLUE NEVUS: Low-power photomicrograph, showing a tumor in the dermis that extends into the subcutaneous fat. Pigmentation is sparse in this tumor. (40×)

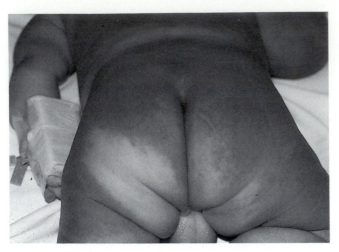

8-7-1 MONGOLIAN SPOTS: Macular hyperpigmentation of the sacrum, buttocks, and lateral thighs in a male infant.

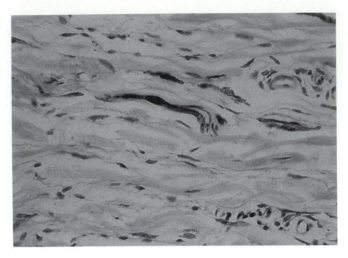

8-7-3 MONGOLIAN SPOTS: High-power photomicrograph of a bipolar pigmented melanocyte in the dermis. (400×)

is usually thinned and uninvolved in the process. The dermal melanocytes are thin, elongated, and bipolar; they lie between collagen bundles, usually in the lower one-half of the dermis (Figure 8-7-2), with the long axis parallel to the epidermal surface. These cells contain cytoplasmic melanin pigment (Figure 8-7-3). The presence or absence of immature sweat glands indicates the age of the patient and helps differentiate this lesion from the usual blue nevus. The dendritic cells are S-100-, and in some cases HMB 45-positive.

Differential Diagnosis
Blue nevus
Nevus of Ito

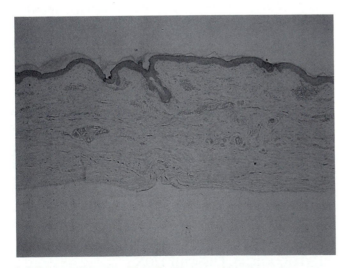

8-7-2 MONGOLIAN SPOTS: Pigmented bipolar melanocytes seen in the mid- and lower reticular dermis. There is a patchy lymphocytic infiltrate. (40×)

8-8 OTA'S AND ITO'S NEVUS

CLINICAL DESCRIPTION

Etiology and Incidence
Ota's and Ito's nevi occur as congenital lesions in about 45% to 50% of cases. They are seen most commonly in Asians but also occur in African Americans. About 75% to 80% of cases are in females. These pigmentary lesions are derived from dermal melanocytes.

Clinical Features
Ota's and Ito's nevi are blue-black to slate gray discolorations of the skin over the lateral aspect of the face and sclera on the affected side (Plate 8-8-1A). These discolorations are most commonly found in the distribution of the second division of the trigeminal nerve. Although the slate gray color usually occurs at birth, some patients develop the discoloration later in life. It persists throughout life and, as with other congenital pigmentation, may darken at puberty.

Ito's nevus is similar in appearance to Ota's nevus but more extensive in distribution. In addition to the face, Ito's nevus may involve the shoulder, side of the neck, deltoid areas, upper arm, and supraclavicular region. Malignant transformation is uncommon in Ota's nevus.

Differential Diagnosis
Nevus flammeus

HISTOLOGICAL DESCRIPTION

Both of these conditions show delicate bipolar pigmented dermal dendritic cells in the superficial dermal collagen. There are more dendritic cells than in the mongolian spot, and they may be found in the papillary dermis as well as in the upper reticular dermis (Plate 8-8-1B). These cells also contain cytoplasmic pigmentation and are S-100-, and sometimes HMB 45-positive. The epidermis is usually thinned, and there is no associated inflammatory reaction.

Differential Diagnosis

Mongolian spot

Blue nevus

8-9 MELANOMA

CLINICAL DESCRIPTION

Malignant melanoma is rare in childhood. Melanoma in childhood may be superficial spreading type, nodular, or acral lentiginous. Melanomas in only the radial growth phase are considered zero-risk melanomas with an excellent prognosis, even though atypical cells are found in the papillary dermis (level II).

Etiology and Incidence

Melanomas occur at any age, but less than 1% occur before puberty. They are most commonly found on the extremities, in the nailbeds, or on the palms, soles, or mucous membranes. Melanomas in children have the same prognosis as in adults when compared with the level of invasion, tumor thickness, number of mitoses, and site. Melanomas are rare in black skin.

Clinical Features

Melanomas are tumors with colors varying from rose-brown to blue-black over the surface of the lesion. The borders are irregular, with a faint halo of erythema and indefinite margins (Plate 8-9-1). Melanomas lose their normal skin markings as proliferation continues. Superficial spreading melanomas are only slightly raised above the skin surface and exhibit a play of colors as previously described. Nodular melanomas are dome-shaped; they arise and grow rapidly and often ulcerate. Ulceration and rapid growth are a poor prognostic sign.

Not all melanomas are pigmented. Amelanotic melanomas present a difficult and often diagnostic dilemma. Any lesion, pigmented or not, with growth change characteristics, erythema, and/or pigment changes should be biopsied.

Acral lentiginous melanoma may present early as pigmented bands of the nailbeds or macular pigmentation on the palms or soles. As these tumors progress pigmentation increases, with leeching of pigment from the tumor to the surrounding skin. Pigmentation of the posterior nailfold (Hutchinson's sign) indicates tumor growth. Lesions of the palms or soles can exhibit nodularity with loss of skin markings. The striking feature in all of these tumors is marked production of pigment.

Differential Diagnosis

Dysplastic nevi

Pigmented nodules

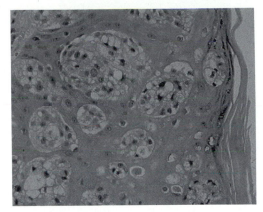

8-9-1 SUPERFICIAL SPREADING MELANOMA: Nested and pagetoid atypical melanocytes within the epidermis at all levels. In other areas (see Figure 8-9-2) atypical melanocytic nests could also be seen in the dermis. (100×)

Spitz nevus

Blue nevus

Junctional nevus

HISTOLOGICAL DESCRIPTION

Superficial Spreading Melanoma

The striking histological feature in superficial spreading melanoma is pagetoid melanoma cells at the dermal-epidermal interface and scattered in the upper epidermis (Figure 8-9-1). There is usually associated focal discrete parakeratosis, which may be pigmented. The melanoma cells are large, with abundant smoky brown cytoplasm and a hyperchromatic nucleus. Extending some distance from the main area of involvement are scattered large single melanocytic cells in the epidermis. There is usually a patchy lymphocytic infiltrate underlying the typical pagetoid melanocytes. This lesion is considered in situ when dermal involvement cannot be found. When there is invasion (vertical growth phase) it is of similar cell types, and there is an associated lymphocytic inflammatory response as well as melanophage pigmentation (Figure 8-9-2). The lymphocytic response diminishes with the duration of dermal invasion.

Nodular Melanoma

In nodular melanoma there is a proliferation of atypical cells in the dermis (Figure 8-9-3). These cells are usually large, with amphophilic cytoplasm, containing pigment. The nuclei vary in size, shape, and chromatin pattern. Mitoses are usually found but vary in number. There may be a patchy peripheral lymphocytic infiltrate. A radial growth phase is absent in these tumors.

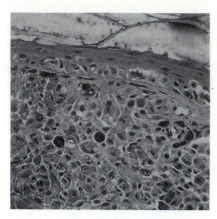

8-9-2 SUPERFICIAL SPREADING MELANOMA: High-power photomicrograph of the dermal component, with nests of atypical melanocytes, with marked cytologic pleomorphism. (400×)

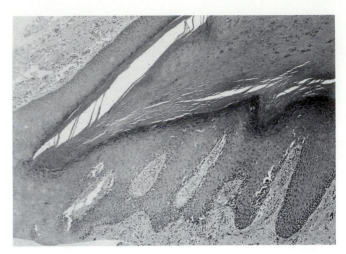

8-9-4 ACRAL LENTIGINOUS MELANOMA: Nailfold with a confluent proliferation of melanocytes at the dermal-epidermal junction. (20×)

The overlying epidermis is thinned, usually with a parakeratotic scale. The cells in some nodular melanomas may be so bizarre and atypical and without pigment that the initial assessment on hematoxylin and eosin sections is difficult. A battery of immunoperoxidase stains is helpful and should include S-100 protein (Plate 8-9-2), HMB 45, keratin, and alpha-1-antitrypsin.

Differential Diagnosis
Acquired congenital nevus
Atypical fibroxanthoma

Acral Lentiginous Melanoma
Acral lentiginous melanoma or acral melanoma can arise on the palm, sole, toes, fingers, or nailbeds. The process is composed of lentiginous epidermal hyperplasia in some cases, with the presence of spindled melanocytes in the basal layer of the epidermis. Early in the disease there may be only an increase in basilar melanocytes, a picture similar to that in lentigo maligna. In addition to the atypical spindle melanocytes, pagetoid atypical melanocytes of the type seen in superficial spreading melanoma can be found. Either type of cell can predominate. A striking finding is the pigmentation produced, which is found in the epidermis as well as the dermis (Figures 8-9-4 and 8-9-5).

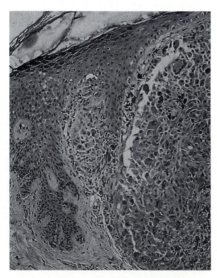

8-9-3 NODULAR MELANOMA: Atypical melanocytic cells in the dermis without an epidermal connection. Many of these cells are epithelioid in character and show significant variation in cell size and configuration. (40×)

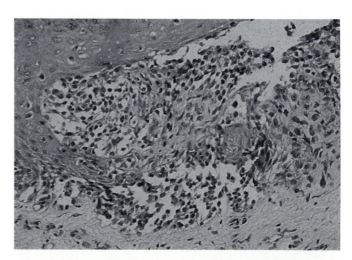

8-9-5 ACRAL LENTIGINOUS MELANOMA: Nailfold with a large collection of atypical melanocytes at the dermal-epidermal junction. There is some suggested pagetoid growth. (200×)

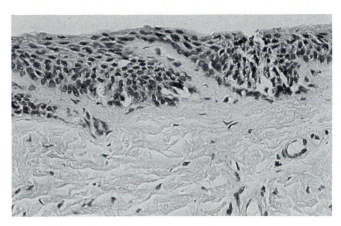

8-10-1 MELANONYCHIA STRIATA: This pigmentation was due to a junction nevus. Nests of melanocytic cells are seen at the dermal-epidermal interface in this nailbed. Pigmentation is seen within the cytoplasm of these melanocytic cells. There is no inflammatory infiltrate. (200×)

8-10 MELANONYCHIA STRIATA

CLINICAL DESCRIPTION

Etiology and Incidence

Melanonychia striata is uncommon in Caucasians but found frequently in the pigmented races. These pigmented nail bands are secondary to nevi, melanoma, or excessive pigment production from within melanocytes in the germinative layer of the epidermis at the posterior nailfold.

Clinical Features

Linear pigmented stripes occur most commonly in the central portion of the nail (Plate 8-10-1). These bands are not usually associated with pigmentation at the distal tip of the finger but may be associated with a rim of pigmentation at the posterior nailfold. These pigmented bands do not usually exhibit erythema or tenderness.

Differential Diagnosis

Acral lentiginous melanoma
Hemorrhage

HISTOLOGICAL DESCRIPTION

There are a variety of melanocytic changes. These lesions can be junction, dermal, or compound nevi (Figure 8-10-1). The clinical hyperpigmentation may result from histological hyperpigmentation. Nevi are most common in Caucasian children and hyperpigmentation is most common in black children. The pigmented bands of the nails may represent acral lentiginous melanoma. Clinical differentiation of a benign pigmented band from one caused by a malignant tumor is impossible, therefore biopsy study is essential.

Differential Diagnosis

Melanocytic nevus
Melanoma

8-11 CONGENITAL NEVUS WITH NODULES (CONGENITAL PSEUDOMELANOMA)

CLINICAL DESCRIPTION

Etiology and Incidence

Congenital nevi in some instances grow rapidly and develop nodules that are present at birth or in the first six months of life. This clinical scenario occurs in less than 1% of congenital nevi. These nodules simulate melanoma clinically and histologically but act biologically benign.

Clinical Features

Pigmented blue-black nodules may be present at birth or develop rapidly shortly after birth (Figure 8-11-1). These nodules may attain a large size, measuring greater than 4 cm in diameter, and ulcerate. They occur in any portion of the congenital nevus. Although they may appear alarming on histological study, the biological behavior of those developing in children less than six months of age is not that of an aggressive malignant melanoma.

Differential Diagnosis

Melanoma
Atypical nevus

HISTOLOGICAL DESCRIPTION

There are several histological patterns of nevus nodules that develop in the milieu of a congenital nevus. Nodular melanoma shows a proliferation of atypical melanocytic cells into

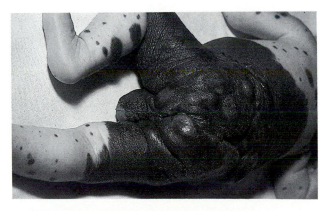

8-11-1 CONGENITAL NEVUS WITH NODULE: Garment type, covering most of the lower trunk and upper thighs. There is within this area a nodule that has some loss of pigment at one margin.

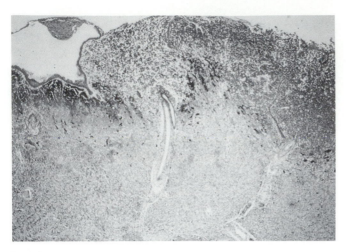

8-11-2 CONGENITAL NEVUS WITH NODULES: Low-power photomicrograph, showing surface ulceration with an inflammatory crust. The pigmentation in the superficial portion is lost. At the margins of this nodule there is dense pigmentation of cells within the papillary dermis. (40×)

the dermis, with marked cellular atypia and mitoses (Figure 8-11-2). A well-defined radial growth phase is not evident, although there may be pagetoid spread in the epidermis.

In superficial spreading melanoma there are nests of atypical epithelioid melanocytes in the epidermis and the dermis. Dyskeratotic cells, mitoses, and cellular necrosis can be found in the dermal portion of this tumor. In malignant melanoma there are changes of the usual type, without epithelioid melanocytes. Finally, there are nodules with some histological features of a superficial spreading melanoma and a dermal component of more spindle atypical melanocytes. The dermal component is associated with desmoplasia and extends into the subcutis (Figure 8-11-3). This tumor, like others, blends into the existing congenital nevus.

8-12 COCKARDE NEVUS

CLINICAL DESCRIPTION

Etiology and Incidence
Cockarde nevus is rare, with only five to six reports in the literature. It is a variant of a compound nevus and must be distinguished from dysplastic nevi.

Clinical Features
Cockarde nevus can present as multiple sharply delineated black-brown macules with a peripheral rim of pigmentation that is darker than the remainder of the nevus (Figure 8-12-1). In the center of the lesion is a dome-shaped, yellow-brown to pink papule, which represents the melanocytic nevus. The color variation makes it difficult to differentiate this nevus from a dysplastic nevus. Dysplastic nevi usually do not have sharply defined borders, unlike Cockarde nevi, or targetoid configurations.

Differential Diagnosis
Dysplastic nevus
Halo nevus
Melanoma

HISTOLOGICAL DESCRIPTION
Cockarde nevi are essentially compound and junctional nevi. Often the central papule is a compound nevus with nevus cell nests in the lower epidermis and dermis (Figure 8-12-2). The peripheral portion of the lesion, from the central papule to the surrounding target area, is a junction nevus with the presence of single as well as grouped melanocytes in the epidermis at the dermal-epidermal interface (Figure 8-12-3). The pigment at the periphery of the lesion is the result of increased

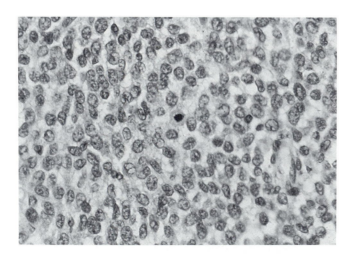

8-11-3 CONGENITAL NEVUS WITH NODULES: High-power photomicrograph, showing the cellular architecture and mitotic activity of the nodules within the congenital nevus. (400×)

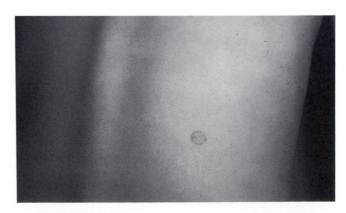

8-12-1 COCKARDE NEVUS: Pigmented annular lesion of the back, showing a peripheral rim of more dense brown pigment surrounding an area of slight erythema with a central small papule.

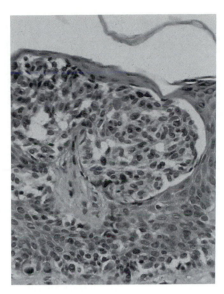

8-12-2 COCKARDE NEVUS: Epidermal nested melanocytes and sparse dermal nests. (400×)

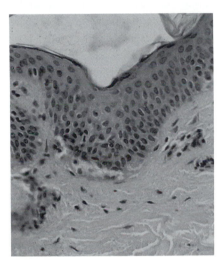

8-12-3 COCKARDE NEVUS: The margin of the nevus, showing small junctional nests and basilar pigmentation. (400×)

melanogenesis, and rarely are there nevus cells. S-100 and HMB 45 stains confirm the presence of melanocytic cells at the periphery. This lesion does not have atypia, as is seen in dysplastic nevus.

Differential Diagnosis
Dysplastic nevus

8-13 NEUROFIBROMATOSIS AND CAFÉ-AU-LAIT SPOTS

CLINICAL DESCRIPTION

Etiology and Incidence
Neurofibromatosis is a hereditary disease transmitted as an autosomal dominant condition and occurring in approximately 1

8-13-1 Neural Tumors

Neurofibromas	Granular cell tumors
Café-au-lait spots	Nasal gliomas
Neurilemomas	Neuromas

per 3,000 to 4,000 births. About one-half of patients have affected relatives. This condition is the result of a genetic defect (on chromosome 17) that causes abnormal function or production of Schwann cells and melanocytes. It appears that only neural-derived cells are affected (Table 8-13-1).

Clinical Findings
The distinctive clinical features of neurofibromatosis include neural tumors and cutaneous pigmentation (Figure 8-13-1). The major pigmentary lesions are the café-au-lait spots, which, when they occur in the axilla (axillary freckle) or inguinal regions, are pathognomonic for neurofibromatosis (Plate 8-13-1). Multiple cutaneous tumors may occur at any site after puberty. Solitary neurofibromas can be found in children but are most commonly seen in adults. Table 8-13-2 lists the criteria necessary to make a diagnosis of neurofibromatosis. Pigmentary changes other than café-au-lait macules that may be seen in neurofibromatosis include diffuse bronzing, macular hypopigmentation or vitiligolike change, vitiligo, and hypopigmented ash-leaf-like macules.

Differential Diagnosis
Epidermoid cyst
Lipoma

HISTOLOGICAL DESCRIPTION

Neurofibromas
Neurofibromas are characterized by the presence of spindle-shaped cells in a loose, almost myxoid mixture of collagen

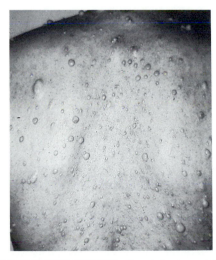

8-13-1 NEUROFIBROMATOSIS: An adolescent with multiple well-defined neurofibromas.

8-13-2   Diagnostic Criteria for Neurofibromatosis Type 1
(two or more of the following)

1. 6 café-au-lait macules, > 5 mm in greatest diameter in prepubertal individuals and > 15 mm in greatest diameter in postpubertal individuals
2. 2 neurofibromas of any type or one plexiform neuroma
3. Freckling in the axillary or inguinal regions
4. Optic glioma
5. Sphenoid dysplasia or thinning of long bone cortex with or without pseudoarthrosis
6. Lisch nodules (iris hamartomas)
7. A first-degree relative (parent, sibling, or offspring) with type I by the above criteria

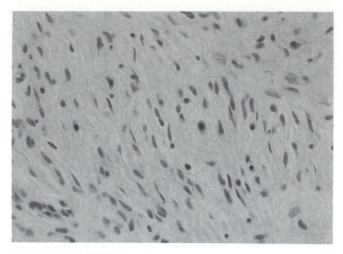

8-13-3 NEUROFIBROMAS: Higher-power photomicrograph, showing spindle-shaped cells. Within the tumor are small, thin-walled blood vessels and mast cells. (200 ×)

(Figure 8-13-2). Although not encapsulated, the cellular mass is distinctly separated from the surrounding dermis. The nuclei in this tumor are bipolar and spindle-shaped (Figure 8-13-3). Nuclei can also be found in wavy parallel rows resembling Verocay bodies, as seen in neurilemomas. Mast cells are frequently found. Neurofibromas often extend into the subcutaneous tissue. Large tumors often have mucinomyxoid degeneration, characterized by the presence of basophilic granular material, which is colloidal iron-positive, and hyaluronidase-labile (hyaluronic acid). Very large tumors are uncommon in children. Histological variations of neurofibroma are storiform neurofibroma and Pacinian neurofibroma. Storiform neurofibroma is composed of spindle-shaped Schwann cells and dendritic melanocytes. Cartwheel-like arrangements may be noted, a feature also seen in dermatofibrosarcoma protuberans. The dendritic melanocytes of the storiform variety show significant pigmentation. It is thought that this tumor may represent a variation of a blue nevus, not a neurofibroma at all. Pacinian neurofibromas are uncommon but may occur in children. This tumor is a well-circumscribed

encapsulated dermal mass containing a multilobular structure showing acellular eosinophilic material surrounded by concentric lamellae of collagen-like material. This structure resembles that of the Pacinian corpuscle. Nervelike bundles and/or nerve trunks can be seen associated with these Pacinian-like lobules. In these areas there are numbers of bipolar and/or spindle-shaped cells that resemble neural cells. Mucinous degeneration alteration may also occur.

Café-au-Lait Spots

The characteristic histological findings on routine hematoxylin and eosin-stained sections occur at the epidermal-dermal interface, where there is basal layer pigmentation and clear cells. On thin sections (1 μm) macromelanosomes may be seen within the clear cells.

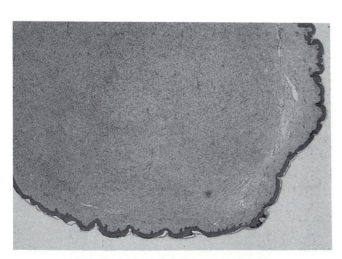

8-13-2 NEUROFIBROMAS: Low-power photomicrograph, showing pale-staining cells occupying the entire dermis. The overlying epidermis is effaced. (40 ×)

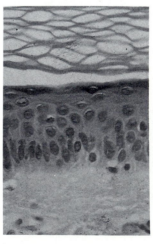
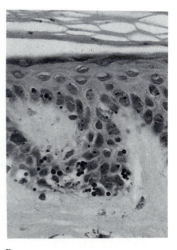

A   B

8-13-4 CAFÉ-AU-LAIT SPOTS: (A) Skin with normal-sized melanocytes and melanosomes. (200 ×) (B) Giant (macromelanosomes) pigment granules within epidermal melanocytes. (400 ×)

Dopa-stained, inverted epidermal whole mounts show increased numbers of melanocytes (per square millimeter) as well as macromelanosomes within the melanocytes (Figure 8-13-4).

Differential Diagnosis

Neurofibroma
Dermatofibroma
Blue nevus
Neurotized dermal nevus

Café-au-Lait Spots
Hyperpigmentation (other causes)

8-14 NEURILEMOMA

CLINICAL DESCRIPTION

Etiology and Incidence

Neurilemomas occur most often as single isolated tumors, although they can be seen in association with neurofibromatosis. They are tumors of Schwann cells, the single variety usually occurring on cranial or cutaneous nerves. Multiple neurilemomas are usually dermal tumors. They rarely develop malignancy.

Clinical Features

Neurilemomas are single or multiple dermal tumors that occur most commonly on the head and neck or on the extremities. This tumor has been associated with neurofibromatosis. Clinically, they are asymptomatic firm, flesh-colored nodules without specific clinical findings.

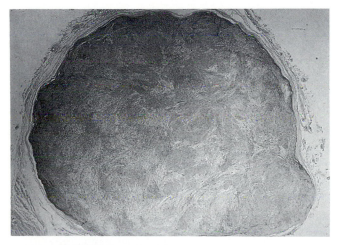

8-14-1 NEURILEMOMAS: Low-power photomicrograph, showing a well-encapsulated tumor with denser and less dense areas within the tumor representing Antoni A and Antoni B tissue. (20×)

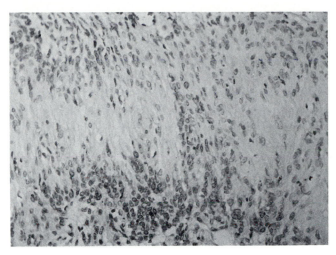

8-14-2 NEURILEMOMAS: Antoni A tissue, showing parallel rows of nuclei separated by a core of amorphous collagen. This is the Verocay body. (400×)

Differential Diagnosis

Neuromas
Neurofibroma
Any flesh-colored dermal nodule

HISTOLOGICAL DESCRIPTION

Neurilemomas are deeply placed encapsulated dermal tumors composed of two types of tissue. The peripheral tissue is loose, reticular, and mucinous and contains few nuclei. It is called Antoni B tissue. This material surrounds the cellular portion containing nuclei, which are bipolar, spindle-shaped, and closely set together (Figure 8-14-1). These nuclei line up in parallel rows separated by portions of amorphous collagen Antoni A tissue. The configuration of nuclei arranged about a core of amorphous collagen is called a Verocay body (Figure 8-14-2). Vessels within the tumor may show surrounding amorphous eosinophilic homogenized collagen. Mast cells may also be seen in this tumor as well as in neurofibromas.

Differential Diagnosis

Neurofibroma
Dermatofibroma

8-15 GRANULAR CELL TUMORS

CLINICAL DESCRIPTION

Etiology and Incidence

Granular cell tumors are uncommon in children but may occur. The most common site is the tongue, although these tumors have been described on all body surfaces as well as internal organs. Granular cell tumors are usually solitary but may occur in multiple sites.

Clinical Findings

Granular cell tumors are firm, nontender dermal tumors that vary in size from 1 to 2 cm. They may have a hyperkeratotic surface when occurring on the skin and are usually darker in color than the surrounding skin (Figure 8-15-1).

Differential Diagnosis

Fibroma
Verruca (tongue lesion)
Dermatofibroma

HISTOLOGICAL DESCRIPTION

The distinctive histological features are acanthosis to the point of pseudoepitheliomatous hyperplasia and an infiltrate of large, pale-staining cells with cytoplasm filled with eosinophilic granules (Figure 8-15-1). These cells have well-defined nuclei, usually located centrally; some cells may be multinucleated. Individual cells are large, varying 40 to 70 μm (Plate 8-15-1A). The granules within these cells are PAS-positive and diastase-resistant. The cells are also S-100-positive (Plate 8-15-1B). Also seen are clusters of cells surrounded by periodic acid-Schiff-positive, diastase-resistant membrane associated with strands of collagen and stellate fibroblasts (flattened fibroblasts). The inflammatory response in these tumors is minimal. Occasional flattened, bipolar cells thought to be a fibroblast may be also seen. Mitoses are uncommon and when seen indicate the possibility of malignant change. Malignant varieties of this tumor do occur but are rare in children.

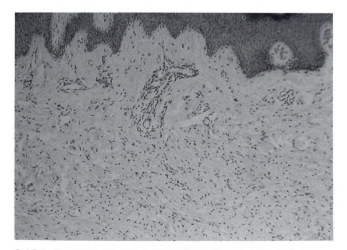

8-15-1 GRANULAR CELL TUMORS: The epidermis is acanthotic with basilar pigmentation. The dermis is filled with a cellular infiltrate composed of large, pale-staining cells with a granular cytoplasm. (40×)

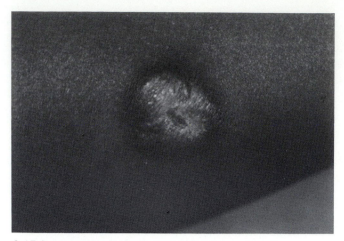

8-15-2 GRANULAR CELL TUMOR: A granular cell tumor on the thigh of a 12-year-old child. Note the central biopsy site.

Differential Diagnosis

Xanthoma
Squamous cell carcinoma (pseudoepitheliomatous hyperplasia)

8-16 NEUROMAS

CLINICAL DESCRIPTION

Etiology and Incidence

Neuromas occur in childhood in three forms: accessory digits, traumatic neuromas, and mucosal neuroma syndrome. Accessory digits in children are common, occurring at birth on the lateral aspects of fingers. Traumatic neuromas vary in incidence but are common in the accident-prone years. The mucosal neuroma syndrome is rare.

Clinical Findings

Accessory digits are small projections seen at the lateral margin of the fifth finger near its base. They are usually small papulonodules and are asymptomatic.

Traumatic or amputation neuromas occur at sites of injury or trauma and present as tender papulonodules that may exhibit spontaneous pain (Figure 8-16-1). Spontaneous true neuromas are rare but have been reported. They may or may not be painful.

Neuromas of the mucosal neuroma syndrome occur in multiples. They begin in childhood as smooth, dome-shaped nodules on the tongue, lips, oral mucosa, or mucosal surfaces or in the gastrointestinal tract. These neuromas are associated with thyroid carcinoma and pheochromocytoma. As these tumors proliferate they cause significant distortions of the tissue and may produce a grotesque facial appearance. When

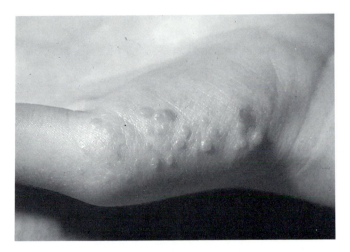

8-16-1 NEUROMAS: Multiple nodules on thenar eminence diagnosed on histological basis.

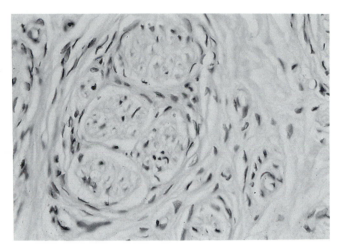

8-16-3 NEUROMA: High magnification, showing nerve bundles in the dermis. (400×)

located in the gastrointestinal tract they may lead to obstruction and failure of growth. Patients with the mucosal neuroma syndrome have a distinctive Marfan-like habitus.

Differential Diagnosis

Blue rubber-bleb nevus
Angiolipoma
Neuroma
Glomus tumor
Leiomyoma

HISTOLOGICAL DESCRIPTION

The histological features of the three clinical varieties of cutaneous neuromas are similar. All show in the dermis large, irregular bundles of nerve tissue, which may be surrounded by a sclerotic or hyalinized collagen. In accessory

digits, the neural elements are in the central portion of the specimen surrounded by a dense collagen (Figures 8-16-2 and 8-16-3). Traumatic neuromas have more dermal fibrosis and scar formation.

There is usually minimal inflammatory response. Vascular dilatation may be seen in the superficial dermis. Neuromas of the multiple neuroma syndrome do not have special features to distinguish them from other neuromas. All of these tumors are S-100 protein-positive, which helps to differentiate them from fibrous tissue tumors.

Differential Diagnosis

Neurofibroma
Scar tissue

REFERENCES

Nevi

Brownstein MH, Kazam BAB, Hashimoto K: Halo congenital nevus. Arch Dermatol 1977; 113:1572.

Cohen HJ, Minkin W, Frank SB: Nevus spilus. Arch Dermatol 1970; 102:433.

Eichenfield LF, Honig PJ: Difficult diagnostic and management issues in pediatric dermatology. Pediatr Clin North Am 1991; 38:687.

Elder DE, Goldman LI, Goldman SC, et al.: Dysplastic nevus syndrome. Cancer 1980; 46:1787.

Everett MA: Histopathology of congenital pigmented nevi. Am J Dermatopathol 1989; 11:11.

Findlay GH: The histology of Sutton's nevus. Br J Dermatol 1957; 69:389.

Gari LM, Rivers JK, Kopf AW: Melanomas arising in large congenital neurocytic nevi: A prospective study. Pediatr Dermatol 1988; 5:145.

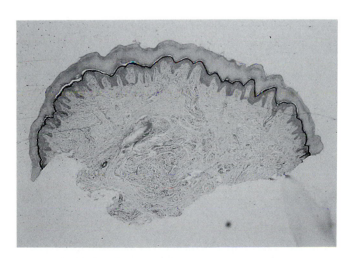

8-16-2 NEUROMA: Low magnification, showing a dermal proliferation of neural tissue. (20×)

Glinick SE, Alper JC, Bogaars H, et al.: Becker's melanosis: Associated abnormalities. J Am Acad Dermatol 1983; 9:509.

Huson SM: Recent developments in the diagnosis and management of neurofibromatosis. Arch Dis Child 1989; 64:745.

Kamino H, Misheloff E, Ackerman AB, et al.: Eosinophilic globules in Spitz's nevi: New findings and a diagnostic sign. Am J Dermatopathol 1979; 1:319.

Lund HZ, Stobbe GD: The natural history of pigmented nevus: Factors of age and anatomic location. Am J Pathol 1949; 25:1117.

Maize JC, Foster G: Age-related changes in melanocytic naevi. Clin Exp Dermatol 1979; 4:49.

Obringer AG, Meadows AT, Zackai EH: The diagnosis of neurofibromatosis-1 in the child under the age of 6 years. Am J Dis Child 1989; 143:717.

Pallor AS, Pensler JM, Tomita T: Nasal midline masses in infants and children. Dermoids, encephaloceles, and gliomas. Arch Dermatol 1991; 127:362.

Pennys NS, Mayoral F, Braunhill R, et al.: Delineation of nevus cell nests in inflammatory infiltrates by immunohistochemical staining for the presence of S-100 protein. J Cutan Pathol 1985; 12:28.

Renfro L, Grant-Vels JM, Brown SA: Multiple agminate Spitz nevi: A prospective study. Pediatr Dermatol 1989; 6:114.

Rhodes AR: Pigmented birthmarks and precursor melanocytic lesions of cutaneous melanoma identifiable in childhood. Pediatr Clin North Am 1983; 30:435.

Rothman KF, Esterle NB: Dysplastic nevi in children (special symposium). Pediatr Dermatol 1990; 7:218.

Silvers DN, Helwig EB: Melanocytic nevi in neonates. J Am Acad Dermatol 1981; 4:166.

Smalek JE: Significance of mongolian spots. J Pediatr 1980; 97:504.

Spitz S: Melanomas of childhood. Am J Pathol 1948; 24:591.

Walton RG, Jacobs AH, Cox AJ: Pigmented lesions in newborn infants. Br J Dermatol 1976; 95:389.

Weddon O, Little JH: Spindle and epithelioid cell nevi in childhood and adults: A review of 211 cases of the Spitz nevus. Cancer 1977; 40:217.

Blue Nevi and Variants

Avidor I, Kessler E: "Atypical" blue nevus, a benign variety of cellular blue nevus. Dermatologica 1977; 154:39.

Dorsey CS, Montgomery H: Blue nevus and its distinction from Mongolian spot and the nevus of Ota. J Invest Dermatol 1954; 22:225.

Hidano A, Kajima H, Ikeda S, et al.: Natural history of nevus of Ota. Arch Dermatol 1967; 95:187.

Kikuchi I, Inoue S: Natural history of Mongolian spot. J Dermatol 1980; 7:449.

Rodriguez HA, Ackerman LV: Cellular blue nevus. Cancer 1968; 21:393.

Melanoma

Ackerman AB, David KM: A unifying concept of malignant melanoma. Hum Pathol 1986; 17:438.

Clark WH Jr: A classification of malignant melanoma in man correlated with histogenesis and biological behavior. In Montagna W, Hu F, eds: Advances in biology of skin, Vol. 8: The pigmentary system. New York: Pergamon Press, 1966: 621.

Kopf AW, Waldo E: Melanonychia striata. Aust J Dermatol 1980; 21:59.

Mancianti ML, Clark WH, Hayes FA, Helwyn M: Malignant melanoma simulants rising in congenital melanocytic nevi do not show experimental evidence for a malignant phenotype. Am J Pathol 1990; 136:817.

Prose NS, Laude TTA, Heilman ER, Coren C: Congenital melanoma. Pediatrics 1987; 79:967.

Stromberg BV: Malignant melanoma in children. J Pediatr Surg 1979; 14:825.

Cockarde Nevus

Guzzo CA, Johnson B, Honig P: Cockarde nevus: A case report and review of the literature. Pediatr Dermatol 1988; 5:250.

Happle R: Kokarden naevus. Hautarzt 1974; 25:594.

Neurofibromatosis

Aparicio SR, Lumsden CE: Light and electron microscopic studies in the granular cell myoblastoma of the tongue. J Pathol 1969; 97:339.

Apisarnthanarax P: Granular cell tumor (review). J Am Acad Dermatol 1981; 5:171.

Crow FW, Schull WJ, Neel JV, eds: Clinical, pathological, and genetic study of multiple neurofibromatosis. Springfield, IL: Charles C. Thomas, 1956.

Johnson BL, Charneco DR: Café-au-lait spot in neurofibromatosis and in normal individuals. Arch Dermatol 1970; 102:442.

Nishio K, Kooa H: A case of storiform neurofibromas. J Dermatol (Tokyo) 1975; 2:143.

Shishiba T, Nillmura M, Ohtsuka F, et al.: Multiple cutaneous neurilemmomas as a skin manifestation of neurofibromatosis. J Am Acad Dermatol 1984; 10:744.

Stout AP: The peripheral manifestations of the specific nerve sheath tumor (neurilemmoma). Am J Cancer 1935; 24:751.

Nasal Glioma

Christianson HB: Nasal glioma. Arch Dermatol 1966; 93:68.

Mirra SS, Pearl GS, Hoffman JC, et al.: Nasal "glioma" with prominent neural component. Arch Pathol 1981; 105:540.

Neuroma

Holm TW, Prawer SE, Sahl WJ Jr, et al.: Multiple cutaneous neuromas. Arch Dermatol 1973; 107:608.

Shapiro L, Jublin EA, Braunstein HM: Rudimentary polydactyly. Arch Dermatol 1973; 108:223.

9

Epidermal and Adnexal Tumors

Contents

9-1 ACTINIC KERATOSIS

CLINICAL DESCRIPTION

Etiology and Incidence
Actinic (solar) keratosis is the result of the cumulative effect of sun exposure over many years. It is therefore uncommon in children unless associated with photosensitive skin disorders (e.g., xeroderma pigmentosum) or radiation for malignancies.

Clinical Features
Rough, erythematous, scaly papules appear in sun-exposed areas, especially on the face.

Differential Diagnosis
Discoid lupus
Seborrheic keratosis (usually not seen in childhood)

HISTOLOGICAL DESCRIPTION
Solar keratoses are precancerous lesions of squamous cell carcinoma in situ. The histological features are hyper- and parakeratosis overlying an epidermis with a variety of atypical changes (Figure 9-1-1). The epidermis may be acanthotic (hypertrophic variety of solar keratosis) with cellular atypia of keratinocytes at the basal cell zone and in upper layers. Atypia that involves the full thickness of the epidermis is known as bowenoid actinic keratosis. Atrophic actinic keratosis is the most common of the actinic keratoses. There is thinning of the atypical epidermis with cytologic atypia of basal and supravasalar keratinocytes. Epidermal atypia is defined by (1) crowding of basal keratinocytes; (2) increased mitotic activity at multiple levels in the epidermis; (3) dyskeratosis; and (4) basal cells that take on the characteristics of squamous cells and proliferate as buds into the papillary dermis. This prolif-

eration is sometimes associated with acantholysis of the cells above the atypical basal cells. This finding is more common at follicular ostia. These types of actinic keratoses are called acantholytic actinic keratoses or adenoacanthomas.

The dermis has a variable inflammatory infiltrate that may vary from lichenoid to patchy perivascular and periadnexal. Solar elastosis and superficial vascular ectasia are usually present.

Differential Diagnosis
Superficial squamous cell carcinoma
Lichenoid keratosis
Lupus erythematosus
Lentigo maligna

9-2 APOCRINE HIDROCYSTOMA

CLINICAL DESCRIPTION

Etiology and Incidence
Tumors of apocrine glands are very rare in children but are, on occasion, present at birth.

Clinical Features
Apocrine hidrocystomas are blue-black to purple, dome-shaped, cystic nodules that occur most commonly on the face at the lateral canthi or in a pretemporal location (Figure 9-2-1).

Differential Diagnosis
Cavernous hemangioma

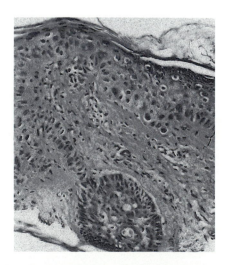

9-1-1 ACTINIC KERATOSIS: Atypical keratinocytes at the basal layer with overlying parakeratosis. (100 ×)

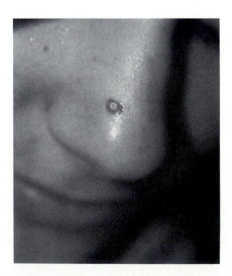

9-2-1 APOCRINE HIDROCYSTOMA: A dome-shaped nodule with a central depression and peripheral hemorrhage on the nose.

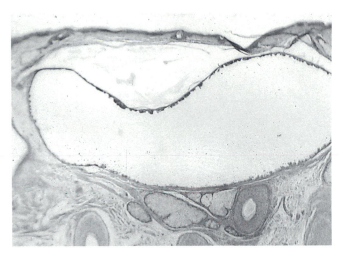

9-2-2 APOCRINE HIDROCYSTOMA: Low-power magnification, showing the cystic structure in the dermis. Prominent cells are seen at the luminal surface. (20 ×)

HISTOLOGICAL DESCRIPTION

The characteristic histological feature is a dilated cystic structure in a mildly inflammatory, fibrocellular dermis (Figure 9-2-2). The cyst is composed of two cell layers. The luminal cell is tall and columnar with abundant eosinophilic cytoplasm that projects into the lumen (Figure 9-2-3). Portions of these projections may be seen within the lumen (decapitation secretion). The peripheral cell is a small cuboidal cell with scanty cytoplasm. Some cysts may show luminal cell proliferation along papillary projections into the luminal space. The stroma may be dense and fibrocellular and contain chronic inflammatory cells. This condition resembles eccrine hidrocystoma, but the latter does not show columnar, tall projecting luminal cells.

Differential Diagnosis
Eccrine hidrocystoma
Syringocystadenoma papilliferum
Median raphe cysts of the penis

9-3 BASAL CELL CARCINOMA

CLINICAL DESCRIPTION

Etiology and Incidence
Basal cell carcinomas (basal cell nevus syndrome) are rare in children; when they occur they are most often as a part of the basal cell nevus syndrome or nevus sebaceus of Jadassohn. Basal cell carcinoma also occurs in children with xeroderma pigmentosum, albinism, and vitiligo and in sites of chronic radiation damage.

Clinical Features
Basal cell nevus syndrome, a genetic form of basal cell carcinoma, has an autosomal dominant mode of inheritance. In addition to basal cell tumors, patients may have jaw cysts, fibromas, ovarian tumors, and fibrosarcomas of the jaw and ovary. Medulloblastomas have been reported. The other clinical manifestations are palmar and plantar pits, which also show basal cell tumor on histological study. Tumors in this syndrome occur most prevalently in sun-exposed areas but do occur in other sites (Figure 9-3-1). Tumors that are a part of the basal cell nevus syndrome do not show the clinical features of the usual adult type of basal cell carcinoma. They have a wide variety of clinical appearances and may resemble keratoses, papillomas, and nevi.

Differential Diagnosis
Multiple trichoepithelomas
Adenoma sebaceum

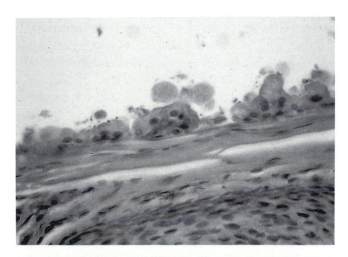

9-2-3 APOCRINE HIDROCYSTOMA: Higher magnification of the wall of the cyst in Figure 9-2-2, showing tall columnar cells exhibiting decapitation secretion. (400 ×)

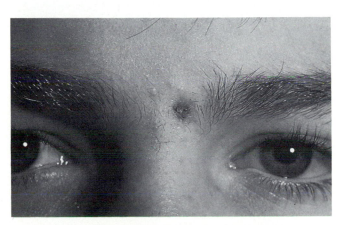

9-3-1 BASAL CELL CARCINOMA: Note typical basal cell carcinoma near the medial aspect of patient's left eyebrow. Typical rolled margins are seen.

HISTOLOGICAL DESCRIPTION

Basal cell carcinomas are characterized by the proliferation of hyperchromatic basaloid tumor islands, which infiltrate the dermis (Plate 9-3-1A), attach to the overlying epidermis, or extend from the follicular adnexae. Tumor lobules are characterized by peripheral palisading (Plate 9-3-1B), nuclear hyperchromasia, and occasional mitotic figures. The stroma has increased mucin (ground substance) and a variable inflammatory response. There are usually retraction spaces that separate the tumor from the stroma. Ulceration, if it occurs in these tumors, has an inflammatory response that is reflective of the ulceration and is usually acute as well as chronic. There is essentially no difference in basal cell carcinomas that arise de novo and those associated with basal nevus syndrome or nevus sebaceus.

Differential Diagnosis

Trichoepithelioma
Desmoplastic trichoepithelioma
Squamous cell carcinoma

9-4 ECCRINE CYLINDROMA

CLINICAL DESCRIPTION

Etiology and Incidence

Eccrine cylindromas are rare in childhood. They most commonly occur after puberty, but have been reported in children as young as four years of age.

Clinical Features

Eccrine cylindromas are smooth, dome-shaped tumors, most commonly on the scalp, are devoid of hair and are firm in consistency (Figure 9-4-1). They are usually asymptomatic.

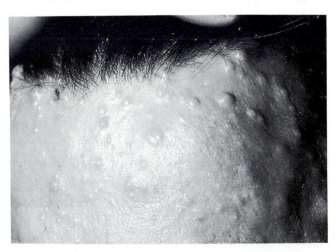

9-4-1 ECCRINE CYLINDROMA: Multiple flesh-colored nodules of varying sizes studding the forehead and extending into the scalp.

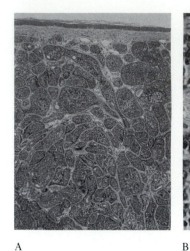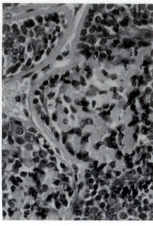

A   B

9-4-2 ECCRINE CYLINDROMA: (A) Basaloid cells in the dermis arranged in a "jigsaw puzzle" pattern. (20×) (B) Homogeneous eosinophilic cuticle outlining the tumor lobules. Eosinophilic droplets are present within the lobules. (200×)

Differential Diagnosis

Sebaceous cyst
Juvenile xanthogranuloma

HISTOLOGICAL DESCRIPTION

The epidermis is thinned over a dermal tumor consisting of multiple irregularly shaped islands of basophilic, epithelial-appearing cells. These tumor islands are surrounded by eosinophilic hyalinized material as well as compressed fibrous connective tissue (Figure 9-4-2A). Within the tumor lobules similar eosinophilic material may be seen, in droplet form. This hyalinlike material is periodic acid Schiff-positive and diastase-resistant and does not stain with stains for sulfated mucopolysaccharides (Figure 9-4-2B). Eccrinelike ducts can be seen within the tumor lobules; they have a periodic acid Schiff-positive, diastase-resistant luminal cuticle. There are two cell types within the tumor lobules: a small dark cell that palisades at the periphery of the lobules and a larger, paler cell that occupies the central portion of the lobules.

Differential Diagnosis

Basal cell carcinoma
Eccrine spiradenoma

9-5 ECCRINE POROMA

CLINICAL DESCRIPTION

Etiology and Incidence

Eccrine poromas are rare in young children but have been reported in adolescence. They occur most commonly on plantar and palmar skin but have been reported in other sites.

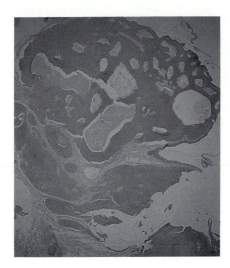

9-5-1 ECCRINE POROMA: Low-power magnification, showing interconnecting basaloid proliferation extending from the epidermal surface. There is hyperkeratosis. (20×)

Clinical Features

These tumors are smooth, dome-shaped pink to red papulo-nodules. They can be verrucous and bleed easily. Some may have a surrounding collarette with the tumor growing from the center. These tumors rarely ulcerate and are asymptomatic.

Differential Diagnosis

Verruca vulgaris
Pyogenic granuloma
Intradermal nevus

HISTOLOGICAL DESCRIPTION

Eccrine poromas arise as a proliferation of poral epithelium within the lower portions of the epidermis (Figure 9-5-1). This proliferation extends into the dermis in interconnecting sheets and cords of cells. There is often a sharp line of demar-

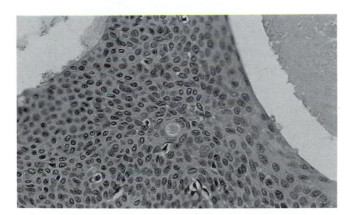

9-5-2 ECCRINE POROMA: Higher-power magnification of eccrine poroma, showing a duct in the center. Eosinophilic material is seen within an ectatic duct that is surrounded by basaloid cells. (200×)

cation between the growing poral cells and the normal epidermis. The surface may show hyper- and parakeratosis as well as hypergranulosis. The poroma cells are uniform in appearance, cuboidal in shape, and have round to oval basophilic nuclei. Granular melanin pigment can be found in poromas, the cells of which have intercellular bridges. Distinct (luminal) ductal structures with an eosinophilic cuticular border are frequently found throughout the tumor (Figure 9-5-2). They may be found in whorls of keratinizing cells. Ductal structures are a hallmark in this tumor. Ulceration is uncommon. The dermis usually shows a chronic mononuclear cell infiltrate and may be fibrocellular. These tumors contain significant amounts of glycogen that is periodic acid-Schiff-positive and diastase-labile. The cuticle of the ductal structures is periodic acid-Schiff-positive and diastase-resistant.

Differential Diagnosis

Seborrheic keratosis
Basal cell carcinoma

9-6 ECCRINE SPIRADENOMA

CLINICAL DESCRIPTION

Etiology and Incidence

Eccrine spiradenomas are uncommon in childhood, occurring in late adolescence. These painful tumors may occur on any part of the body.

Clinical Features

Eccrine spiradenomas are nondescript papulonodules, usually less than 1 cm in diameter and the color of the patient's skin or reddish blue. The main symptom is pain, either spontaneous or secondary to pressure, touching, or injury. Ulceration is uncommon.

Differential Diagnosis

Blue rubber-bleb nevus
Angiolipoma
Neuroma
Glomus tumor
Leiomyoma

HISTOLOGICAL DESCRIPTION

Characteristic histological features of eccrine spiradenomas are multiple basophilic, sharply circumscribed nodules in the dermis (Figure 9-6-1) surrounded by compressed connective tissue and associated with chronic inflammation. Within the lobules there are two types of cells. The larger type has a large, irregular to ovoid or spherical well-defined nucleus with a nucleolus (Figure 9-6-2). The cytoplasm is faintly basophilic.

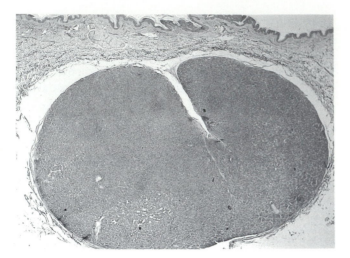

9-6-1 ECCRINE SPIRADENOMA: Low-power magnification, showing a typical configuration: a large nodule of basophilic-staining cells. (20×)

The smaller of the two types has a hyperchromatic nucleus and scanty cytoplasm; it is somewhat basophilic and resembles a lymphocyte. This type of cell is seen mainly at the periphery of the lobules, but there is enough admixture of the two types of cells within the lobules to produce a "salt and pepper" effect at low magnification. Eccrine duct-like lumina can be noted within the lobules. The luminal border contains an eosinophilic, periodic acid-Schiff-positive, diastase-resistant cuticle.

Differential Diagnosis
Basal cell carcinoma
Eccrine cylindroma
Lymphocytic infiltrative processes

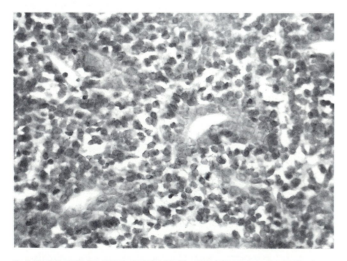

9-6-2 ECCRINE SPIRADENOMA: Higher-power magnification, showing the ductal structures within the lobules and an admixture of two cell types: smaller dark cells admixed with a larger cell with a more eosinophilic and vesicular nucleus. (200×)

9-7 FORDYCE'S DISEASE
CLINICAL DESCRIPTION

Etiology and Incidence
Fordyce's disease is uncommon in children.

Clinical Features
Fordyce's disease presents as asymptomatic, small, yellowish papules on the mucosal surface. The oral mucosa is most commonly affected, although they can occur on other mucosal surfaces.

Differential Diagnosis
Mucous cyst

HISTOLOGICAL DESCRIPTION

Mature sebaceous glands are found in a well-vascularized stroma, without surrounding inflammation. The epithelium shows the changes characteristic of mucosa (Figure 9-7-1). Multiple sections may reveal a sebaceous duct that connects to the epithelial surface.

Differential Diagnosis
Sebaceous hyperplasia

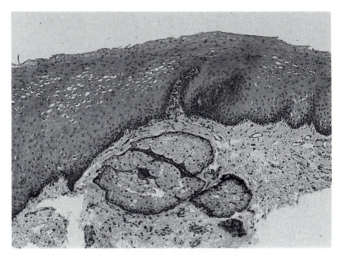

9-7-1 FORDYCE CONDITION: Low-power magnification, showing mucosal epithelium and a mature-appearing sebaceous gland within the stroma. (20×)

9-8 KERATOACANTHOMA
CLINICAL DESCRIPTION

Etiology and Incidence
Keratoacanthomas are not common in childhood but can occur in this age group and have been seen in infancy. The usual time of development is postpuberty. In individuals with

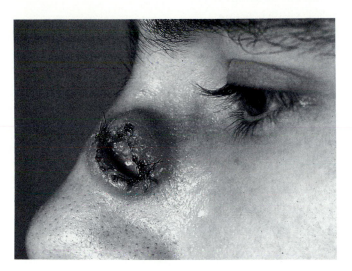

9-8-1 KERATOACANTHOMA: Dome-shaped nodule with keratotic plug and crust on bridge of this young man's nose.

increased susceptibility to ultraviolet light (i.e., xeroderma pigmentosum, albinism, chronic exposure to radiation), keratoacanthomas may occur at any age.

Clinical Features

These lesions appear as tumor nodules that vary in size from 0.5 to 2 cm. They are usually domed-shaped and have a well-defined, distinct keratotic plug, which may or may not be covered with a crust (Figure 9-8-1). These nodules appear suddenly and grow rapidly and sometimes alarmingly to a large size and then stabilize. They may then regress spontaneously, leaving a depressed white or violaceous scar.

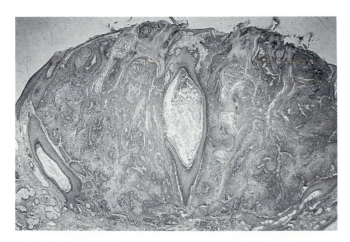

9-8-2 KERATOACANTHOMA: Low-power magnification, showing a cuplike configuration that contains proliferations of hyalinized and eosinophilic-appearing squamous cells. (20×)

Differential Diagnosis

Squamous cell cancer

Verruca vulgaris

HISTOLOGICAL DESCRIPTION

The histological features are a central crateriform area filled with keratin in which there are parakeratotic cells and micro-abscesses filled with polymorphonuclear leukocytes (Figure 9-8-2). Underlying this keratin mass there is epidermal proliferation of atypical squamous cells that have a distinct eosinophilic, hyalinlike, and/or ground glass appearance. At the interface of the dermis and the proliferating atypical epidermis there is frequently a dense cellular inflammatory infiltrate that obscures the dermal-epidermal junction and permeates the proliferating epidermis. It is in this area that significant cytologic atypia occurs and the proliferation has the appearance of invasion. The overall configuration of this tumor is that of a cup-shaped proliferating epidermis filled with keratin whose lower borders show rather marked cellular atypia and exocytosis. The stroma has an inflammatory infiltrate of lymphocytes, histiocytes, polymorphonuclear leukocytes, and eosinophils. There may be dermal fibrosis. Keratinization continues within this proliferation; keratin pearls with fully keratinized centers are sometimes seen. Cytologic atypia at varying levels within the proliferating mass is uncommon, which helps to differentiate this tumor from squamous cell carcinoma. Most of the cytologic atypia occurs at the dermal-epidermal interface, where many mitoses may be seen.

The architectural change and historical correlation of rapid growth are important in the diagnosis of keratoacanthoma. As these lesions involute, proliferation at the dermal-epidermal interface ceases and eosinophilic homogenized hyalinlike cells occur almost throughout the entire lesion. Well-defined keratoacanthomas rarely extend below the level of the sweat glands.

Differential Diagnosis

Squamous cell carcinoma

Verrucous carcinoma

9-9 NEVUS SEBACEUS OF JADASSOHN

CLINICAL DESCRIPTION

Etiology and Incidence

Nevus sebaceus of Jadassohn occurs at birth as a solitary yellowish plaque that is devoid of hair and usually smooth on the surface. It is most commonly located on the scalp but can be found in other sites.

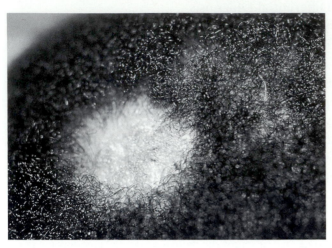

9-9-1 NEVUS SEBACEUS OF JADASSOHN: Yellow, cobble-stoned, circular bald area on infant's scalp.

Clinical Features

These lesions become cobblestone and verrucous in appearance and may develop basal cell carcinoma or syringocystadenoma at or after puberty (Figure 9-9-1). Nevus sebaceus may be associated with squamous cell carcinoma and apocrine carcinoma in addition to the more frequently associated basal cell carcinoma and syringocystadenoma. Nevus sebaceus may be associated with neuroectodermal defects. These include neurologic abnormalities (seizures, mental deficiency, intracerebral masses), hamartomatous lesions of the kidney, eye (lipodermoid cyst of conjunctiva, microophthalmia, ectopic displacement of the pupils, and ocular hemangiomas), and skeletal system.

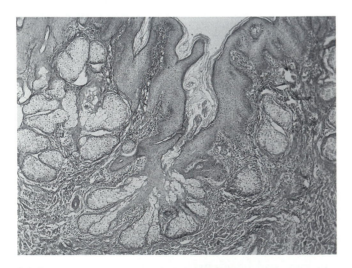

9-9-2 NEVUS SEBACEUS OF JADASSOHN: Low-power magnification, showing verrucous epidermal hyperplasia with the presence of sebaceous lobules closely approximating epidermis. Numerous sebaceous glands are seen within the fibrocellular stroma. (20×)

Differential Diagnosis

Aplasia cutis congenita
Epidermal nevus
Verruca plana
Scar
Normal skin

HISTOLOGICAL DESCRIPTION

The histological features during childhood and infancy may not be characteristic. Sebaceous glands are not enlarged and appear small and underdeveloped. The epithelial changes are not significant until after puberty. Hair structures appear rudimentary, and there may be cords or islands of basaloid follicular epithelial cells without hair. Small, keratin-filled, dilated follicular infundibula can be found. Sweat glands in this stage appear rudimentary, as in the skin of infants and young children. Ectopic or dilated apocrine glands are not noted. The dermis may be quite cellular.

After puberty there are the characteristic features of hyperkeratosis, acanthosis, and papillomatous and follicular hyperkeratosis (Figure 9-9-2). Numerous large mature sebaceous glands are seen in the dermis associated with sebaceous follicles. The stroma may show chronic inflammation, mainly of mononuclear cells. Deep to the sebaceous proliferation in the lower dermis there are dilated apocrine glands. In order of frequency, tumors arising in nevus sebaceus of Jadassohn include basal cell carcinoma (40%), adnexal and pilar tumors (40%), and apocrine tumors (20%).

Differential Diagnosis

Postpubertal sebaceous hyperplasia
Lichen simplex chronicus
Prepubertal hamartoma
Normal skin

9-10 OSTEOMA CUTIS

CLINICAL DESCRIPTION

Etiology and Incidence

Osteoma cutis refers to spontaneous new bone formation in the skin. It may be primary or secondary. Causes of osteoma cutis include pseudohypoparathyroidism and pseudopseudohypoparathyroidism inherited conditions (X-linked or autosomal dominant). Another form of primary osteoma cutis has no features of these two conditions but shows ectopic bone formation in the skin at various locations. This condition occurs in a sporadic fashion. Secondary osteoma cutis arises in tumors (e.g., pilomatricoma) or inflamed skin (e.g., patients with dermatomyositis). These conditions occur at any age, including birth.

Clinical Features

Short stature, round facies, and multiple skeletal anomalies [especially shortened metacarpals, (mainly the fourth) and metatarsals] are found in pseudohypoparathyroidism (PHT) and pseudopseudohypoparathyroidism (PPHT). Patients with PHT have low serum calcium levels that do not respond to parathyroid hormone (PTH) (an end organ problem). Those with PPHT do not have abnormalities of calcium and phosphorous.

The tumors of osteoma cutis are firm, indurated, sharply marginated dermal masses (Plate 9-10-1). They vary in size from 0.5 to 7 mm. Inflammation or ulceration of the overlying skin is frequently present. At times, bony particles are extruded.

Differential Diagnosis

Subungual exostosis of digit
Pilomatrixoma (calcifying epithelioma)
Calcified acne lesions

HISTOLOGICAL DESCRIPTION

There are areas of bone formation of varying size in the dermis that may extend into the subcutaneous tissue (Plate 9-10-2). The small sheets or plates of bone show numerous osteocytes, with or without cement lines (Figure 9-10-1). Polarized light is helpful in viewing the cement lines. At the margins of the bone and connective tissue, cells with elongated nuclei can be seen. These are thought to represent osteoblasts. The multinucleated cells within the bone are thought to represent osteoclasts. The surrounding stroma may show a mixed inflammatory reaction that varies from granulomatous to chronic.

Differential Diagnosis

Calcinosis cutis

9-11 PILOMATRIXOMA

CLINICAL DESCRIPTION

Etiology and Incidence

Pilomatrixoma (calcifying epithelioma of Malherbe) is a benign lesion that occurs most frequently in the first two decades of life (80%). It accounts for 10% of superficial lumps in childhood. Multiple lesions occur in 3.5% of patients. The nodule is thought to be derived from the hair matrix. Females with this lesion outnumber males. There have been familial cases reported.

Clinical Features

Most often this nodule appears on the head and neck (50%) (Figure 9-11-1). The upper extremities are also frequently involved. It is subcutaneous in location, firm, and frequently covered by reddish blue skin. The nodules vary in size from 0.5 to 3 cm in diameter. The lesion may be tender.

Differential Diagnosis

Sebaceous cyst
Dermoid cyst
Epidermoid cyst

HISTOLOGICAL DESCRIPTION

This is a dermal tumor, often located in the deep dermis. It is often surrounded by a compressed connective tissue capsule. In the tumor mass there are cells of two types: basophilic cells and eosinophilic keratinized cells with well-defined cell borders without central nuclei (shadow cells) (Figure 9-11-2). The quantities of both cell types are variable within tumors.

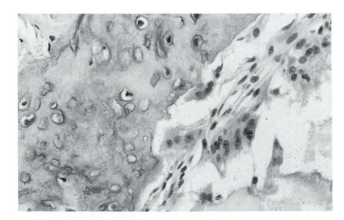

9-10-1 OSTEOMA CUTIS: High magnification shows multinucleated cells (osteoclasts) closely apposed to the osteoma. (400×)

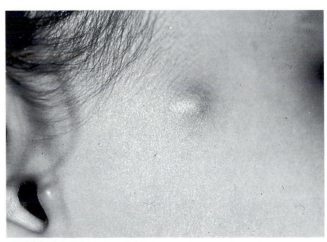

9-11-1 PILOMATRIXOMA: Flesh-colored nodule on the side of a young girl's face.

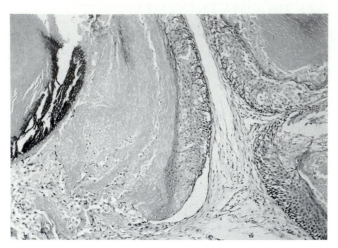

9-11-2 PILOMATRIXOMA: Low-power magnification, showing cornified cells surrounded by basophilic-staining cells in a fibrocellular stroma. Basophilic-staining shadow cells are seen within the center of the lobules. (40×)

Basophilic cells are commonly present in tumors of recent onset, but are noticeably absent in long-standing lesions. Shadow cells are commonly seen in both types of tumors. There is a transition from the basophilic cells to the shadow cells and finally to calcified keratinocytes. Bone formation can occur in these tumors. Pilomatrixoma may contain melanin.

Differential Diagnosis
Proliferating trichilemmal cyst
Trichilemmal cyst
Osteoma cutis

9-12 SQUAMOUS CELL CARCINOMA

CLINICAL DESCRIPTION

Etiology and Incidence
Squamous cell carcinoma (SCC) is rare in children. It does occur in those children whose skin has been damaged either on the basis of a genetic defect (e.g., xeroderma pigmentosa) or from chronic exposure to radiation (thermal, ultraviolet, or x-ray) or who have other syndromes associated with SCC (e.g., epidermolysis bullosa, Bloom's syndrome, Rothmund-Thomson syndrome, dyskeratosis congenita, Keratitis, Ichthyosis, Deafness (KID) syndrome, hidrotic ectodermal dysplasia). Squamous cell carcinoma also occurs in albino children, who have lost their protection from ultraviolet radiation.

Clinical Features
Squamous cell carcinoma develops as a nodule in the skin (Figure 9-12-1), most commonly on sun-exposed areas. The nodules grow rapidly, are indurated, develop a central crust, and then ulcerate. Squamous cell carcinoma can resemble basal cell carcinoma, but squamous cell carcinomas grow more rapidly, are indurated, and are larger. Squamous cell carcinomas can develop from actinic keratoses in children who are especially susceptible to actinic radiation. They may be verrucous or papillary. Their clinical features can be similar or identical to those of keratoacanthoma, although the latter grow more rapidly and instead of ulceration have a central keratotic crater. Squamous cell carcinomas that arise on mucosal surfaces have a greater potential for metastasis. These tumors require early diagnosis and treatment.

Differential Diagnosis
Verruca vulgaris
Persistent ulcer
Keratoacanthoma
Basal cell carcinoma

Reference
See Xeroderma Pigmentosum

HISTOLOGICAL DESCRIPTION

Squamous cell carcinoma represents a tumor proliferation of atypical squamous epidermal cells that proliferate downward into the underlying stroma (Figure 9-12-2A). Individual cells within this proliferation show a varying degree of cytological

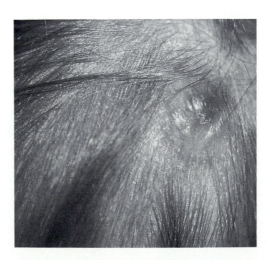

9-12-1 SQUAMOUS CELL CARCINOMA: An exophytic crusted nodule on a background of severe solar elastosis in an adolescent with xeroderma pigmentosum.

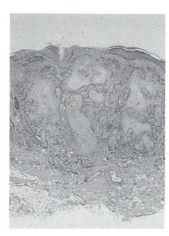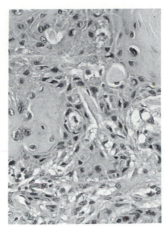

A   B

9-12-2 SQUAMOUS CELL CARCINOMA: (A) Low magnification shows proliferation of atypical squamous cells into the dermis. Note the prominent solar elastosis. (20×) (B) High magnification shows atypical squamous proliferation with the presence of dyskeratotic cells and mitotic figures. (200×)

atypia, dyskeratosis, and atypical mitotic figures (Figure 9-12-2B). There is great variation in cell size and shape of the proliferating cells. Keratinization continues within this process, and keratin pearls are produced within the proliferating atypical epidermis. Individual cell keratinization also occurs and has been referred to as malignant dyskeratosis. There are several variations in the cytological and architectural patterns of squamous cell carcinomas. In the adenoid (acantholytic) variety, there are glandularlike structures produced within the proliferating atypical masses of cells. The clear cell and spindle cell varieties occur with less frequency than do other varieties. In these two types differentiation from other spindle cell tumors and melanoma is often difficult. Immunoperoxidase stains are of assistance in separating atypical varieties of squamous cell carcinomas from other types of spindle cell and clear cell tumors.

Differential Diagnosis
Keratotic Squamous Cell Carcinoma
Keratoacanthoma
Clear cell squamous cell carcinoma
Melanoma

Spindle Cell Squamous Cell Carcinoma
Melanoma
Malignant fibrous histiocytoma

Pseudoglandular Squamous Cell Carcinoma
Metastatic tumor

9-13 SYRINGOCYSTADENOMA PAPILLIFERUM

CLINICAL DESCRIPTION

Etiology and Incidence
Syringocystadenomas can arise at birth (50%) or in early childhood. One-third of patients have an associated nevus sebaceus. It is thought to be of apocrine origin.

Clinical Features
Syringocystadenomas are nondescript, consisting of one or more linear groups of papules commonly associated with nevus sebaceus (Figure 9-13-1). When this tumor is unassociated with nevus sebaceus, it presents as slowly increasing nodules that ooze and become crusted.

Differential Diagnosis
Verruca
Pyogenic granuloma

HISTOLOGICAL DESCRIPTION
The epidermis shows hyperplasia with loss of surface continuity. There are cystic openings that extend from the surface into the tumor lobule. The upper portion of the epidermal opening shows keratinization that is continuous with the glandular proliferation in the lower portion of this tumor. The base of the cystic cavity contains multiple papillary projections (Figure 9-13-2A) that are lined by two rows of cells. The luminal cells are tall and columnar with eosinophilic cytoplasmic projections into the luminal space (Figure 9-13-2B). The cells of the inner row are small and cuboidal, with scant cytoplasm and a hyperchromatic nucleus. The stroma of the papillary projections is filled with plasma cells. The stroma is also

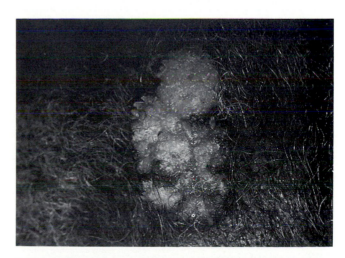

9-13-1 SYRINGOCYSTADENOMA PAPILLIFERUM: Grapelike group of papules and nodules arising from nevus sebaceus of Jadassohn. (Courtesy of Allen Gaisen, M.D.)

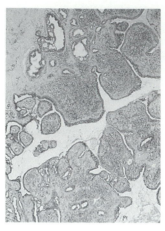
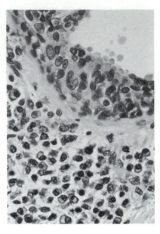
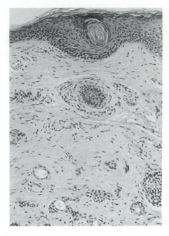
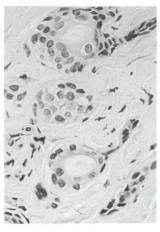

A   B

A   B

9-13-2 SYRINGOCYSTADENOMA PAPILLIFERUM: (A) Low magnification shows papillary projections extending into a cavitylike space with underlying dilated ductal structures. (20×) (B) Higher magnification shows the border of a papillary projection with two cell types: tall columnar luminal cells and an underlying small cuboidal cell. The stroma is filled with plasma cells. (200×)

9-14-1 SYRINGOMA: (A) Low-power magnification, showing ductlike structures in a fibrocellular stroma. The overlying epidermis is somewhat acanthotic. (20×) (B) High-power magnification, showing the eccrine ducts with basaloid proliferation extending from the ducts, producing a commalike figure. (200×)

edematous and may show vascular ectasia. Deep to the tumor there may be dilated apocrine glands, which have been shown to connect with the tumor when multiple sections are studied. Hair and/or sebaceous glands may be found in association with syringocystadenoma. This tumor occurs often with nevus sebaceus, whose changes can also be seen on histological study.

Differential Diagnosis
Tubular apocrine adenoma

9-14 SYRINGOMA

CLINICAL DESCRIPTION

Etiology and Incidence
Syringomas may occur at any age but are most common around the age of puberty. Familial syringomas have been reported occurring as early as five years of age. They have been noted to occur at an early age in mongoloid children at a significantly higher incidence than in the general population.

Clinical Features
Syringomas are small, yellowish, firm papules that may appear angulated and are most commonly located on the lower eyelids. They may also occur in any other location, especially the upper chest and lower abdomen (Plate 9-14-1). Ulceration is infrequent to rare. The tumors are asymptomatic.

Differential Diagnosis
Fordyce's disease
Eruptive vellus hair cyst

Trichoepithelioma
Adenoma sebaceum

HISTOLOGICAL DESCRIPTION

Characteristically syringoma consists of collections of ductal cells in a dense fibrocellular stroma (Figure 9-14-1A). There are two rows of flattened cells with a central luminal opening that contains a periodic acid-Schiff-positive, diastase-resistant cuticle. Luminal cells may be clear and glycogenated in the clear cell variety of this tumor. The lumen may be filled with orthokeratin and amorphous debris. In some areas there are solid cords of cells without a lumen; extending from these ductal lobules are short cords of cells that resemble a comma or tadpole (Figure 9-14-1B). Foreign body reactions may occur secondary to rupture of small tumor ducts that are keratin-filled. The usual inflammatory cell is the lymphocyte with associated histiocytes.

Differential Diagnosis
Trichoepithelioma
Basal cell carcinoma
Microcystic adnexal carcinoma

9-15 TRICHOEPITHELIOMA

CLINICAL DESCRIPTION

Etiology and Incidence
Trichoepitheliomas in children are usually multiple and inherited in an autosomal dominant manner. The solitary type is rarely seen in childhood.

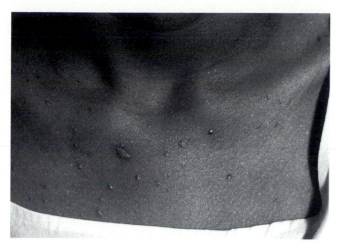

9-15-1 TRICHOEPITHELIOMA: Flesh-colored papules and nodules on a patient's chest.

Clinical Features

Trichoepitheliomas are papulonodules that occur most commonly on the head and neck, and rarely on other sites (Figure 9-15-1). They are flesh-colored and glistening and may have telangiectasias overlying them. They do not ulcerate and usually grow slowly. Trichoepitheliomas can be confused with basal cell carcinoma, both clinically and histologically. Often the differentiation is impossible.

Differential Diagnosis

Syringoma
Adenoma sebaceum
Basal cell epithelioma

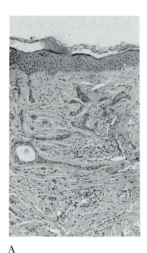

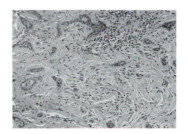

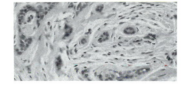

9-15-2 TRICHOEPITHELIOMA: (A) Low magnification shows basaloid cells in chords and occasionally in nests with central collections of keratin. (40×) (B) Small nests in a loose and inflamed stroma. (100×) (C) Thickening of the collagen bundles, as may be seen in desmoplastic variants. (200×)

HISTOLOGICAL DESCRIPTION

Trichoepitheliomas are characterized by the presence of basaloid tumor islands with horn cysts in a rather dense fibrocellular stroma (Figure 9-15-2A). The keratinization is abrupt and there is no keratin pearl formation as in squamous cell carcinoma (Figure 9-15-2B). The tumor islands have peripheral palisading and nuclear hyperchromatism (Figure 9-15-2C). Mitoses are infrequent. The dermis is fibrocellular, with chronic inflammatory cells. There is often granulomatous inflammation secondary to the rupture of horn cysts. One variety of trichoepithelioma has adenoid proliferation with interconnecting cords of basaloid cells. Differentiating basal cell carcinomas from trichoepitheliomas is difficult (Table 9-15-1).

Differential Diagnosis

Basal cell carcinoma
Syringoma

9-15-1

Characteristic	Trichoepithelioma	Basal Cell Carcinoma
Proliferating cell	Basaloid	Basaloid
Horn cysts	Frequent	Rare
Necrosis in tumor islands	Rare	Frequent
Stroma	Fibrotic	Mucinous
Peripheral retraction space	Rare	Common
Ulceration, hemorrhage	Rare	Common

REFERENCES

Actinic Keratosis

Billano RA, Little WP: Hypertrophic solar keratosis. J Am Acad Dermatol 1983; 7:484.

Carapeto FJ, Garcia-Perez A: Acantholytic keratosis. Dermatologica 1974; 148:233, 239.

Hirsch P, Marmelzat WL: Lichenoid actinic keratosis. Dermatol Int 1967; 6:101.

Lynch HT, Fichot BC, Lynch JF: Cancer control in xeroderma pigmentosum. Arch Dermatol 1977; 113:193.

Pinkus H: Keratosis senilis. Am J Clin Pathol 1958; 29:193.

Apocrine Hidrocystoma

Hassan MD, Khan MA, Krusg TV: Apocrine cystadenoma. Arch Dermatol 1979; 115:194.

Schewach-Millet M, Tran H: Congenital papillated apocrine cystadenoma: A mixed form of hidrocystoma, hidradenoma papilliferum and syringocystadenoma papilliferum. J Am Acad Dermatol 1984; 11:374.

Basal Cell Carcinoma

Asarch RF, Golitz LE, Sausker WF, et al.: Median raphe cysts of the penis. Arch Dermatol 1979; 115:1084.

Coskey R, Chow G: Basal cell epithelioma in children and young adults. Cutis 1973; 12:224.

Goldstein AM, Bale SJ, Peck GL, et al.: Sun exposure and basal cell carcinomas in the nevoid basal cell carcinoma syndrome. J Am Acad Dermatol 1993; 29:34.

Milstone ED, Helwig EB: Basal cell carcinoma in children. Arch Dermatol 1973; 108:523.

Robbins JH, Kramemer K, Lutzner M, et al.: Xeroderma pigmentosum: An inherited disease with sun sensitivity, multiple cutaneous neoplasms and abnormal DNA repair. Ann Intern Med 1974; 80:221.

Taylor WB, Anderson DE, Howell JB, et al.: The nevoid basal cell carcinoma syndrome autopsy findings. Arch Dermatol 1968; 98:612.

Eccrine Cylindroma

Crain RC, Helwig EB: Dermal cylindroma (dermal eccrine cylindroma). Am J Clin Pathol 1961; 35:504.

Heyman AB, Braunstein MH: Eccrine poroma: Analysis of 45 new cases. Dermatologica 1969; 138:29.

Eccrine Poroma

Kersting DW, Helwig EB: Eccrine spiradenoma. Arch Dermatol 1956; 73:199.

Mambo NC: Eccrine spiradenoma: Clinical and pathologic study of 49 tumors. J Cutan Pathol 1983; 10:312.

Naversen DN, Trask DM, Watson FH, et al.: Painful tumors of the skin: "Lend an egg." J Am Acad Dermatol 1993; 28:298.

Pinkus H, Rogin JR, Goldman P: Eccrine poroma. Arch Dermatol 1956; 74:511.

Fordyce's Disease

Miles AEW: Sebaceous glands on the lip and cheek mucosa of man. Br Dent J 1958; 105:235.

Keratoacanthoma

Kim WH, McGray MK: The histopathological differentiation of keratoacanthoma and squamous cell carcinoma of the skin. J Cutan Pathol 1980; 7:318.

Nevus Sebaceus of Jadassohn

Domingo J, Helwig EB: Malignant neoplasms associated with nevus sebaceous of Jadassohn. J Am Acad Dermatol 1979; 1:545, 556.

Feinstein R, Mims L: Linear nevus sebaceous with convulsions and mental retardation. Am J Dis Child 1962; 10:675.

Lentz CL, Altman J, Mopper C: Nevus sebaceous of Jadassohn. Arch Dermatol 1968; 97:294.

Morioka S: The natural history of nevus sebaceous. J Cutan Pathol 1985; 12:200.

Osteoma Cutis

Jewell EW: Osteoma cutis. Arch Dermatol 1971; 103:553.

Monroe AB, Burgdorf WHC, Sheward S: Plate like cutaneous osteoma. J Am Acad Dermatol 1987; 16:481.

O'Donnel TF Jr, Gellar SA: Primary osteoma cutis. Arch Dermatol 1971; 104:325.

Roth SI, Stowell RE, Helwig EB: Cutaneous ossification. Arch Pathol 1963; 76:44.

Pilomatrixoma

Forbis R Jr, Helwig EB: Pilomatrixoma (calcifying epithelioma). Arch Dermatol 1961; 83:606.

Schlechter R, Hartsough NA, Guttman FM: Multiple pilomatricomas (calcifying epitheliomas of Malherbe). Pediatr Dermatol 1984; 2:23.

Squamous Cell Carcinoma

Brodin MB, Mehregan AH: Verrucous carcinoma. Arch Dermatol 1980; 116:987.

Epstein E, Epstein NN, Bragg K, et al.: Metastasis from squamous cell carcinomas of the skin. Arch Dermatol 1986; 97:245.

Gatter KC, Alcock C, Heryet A: The differential diagnosis of routinely processed anaplastic tumors using monoclonal antibodies. Am J Clin Pathol 1984; 82:33.

Syringocystadenoma Papilliferum

Helwig EB, Hackney VC: Syringocystadenoma papilliferum. Arch Dermatol 1955; 71:361.

Syringoma

Butterworth T, Strean LP, Beerman H, et al.: Syringoma and mongolism. Arch Dermatol 1964; 90:483.

Feibelman CE, Maize JC: Clear-cell syringoma. Am J Dermatopathol 1984; 6:139.

Winkelman RK, Muller SA: Sweat gland tumors. Arch Dermatol 1964; 89:827.

Trichoepithelioma

Brownstein MH, Shapiro L: Desmoplastic trichoepithelioma. Cancer 1977; 40:2979.

Gray HR, Helwig EB: Epithelioma adenoides cysticum and solitary trichoepithelioma. Arch Dermatol 1963; 87:102.

Ziprkowski L, Schewach-Millet M: Multiple trichoepithelioma in a mother and two children. Dermatologica 1966; 132:248.

10

Tumors of Fat, Muscle, and Fibrous Tissue

Contents

10-1 ANGIOLIPOMA

CLINICAL DESCRIPTION

These benign subcutaneous tumors suggest a broad clinical differential diagnosis and are usually diagnosed on the basis of histological features.

Etiology and Incidence

The stimulus for the formation of these benign hamartomas is unknown. Angiolipomas are usually found on the trunk or upper extremities. They may be solitary or multiple. Although they are not as common as lipomas, they are seen often in adolescents and may occasionally occur on a familial basis.

Clinical Features

Solitary or multiple tender subcutaneous nodules raise the differential diagnosis of eccrine spiradenoma, neuroma, glomus tumor, leiomyoma, and angiolipoma. The surface overlying angiolipomas is flesh-colored and may or may not be slightly raised. The nodules themselves are usually small and mobile. If they are not tender, angiolipomas may be thought to represent lipomas. The diagnosis becomes readily apparent on histological examination.

Differential Diagnosis

Neuroma
Eccrine spiradenoma
Glomus tumor
Leiomyoma
Lipoma

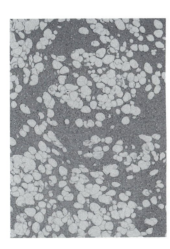
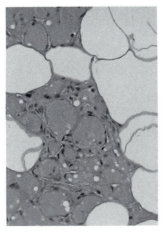

A   B

10-1-1 ANGIOLIPOMA: (A) Low-power view, showing adipocytes surrounded and infiltrated by collagenous stroma. (20×) (B) Closer examination shows the stroma to contain blood vessels congested with erythrocytes. (200×)

HISTOLOGICAL DESCRIPTION

Angiolipomas appear on histological study as circumscribed nodules composed of mature adipocytes and intervening endothelial-lined vascular channels of small caliber enmeshed in delicate fibrous septae (Figure 10-1-1). Angiolipomas differ from lipomas by their prominent vascular component. On the lower extremities angiolipomas may infiltrate muscle. This characteristic should prompt complete removal of such tumors to prevent recurrence.

Differential Diagnosis

Lipoma
Fibrolipoma

10-2 CONGENITAL FIBROMATOSIS

CLINICAL DESCRIPTION

This disorder is known by various other names, including infantile myofibromatosis, diffuse or generalized congenital fibromatosis, and generalized hamartomatosis.

Etiology and Incidence

The etiology of this disorder is unknown. It occurs rarely and most often in a sporadic fashion, although familial cases have been reported. Lesions of congenital generalized fibromatosis are usually present at birth but may appear up to the age of five years.

Clinical Features

Lesions of congenital fibromatosis may be solitary, multiple, or generalized. Cutaneous lesions are deep red to purple, firm to rubbery nodules that range in number from a few to more than seventy-five. They most commonly affect the shoulders, thighs, and trunk. When located superficially, they appear translucent (Plate 10-2-1). If deep-seated, they are firm and may bind the skin to deeper structures, leading to a depression on the skin surface (Figure 10-2-1).

In the multiple and generalized form, bony lesions appear on radiographs as lytic foci and thus suggest a diagnosis of sarcoma. Isolated and multiple lesions restricted to the subcutis, muscles, and bones often spontaneously involute over the course of several years and thus have a good prognosis. By contrast, in the generalized form visceral lesions occur, which may interfere with the digestive, cardiovascular, and respiratory systems and lead to a fatal outcome (Table 10-2-1).

Differential Diagnosis

Juvenile hyaline fibromatosis
Hemanigiomatosis
Lipomatosis

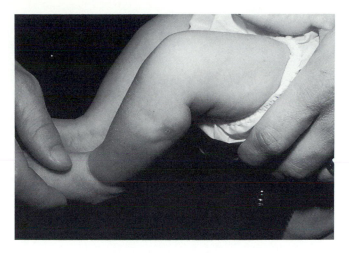

10-2-1 CONGENITAL FIBROMATOSIS: A fibroma on a child's lower leg. Depressions in the center and periphery indicate binding of skin to deeper structures.

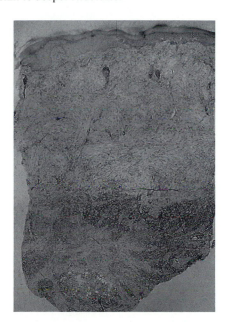

10-2-2 CONGENITAL FIBROMATOSIS: Low magnification shows diffuse replacement of the dermal stroma by proliferating basophilic cells in dense aggregates and in a loose matrix. (50×) (Courtesy of Jane Chatten, M.D., Department of Pathology of Children's Hospital of Philadelphia.)

Spitz nevus
Metastatic neuroblastoma

HISTOLOGICAL DESCRIPTION

Elongate, plump, spindle cells proliferate in bundles in the dermis. They are seen in various planes of section in well-defined zones of the dermis (Figure 10-2-2). Dense bundles of collagen outline the proliferating cells, some of which have features of smooth muscle cells. Peripherally there is a higher degree of cellularity than centrally, where vascular proliferation is more evident (Plate 10-2-2). The spindle cells may proliferate in an intravascular pattern. Variable features include stippled calcifications, hyalinization, and foci of necrosis.

Differential Diagnosis

Fibrosarcoma
Hemangiopericytoma

10-3 DERMATOFIBROMA

CLINICAL DESCRIPTION

A common fibrous tumor of adults, dermatofibromas are rare in children.

Etiology and Incidence

The exact cause of dermatofibroma is unknown. Speculation exists as to the possible role of localized trauma, such as insect bites, in their formation. In a large series examining these benign tumors, only 0.5% were seen in children younger than twelve years. They are much more common in the adult population.

Clinical Features

These discrete lesions are most often found on the lower extremities but can be found on the trunk and upper extremities as well. They show sharp demarcation from surrounding normal skin and are firm to the touch. They may be flat, nodular, or pedunculated. The overlying skin is smooth and frequently shows hyperpigmentation (Plate 10-3-1).

10-2-1 Congenital Fibromatosis

	Solitary	*Multiple*	*Generalized*
Location	Skin, subcutis, muscle	Skin, subcutis, muscle, bone	Skin, subcutis, bone, mucosa viscera
Clinical presentation	Infancy; on head, neck, or upper torso	External lesions almost uniformly at birth	Involves digestive, cardiovascular, ± respiratory tracts
Behavior pattern	Spontaneously involutes with atrophic scar	Often involute spontaneously	Visceral involvement can be fatal

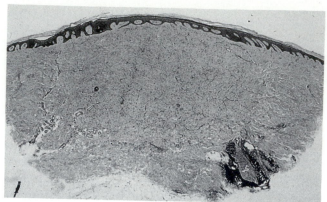

10-3-1 DERMATOFIBROMA: Low-power view shows a centrally hyperplastic epidermis overlying a dermal nodule with increased cellularity, as compared with the peripheral dermal stroma. (40×)

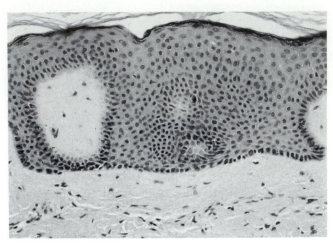

10-3-3 DERMATOFIBROMA: The epidermis overlying the dermatofibroma is hyperplastic and shows basilar hyperpigmentation, likened by some observers to "dirty fingers." (200×)

Differential Diagnosis
Epidermal inclusion cyst
Pilomatrixoma
Scar
Xanthogranuloma
Neurofibroma

HISTOLOGICAL DESCRIPTION

In the dermis there is a fibroblastic proliferation with a vague cartwheel array surrounding small blood vessels (Figure 10-3-1). Along the periphery of this proliferation individual bundles of collagen appear to be outlined by fibroblasts (Figure 10-3-2). Within the proliferation histiocytes are commonly seen, but multinucleated giant cells, lymphocytes, and

plasma cells may be scattered as well. Occasionally, the giant cells may show lipidization of their cytoplasms or incorporation of hemosiderin after local hemorrhage.

The overlying epidermis may be hyperplastic and hyperpigmented along the basilar layer. The elongate hyperpigmented rete have been likened to dirty fingers protruding into the subjacent dermis (Figure 10-3-3). Alternatively, the epidermis may show effacement of the rete ridge pattern and attenuation as it forms a collarette that circumscribes the dermal fibroblastic nodule.

Interesting inductive effects of the dermatofibroma on the overlying epidermis include the epidermal hyperplasia and hyperpigmentation, as discussed above, and basaloid budding along the lower portion of the epidermis, simulating basal cell carcinoma. These buds, however, do not appear to behave as conventional basal cell carcinomas.

Differential Diagnosis
Scar
Juvenile xanthogranuloma
Reticulohistiocytoma
Dermatofibrosarcoma protuberans

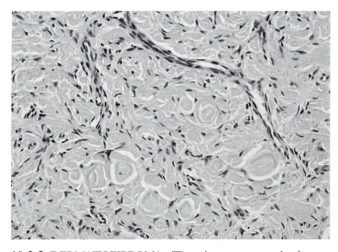

10-3-2 DERMATOFIBROMA: There is a vague cartwheel array to this fibroblastic proliferation. In addition, individual collagen bundles appear outlined by the proliferating basaloid cells. (200×)

10-4 DESMOID TUMOR

CLINICAL DESCRIPTION

Desmoid tumors are deep-seated fibrous tumors that may present in various settings.

Etiology and Incidence
Although the etiology of these tumors is unknown, the lineage of proliferating cells is fibroblastic. Desmoid tumors are rare in children.

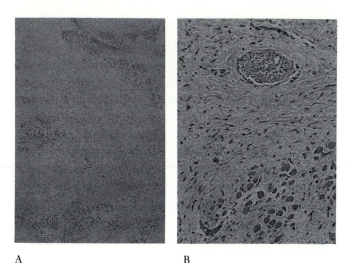

A   B

10-4-1 DESMOID TUMOR: (A) Low-power view of an extensive fibrous proliferation that surrounds skeletal muscle fibers. (20×) (B) This proliferation dissects among skeletal fibers and surrounds nerves. (100×) (Courtesy of Jane Chatten, M.D., Department of Pathology of Children's Hospital of Philadelphia.)

Clinical Features

Abdominal and extraabdominal (e.g., shoulder girdle) desmoids are rarely reported in children. They are usually solitary, firm masses with slow to aggressive growth patterns that attain a size of 5 to 15 cm. They may be fixed to underlying tissues. Desmoid tumors may cause pain if they impinge on nerves or may be fatal if they compromise vital structures. When they occur in the abdomen, desmoids can be found in the pelvis (commonly in young female adolescents and adults), mesentery, or retroperitoneum. The latter presentations are also seen in adolescents with Gardner's syndrome, an autosomally inherited disorder in which osteomas, epidermoid cysts, and gastrointestinal polyps also occur.

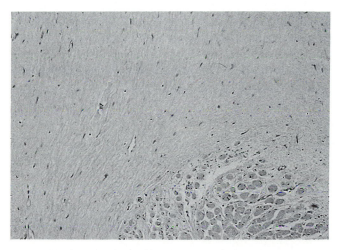

10-4-2 DESMOID TUMOR: Sparse fibroblast nuclei stud thick bands of collagen. (100×) (Courtesy of Jane Chatten, M.D., Department of Pathology of Children's Hospital of Philadelphia.)

Desmoids are usually treated with complete excision to prevent compromise of bodily functions and local recurrence. Recurrence is more common in tumors of children and adolescents arising in the shoulder and pelvis. Spontaneous regression of desmoids has been reported.

Differential Diagnosis
Fibrosarcoma
Dermatofibrosarcoma protuberans

HISTOLOGICAL DESCRIPTION

Elongate spindle cells proliferate in a fibrotic stroma where they are surrounded by abundant collagen. Occasionally fibers are hyalinized, reminiscent of those seen in keloids. The fibrocollagenous matrix becomes more apparent on trichrome staining (Figures 10-4-1 and 10-4-2; and Plate 10-4-1). The tumor has ill-defined borders but minimal atypia and only rare mitoses.

Differential Diagnosis
Reactive fibrosis (secondary to injury or trauma)
Fibrosarcoma

10-5 FIBROUS HAMARTOMA OF INFANCY

CLINICAL DESCRIPTION

This disorder was first described as subdermal fibromatous tumor of infancy.

Etiology and Incidence
This tumor is a localized proliferation of tissue normally seen in the subcutis but is abnormally arranged and present in different quantities than normal. It is not common but characteristically presents at birth (15% to 20% cases) or develops during the first year of life.

Clinical Features
Fibrous hamartoma of infancy is usually a solitary mass in the dermis or subcutis. It is usually freely moveable but can become fixed to underlying muscle or fascia. This tumor occurs more frequently in boys than in girls and is usually asymptomatic. Commonly affected sites include the axillae, proximal extremities, inguinal region, shoulder, and back. The hands and feet are typically spared. Although these hamartomas do not regress, they rarely recur after local excision.

Differential Diagnosis
Lipoma
Fibrolipoma

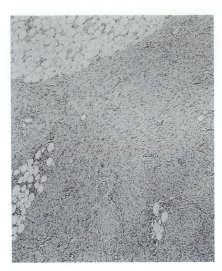

10-5-1 FIBROUS HAMARTOMA OF INFANCY: Bands of fibrous tissue extend to and surround adipose tissue. Lighter-staining areas in this proliferation indicate a stroma containing mucin. (40×)

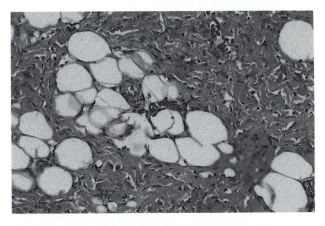

10-5-2 FIBROUS HAMARTOMA OF INFANCY: The collagenous matrix contains relatively few cells. The proliferating cells are surrounded by mature adipocytes. (200×)

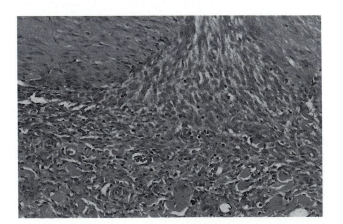

10-5-3 FIBROUS HAMARTOMA OF INFANCY: More cellular areas show a less collagenous stroma impinging on pilar muscle. (200×)

HISTOLOGICAL DESCRIPTION

Several tissue components characterize these localized cutaneous lesions. In the deep dermis to subcutis there are interlacing bundles of fibrous tissue composed of spindle cells within a collagenous matrix (Figure 10-5-1). These are surrounded by mature adipocytes (Figure 10-5-2) and collections of round cells embedded in a mucinous matrix (Figure 10-5-3). Ultrastructural analysis has shown the spindle cells to have features of myofibroblasts and fibroblasts. Although highly fibrous areas may appear neurofibromalike, the fibrous bundles and organoid pattern of this proliferation are rather characteristic.

Differential Diagnosis

Neurofibroma (in more fibrotic areas)

10-6 HYPERTROPHIC SCAR AND KELOID

CLINICAL DESCRIPTION

Both hypertrophic scars and keloids represent a localized overgrowth of scar tissue.

Etiology and Incidence

Most often hypertrophic scars and keloids arise after localized trauma. They are seen in adolescents and only rarely in prepubertal children. In particular, the tendency to formation of keloids may have a hereditary predisposition and occurs more commonly in deeply pigmented individuals. Both processes occur in males and females alike.

Clinical Features

A hypertrophic scar is clinically appreciated as a thick fibrous band raised above the surface of the skin. It is characteristically confined to the site of injury. In contrast, a keloid extends beyond the site of trauma: its extension onto normal skin gives the border a clawlike appearance.

Hypertrophic scars may arise at any site of trauma. Keloids preferentially occur on the upper trunk and arms (Figure 10-6-1), and with high frequency on earlobes after ear piercing.

Hypertrophic scars are initially raised and erythematous. They fade in color over time and flatten. They are usually asymptomatic. Keloids, on the other hand, do not usually flatten on their own and are frequently pruritic or hypersensitive. They may arise subsequent to acne lesions or, in rare instances, spontaneously in areas of skin tension (e.g., chest wall).

Differential Diagnosis

Scar
Dermatofibroma
Dermatofibrosarcoma protuberans

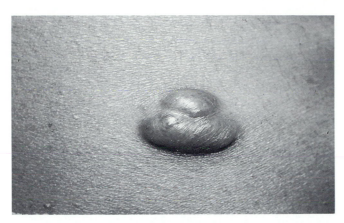

10-6-1 KELOID: A bilobed exophytic nodule on this black child's chest has a variably hyperpigmented smooth surface.

HISTOLOGICAL DESCRIPTION

Hypertrophic scars and keloids have similar histological features in their early stages of evolution: they show dermal fibrosis associated with proliferating blood vessels, increased numbers of mast cells, and a mixed inflammatory infiltrate. As they evolve, hypertrophic scars show collagen bundles arranged in parallel to the epidermis, while the overlying epidermis often has an effaced rete ridge pattern. Keloids characteristically show thick, eosinophilic, hyalinized bands of collagen randomly distributed within a fibroblastic stroma, giving the dermis a zebra stripe pattern (Figure 10-6-2). These hyalinized fibers are rare to absent in hypertrophic scars. The epidermis overlying keloids may be hyperplastic, normal, or attenuated. Electron microscopic study has suggested that keloids are composed of myofibroblasts.

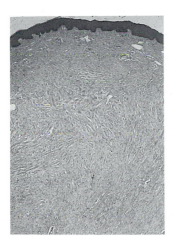
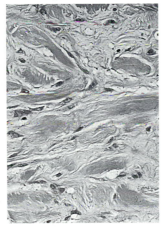

A   B

10-6-2 KELOID: (A) A dermal nodule composed of interlacing bands of collagen. (20×) (B) Thick hyalinized eosinophilic bands of collagen characteristic of keloids course through the stroma. (200×)

Differential Diagnosis
Scar

10-7 JUVENILE HYALINE FIBROMATOSIS

CLINICAL DESCRIPTION

This extremely rare form of childhood fibromatosis may produce severe physical deformities.

Etiology and Incidence

The etiology of this disorder is thought to be localized metabolic disturbances in collagen synthesis. It is extremely rare, and in contrast to infantile myofibromatosis is not seen at birth but becomes noticeable between the ages of two and five years. It occurs in children of consanguineous parents and appears to be transmitted as an autosomal recessive trait. Both males and females have been affected by juvenile hyaline fibromatosis.

Clinical Features

Most lesions arise in childhood, but they may occur in adult life as well. They are multiple flesh-colored papules or nodules, or yellowish plaques. They are seen most often on the nose, ears, scalp, back, and knees. Flexion deformities occur when lesions arise near joints, and excisional surgery may be mutilating. Thickening of the gums, lytic bony lesions on radiographs, and muscle weakness may be present as well. Of note, there is lack of involvement of vocal cords, which helps differentiate this disorder from lipoid proteinosis.

Differential Diagnosis
Lipoid proteinosis
Infantile myofibromatosis

HISTOLOGICAL DESCRIPTION

Lesions of recent onset show a dense proliferation of plump, elongate fibroblasts with ill-defined margins in the dermis. This proliferation is separated from the overlying epidermis by a Grenz zone. In areas there is evidence of amorphous eosinophilic matrix formation. As lesions become established, the cellular component decreases but the hyalinized eosinophilic matrix becomes much more prominent and is highlighted by periodic acid-Schiff staining. Occasionally calcification may be found. Although lipoid proteinosis also has an eosinophilic matrix, it lacks the spindle cell proliferation characteristically seen in juvenile hyaline fibromatosis. Ultrastructural studies suggest there is progressive abnormal collagen synthesis in this disorder.

Differential Diagnosis
Lipoid proteinosis

	Lesion	Site	Symptoms	Origin
Genital	Solitary	Scrotum, labia majora, nipple, or areola	Rarely painful	Scrotal (dartoic), areolar, and mammary smooth muscle
Extragenital	Solitary or multiple	Extremities, trunk and face	Often painful or tender	Arrector pili muscle

10-8 LEIOMYOMA

CLINICAL DESCRIPTION

Localized increases in smooth muscle bundles comprise leiomyomas.

Etiology and Incidence

The stimulus for the proliferation of smooth muscle in skin is unknown. Leiomyomas are uncommon in children, but patients affected at birth and early childhood have been reported. Familial occurrences (possibly autosomal dominant inheritance pattern) have also been reported in the literature. Rarely, multiple leiomyomas can be seen in type I multiple endocrine adenomatosis.

Clinical Features

The clinical features of cutaneous leiomyomas are summarized in Table 10-8-1. Leimyomas are clinically discrete small (1 to 2 mm), skin-colored or pink papules, which over time may increase in size to form nodules. Occasionally they may have a dermatomal distribution or localize to one extremity. They do not appear to involute spontaneously.

Differential Diagnosis

Dermatofibroma

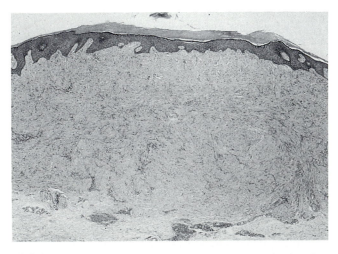

10-8-1 LEIOMYOMA: Low-power view shows that the dermis contains interlacing bundles of smooth muscle in various planes of section. Note the similarity of this proliferation to a dermatofibroma (Figure 10-3-1) on low magnification. (40×)

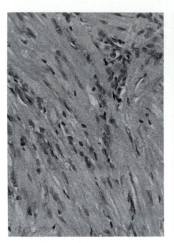 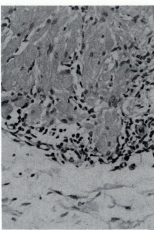

A   B

10-8-2 LEIOMYOMA: (A) In elongate (200×) and (B) cross section (200×), the cytoplasm of cells appears somewhat vacuolated. Note blunt-tipped nuclei when cells are viewed on their long axis.

HISTOLOGICAL DESCRIPTION

In the dermis there are increased numbers of smooth muscle bundles arranged in various planes of section (Figure 10-8-1). Where cells are sectioned longitudinally, their nuclei have blunted ends, giving them a cigarlike appearance (Figure 10-8-2). Bundles of smooth muscle cells often blend with the surrounding dermal stroma and adjacent pilar muscle. If there is doubt as to the lineage of proliferating cell in the dermis, trichrome stains are of value, as they highlight smooth muscle bundles in red. Electron microscopic studies show myofilaments within the cytoplasm of the cells.

Differential Diagnosis

Dermatofibroma

10-9 LIPOMA

CLINICAL DESCRIPTION

Lipomas are benign collections of adipocytes (fat cells).

Etiology and Incidence

The cause of a local proliferation of adipocytes is unknown. Lipomas are uncommon in children and adolescents but common in adults.

Clinical Features

Lipomas commonly present as asymptomatic mobile subcutaneous masses with well-defined margins and a soft consistency. They are most often solitary lesions but can occasionally occur in multiples.

Solitary lesions may be seen on the neck, trunk, and extremities. They may slowly increase in size over time, atrophy, calcify, or infarct subsequent to trauma.

In infants and children solitary lipomas may be seen in the midline of the lumbosacral spine. Such lipomas should raise suspicions of an underlying defect of the spinal lamina. They may connect to the subjacent spinal canal or to a lipoma adjacent to the dura. Early radiologic evaluation and neurosurgical intervention are necessary in such instances.

Multiple lipomas can occasionally be seen in adolescents associated with joints and tendon sheaths, causing local discomfort and contractures. Finally, multiple lipomas may arise on the forearms and thighs after puberty. If there is a familial inheritance pattern it is usually autosomal dominant with variable penetrance. Multiple symmetric lipomatosis (Madelung's disease) is essentially not seen until adult life and is not further addressed here.

Differential Diagnosis

Epidermal or pilar cyst
Lymph node
Benign lipoblastoma
Pilomatrixomas and other appendage tumors

HISTOLOGICAL DESCRIPTION

A large aggregate of mature adipocytes surrounded by a delicate band of fibrous tissue is the histological appearance of a lipoma. Individual adipocytes are uniformly rounded to polygonal cells with an eccentrically placed nucleus and vacuolated cytoplasms (Figure 10-9-1). With trauma, adipocytes become necrotic and their lipid is engulfed by histiocytes, which in turn acquire foamy cytoplasms. As the inflammatory phase subsides, fibrosis and dystrophic calcification may ensue. Lack of primitive-appearing lipocytes or a myxoid stroma differentiates lipomas from benign lipoblastomas, which are seen in infants and young children.

Differential Diagnosis

Angiolipoma
Fibrolipoma

10-10 RECURRENT INFANTILE DIGITAL FIBROMA

CLINICAL DESCRIPTION

This benign fibrous tumor has characteristic clinical and histological findings.

Etiology and Incidence

Although the reason for the occurrence of these tumors is unknown, the cells proliferating in these growths appear to be myofibroblasts. Infantile digital fibromas occur infrequently and sporadically. Lesions are recognized at birth in approximately one-third of cases and by the end of the first year of life in 86%. Males and females are equally affected.

Clinical Features

Infantile digital fibromas appear as single or multiple, flesh-colored to pink, broad-based, asymptomatic nodules. They characteristically occur on the extensor and lateral surfaces of the digits, usually sparing the thumbs and the great toes uniformly (Plate 10-10-1). Up to 61% have been reported to recur after local excision. After nodule growth plateaus, they tend to involute spontaneously. Surgical excision is thus indicated only to correct functional restriction or contractures.

Differential Diagnosis

Fibroma
Leiomyoma
Angiofibroma
Digital mucous cyst
Acquired digital fibrokeratoma
Dermatofibroma

HISTOLOGICAL DESCRIPTION

In the dermis there is a dense, ill-defined proliferation of uniform-appearing fibroblasts surrounded by collagen. The cytoplasm of these fibroblasts contains variable numbers of

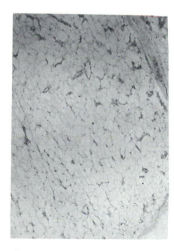
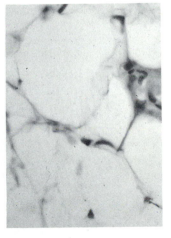

A   B

10-9-1 LIPOMA: (A) Low magnification shows an aggregate of mature adipocytes surrounded by a thin fibrous capsule. (20×) (B) Individual adipocytes have a single eccentrically placed nucleus and appear to have vacuolated cytoplasms. (400×)

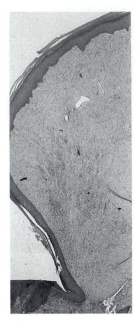
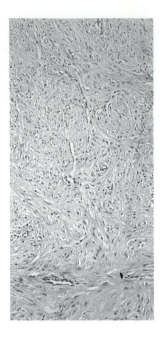

A   B

10-10-1 RECURRENT INFANTILE DIGITAL FIBROMA:
(A) Exophytic nodule surrounded by a collarette of hyperplastic epithelium. (20×) (B) Higher magnification shows a
dermal proliferation of epithelioid-appearing cells arranged in
fascicles in various planes of section. (100×) (Courtesy of Jane
Chatten, M.D., Department of Pathology of Children's Hospital
of Philadelphia.)

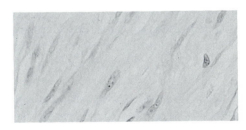

A

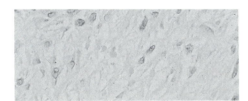

B

10-10-2 RECURRENT INFANTILE DIGITAL FIBROMA:
Eosinophilic intracytoplasmic droplets may be seen in the cytoplasms of these cells when viewed in both elongate (A, 200×)
and cross section (B, 200×). (Courtesy of Jane Chatten, M.D.,
Department of Pathology of Children's Hospital
of Philadelphia.)

small, round eosinophilic inclusions adjacent to the nucleus
(Figures 10-10-1 and 10-10-2). These inclusions are highlighted with trichrome (Plate 10-10-2) and phosphotungstic
acid-hematoxylin stains. Although these inclusions were suspected to be related to viral infection, ultrastructural analysis
has shown them to be abnormally contracted actin filaments
in myofibroblasts.

Differential Diagnosis
Other fibromatoses

10-11 SMOOTH MUSCLE HAMARTOMA

Clinical Description
This is a localized anomaly of smooth muscle of pilar origin.

Etiology and Incidence
This hamartoma is uncommon. When it occurs it is present at
birth or becomes apparent in early infancy. There appears to
be no inheritance pattern to this hamartoma.

Clinical Features
Smooth muscle hamartomas appear as flesh-colored to hyperpigmented plaques on the arms or trunk (Figure 10-11-1).
Vellus or terminal hairs emerging from the surface appear
more prominent than normal hairs. Upon stroking the surface
of these lesions muscle fibers contract, giving them an uneven
surface.

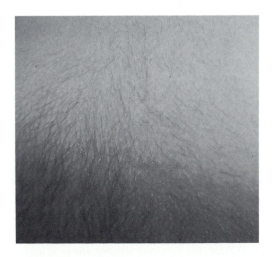

10-11-1 SMOOTH MUSCLE HAMARTOMA: Note hair
growing from "puckered skin" on the back of a child with a congenital smooth muscle hamartoma.

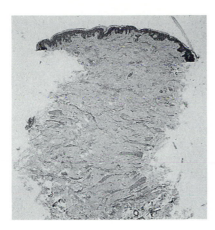

10-11-2 SMOOTH MUSCLE HAMARTOMA: Low magnification shows haphazard bundles of smooth muscle coursing through the dermis. (20×)

Although Becker's nevus may show hyperpigmentation and smooth muscle hyperplasia, it is not a congenital lesion as is the smooth muscle hamartoma. Becker's nevus arises in childhood or adolescence, a feature that allows separation of these two entities.

Differential Diagnosis

Congenital nevus
Mastocytoma
Connective tissue nevus
Becker's nevus

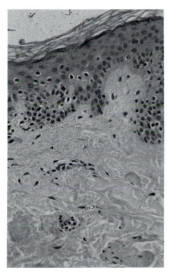
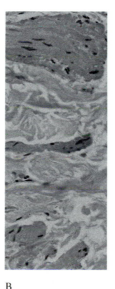

A   B

10-11-3 SMOOTH MUSCLE HAMARTOMA: (A) The epidermis overlying a smooth muscle hamartoma may be hyperplastic and display slight basilar hyperpigmentation. (100×) (B) A loose array of smooth muscle bundles is separated by mature dermal collagen bundles. (200×)

HISTOLOGICAL DESCRIPTION

In the dermis there are large numbers of smooth muscle bundles in a scattered, haphazard array separated by bundles of collagen (Figures 10-11-2 and 10-11-3). If the lesion is nodular, it shows better demarcation of smooth muscle bundles from surrounding dermal stroma than does a leiomyoma. Trichrome stains confirm the presence of increased numbers of smooth muscle bundles (red-staining) among collagen bundles (blue-staining).

Electron microscopy shows discrete, large smooth muscle bundles. Examination of the cytoplasm of such cells reveals many wavy or whorled myofilaments.

Differential Diagnosis

Leiomyoma

REFERENCES

Angiolipoma

Belcher RW, Czarnetzki BM, Carney JF, et al.: Multiple (subcutaneous) angiolipomas. Arch Dermatol 1974; 110:583.

Howard WR, Helwig EB: Angiolipoma. Arch Dermatol 1960; 82:924.

Congenital Generalized Fibromatosis

Mehregan AM: Superficial fibrous tumors in childhood. J Cutan Pathol 1981; 8:321.

Parker RK, Mallory SB, Baker GF: Infantile myofibromatosis. Pediatr Dermatol 1991; 8:129.

Wiswell TE, Davis J, Cunningham BE, et al.: Infantile myofibromatosis: The most common fibrous tumor of infancy. J Ped Surg 1988; 23:315.

Dermatofibroma

Mehregan AM: Superficial fibrous tumors in childhood. J Cutan Pathol 1981; 8:321.

Desmoid Tumor

Enzinger FM, Weiss SW: Soft tissue tumors, 2nd ed. St. Louis: CV Mosby, 1988:135.

Klemmer S, Pascoe L, DeCosse J: Occurrence of desmoids in patients with familial adenomatous polyposis of the colon. Am J Med Genet 1987; 28:385.

Scougall P, Staheli LT, Chew DE, et al.: Desmoid tumors in childhood. Orthop Rev 1987; 16:481.

Fibrous Hamartoma of Infancy

Enzinger FM, Weiss SW: Soft tissue tumors, 2nd ed. St. Louis: CV Mosby, 1988:164.

King DF, Barr RJ, Hirose FM: Fibrous hamartoma of infancy. J Derm Surg Oncol 1979; 5:482.

Maung R, Lindsay R, Trevenen C, et al.: Fibrous hamartoma of infancy. Hum Pathol 1987; 18:652.

Hypertrophic Scar and Keloid

Asboe-Hanson G: Hypertrophic scars and keloids. Dermatologica 1960; 120:178.

Blackburn WR, Cosman R: Histologic basis of keloid and hypertrophic scar differentiation: Clinicopathologic correlation. Arch Pathol 1966; 82:65.

Enzinger FM, Weiss SW: Soft tissue tumors, 2nd ed. St. Louis: CV Mosby, 1988:129.

James WD, Besanceney CD, Odom RB: The ultrastructure of a keloid. J Am Acad Dermatol 1980; 3:50.

Juvenile Hyaline Fibromatosis

Kan AE, Rogers M: Juvenile hyaline fibromatosis: An expanded clinicopathologic spectrum. Pediatr Dermatol 1989; 6:68.

Kitano Y: Juvenile hyaline fibromatosis. Arch Dermatol 1976; 112:86.

Kitano Y, Horiki M, Aoki T, et al.: Two cases of juvenile hyaline fibromatosis: Some histological, EM, and tissue culture observations. Arch Dermatol 1972; 106:877.

Visona A, Ronconi G, Montaguti A, et al.: Juvenile hyaline fibromatosis: Case report and review of the literature. Pathologica 1987; 79:357.

Leiomyoma

Fisher WC, Helwig EB: Leiomyomas of the skin. Arch Dermatol 1963; 88:510.

Mann PR: Leiomyoma cutis: An electron microscope study. Br J Dermatol 1970; 82:463.

Montgomery H, Winkelmann RK: Smooth muscle tumors of the skin. Arch Dermatol 1959; 79:32.

Lipoma

Brasfield RD, Das Gupta TK: Soft tissue tumors: Benign tumors of adipose tissue. Cancer 1969; 19:3.

Recurrent Infantile Digital Fibroma

Beckett IH, Jacobs AH: Recurring digital fibrous tumors of childhood. Pediatrics 1977; 59:401.

Iwasaki H, Kikuchi M, Mori R, et al.: Infantile digital fibromatosis: Ultrastructural, histochemical and tissue culture observations. Cancer 1980; 46:2238.

Zhu WY, Xia MY, Huang YF, et al.: Infantile digital fibromatosis: Ultrastructural human papillomavirus and herpes simplex virus DNA observation. Pediatr Dermatol 1991; 8:137.

Smooth Muscle Hamartoma

Berger TG, Levin MW: Congenital smooth muscle hamartoma. J Am Acad Dermatol 1984; 11:709.

11

Purpuras, Vascular Tumors, and Vascular Disease

Contents

11-1 CRYOGLOBULINEMIA

CLINICAL DESCRIPTION

Precipitation of globulins at cold temperatures is known as cryoglobulinemia.

Etiology and Incidence

Cryoglobulinemia may be caused by a monoclonal or polyclonal increase in immunoglobulins. The monoclonal variety is most often due to an increase in IgG or IgM. The polyclonal variety occurs after infections (hepatitis, poststreptococcal glomerulonephritis) and with immune complex diseases such as Henoch-Schönlein purpura and lupus erythematosus. Cryoglobulinemia has rarely been reported in children and adolescents.

Clinical Features

Cryoglobulinemia may be asymptomatic or show peripheral vascular changes. The latter include purpuric lesions, thrombosis, and ulcerations, which may be localized to the extremities or widespread. If the digits are affected, ulceration and gangrene may occur. Visceral thrombosis may affect the kidneys, lungs, and brain.

Differential Diagnosis

Leukocytoclastic vasculitis
Embolic phenomenon
Purpura fulminans
Sepsis

HISTOLOGICAL DESCRIPTION

The striking histological features are changes within the papillary blood vessels. The dermal papillary vessels contain in their lumen distinctly eosinophilic amorphous material (pre-

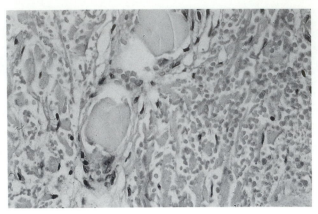

11-1-2 CRYOGLOBULINEMIA: Plugging of dermal vessels by homogeneous eosinophilic material. (200×)

cipitated cryoglobulin) in association with numerous red blood cells. These vascular changes may also be found in the midreticular dermis and subcutaneous tissue (Figures 11-1-1 and 11-1-2). The adjacent dermis may show extensive hemorrhage and a chronic inflammatory infiltrate of mononuclear cells, mainly lymphocytes. There is no leukocytoclastic vasculitis (Figure 11-1-3). Although the precipitated cryoglobulin is well visualized on hematoxylin and eosin-stained sections, it is best demonstrated with periodic acid-Schiff stains. IgG or IgM can be demonstrated by immunodiagnostic tests. The mixed cryoglobulinemias show leukocytoclastic vasculitis in addition to the precipitated material within the blood vessels.

Differential Diagnosis

Henoch-Schönlein purpura
Vasculitis of other causes

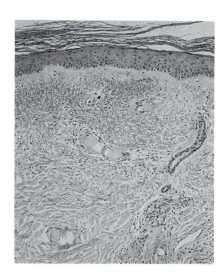

11-1-1 CRYOGLOBULINEMIA: There is superficial dermal hemorrhage. Low power shows plugging of vessel lumina in superficial and deep dermal vessels. (40×)

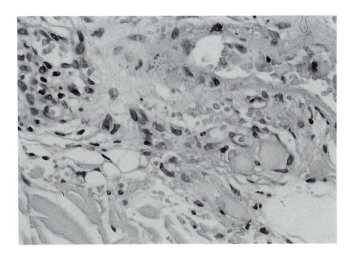

11-1-3 CRYOGLOBULINEMIA: Although there is modest inflammation around involved vessels, vessel endothelial cells remain intact. Changes of leukocytoclastic vasculitis are not present. (200×)

11-2 HENOCH-SCHÖNLEIN PURPURA

Etiology and Incidence

Henoch-Schönlein purpura is a systemic vasculitis of children and young adults. The vasculitis may be triggered by many events, including infection, allergens, or toxins, but infection appears to be the most significant cause of this condition. It occurs most commonly in children between the ages of four and ten years.

Clinical Features

Patients develop successive crops of erythematous macules, papules, or wheals. They are frequently found on the buttocks and the extensor surfaces of the extremities (Plate 11-2-1). These lesions become purpuric (palpable purpura); when severe, necrosis occurs. As the lesions resolve they leave brown-red macules or macular areas of purpura. The face and mucosa may be affected, but this is not a frequent occurrence. Young children (younger than two years) often have striking edema of the face, scalp, scrotum, hands, and feet. The skin findings are associated with systemic disease in 75% of cases. This is manifested by gastrointestinal disease (bloody diarrhea, intussusception), renal disease, arthritis, and hepatosplenomegaly. The usual course in the disease is recovery.

Differential Diagnosis

Drug eruption
Erythema multiforme
Rocky Mountain spotted fever
Rickettsial disease

HISTOLOGICAL DESCRIPTION

The histological features of Henoch-Schönlein purpura are leukocytoclastic vasculitis with rather marked hemorrhage. The vessels of the papillary and reticular dermis show a dense perivascular inflammatory infiltrate of lymphocytes, histiocytes, and neutrophils with fragmentation of neutrophils in the dermis and about vessel walls (Plate 11-2-2). The vessels within this infiltrate show endothelial swelling and may show total vascular occlusion. Deposition of fibrin may occur about these altered vessels and may also be found in the intervening dermis associated with a neutrophilic infiltrate. Frequently the collagen appears indistinct, with loss of its normal fibrillar quality. This is due to the deposition of fibrin and edema that extends from the perivascular area. Subepidermal blisters and/or vesicles may occur and are often associated with epidermal necrosis. Dermal necrosis is rarely seen in this condition; when present, it is usually secondary to ulceration. Older lesions show a less intense reaction with the presence of a

vasculitis and hemorrhage. Direct immunofluorescence of lesions less than forty-eight hours old characteristically show granular deposits of IgA in blood vessel walls (Plate 11-2-2).

Differential Diagnosis

Drug reaction
Cryoglobulinemia

11-3 CHRONIC PIGMENTED PURPURA

CLINICAL DESCRIPTION

Purpura refers to the purplish discoloration of skin and indicates leakage of erythrocytes from cutaneous blood vessels.

Etiology and Incidence

The cause of chronic pigmented purpuras is inflammation of the capillaries, or capillaritis. It most commonly affects the lower limbs, where hydrostatic pressure is the greatest. This disorder is usually not seen in young children but more often in adolescents.

Clinical Features

Chronic pigmented purpuras are most commonly seen on the lower legs as grouped erythematous macules that become brownish over time (Plate 11-3-1). This change results from extravasation of erythrocytes into dermis and subsequent breakdown into hemosiderin. A new crop of macules arises as an old one resolves. This cycle may lead to chronic discoloration of affected skin. Pruritus may or may not accompany the eruptions. Clinical variations of this process include lichenoid purpuric dermatitis (Gougerot and Blum disease), eczematous purpuric dermatosis (Doucas and Kapetanakis), purpura annularis telangiectodes (Majocchi's disease), and progressive pigmentary dermatosis (Schamberg's disease).

Differential Diagnosis

Leukocytoclastic vasculitis
Wiskott-Aldrich syndrome
Factitial purpura

HISTOLOGICAL DESCRIPTION

The histological features are essentially a perivascular lymphocytic inflammatory infiltrate about the papillary dermal capillaries. There is no true vasculitis, in that there is no leukocytoclasis, endothelial swelling, and/or vascular occlusion. There is microhemorrhage noted within the papillary dermis (Figures 11-3-1 and 11-3-2). The epidermis overlying these changes may show basal layer hyperpigmentation. Hemosiderin deposition is often found in the papillary dermis,

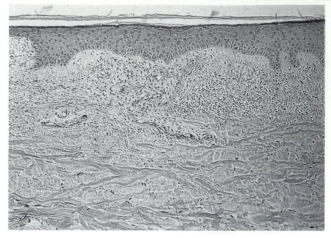

11-3-1 CHRONIC PIGMENTED PURPURA: Prominent extravasation of erythrocytes around superficial dermal vessels. (100×)

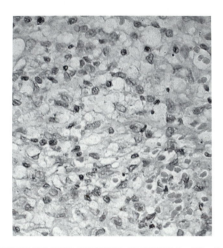

11-3-2 CHRONIC PIGMENTED PURPURA: The inflammatory infiltrate is mononuclear (mainly lymphocytes). Extravasated red blood cells are prominent. (400×)

and in conjunction with the dermal melanocytic pigmentation accounts for the color change seen clinically. All clinical varieties of the pigmented purpura have essentially similar features except for the pigmented purpuric lichenoid dermatitis, which shows, in addition to a lichenoid inflammatory infiltrate, focal areas of parakeratosis and exocytosis of mononuclear cells.

Differential Diagnosis

Stasis dermatitis

11-4 PURPURA FULMINANS

CLINICAL DESCRIPTION

This life-threatening illness is a rapidly progressive form of disseminated intravascular coagulation.

Etiology and Incidence

Purpura fulminans may be a manifestation of congenital or acquired protein C deficiency. More often, however, it occurs in association with a febrile illness (meningococcemia) and represents an immune complex-mediated disorder. Although purpura fulminans is rare, affected patients are predominantly children younger than six years of age. It has been reported infrequently in neonates. Boys and girls are both affected.

Clinical Features

One to four weeks after a bacterial (*Streptococcus pyogenes*, meningococcal), viral (varicella), or fungal (*Candida* sepsis) infection, the appearance of large symmetric ecchymoses heralds the onset of purpura fulminans (Plate 11-4-1). The ecchymoses are characteristically on the lateral thighs, buttocks, and ankles but may be present on the abdomen and upper extremities as well. They may progress to form bullae. Affected areas become necrotic and gangrenous. If tissue damage is extensive, shock may ensue.

Consumption of clotting factors becomes evident as increased levels of fibrin-split products, decreased levels of fibrinogen, factors V and VIII, and prolonged prothrombin and partial thromboplastin times occur. The mortality rate is high. Survivors may require grafting or amputation.

Differential Diagnosis

Sepsis
Coumarin necrosis

HISTOLOGICAL DESCRIPTION

Purpura fulminans is a noninflammatory purpura with the striking histological feature of massive areas of hemorrhage without associated inflammation (Figure 11-4-1). Small ves-

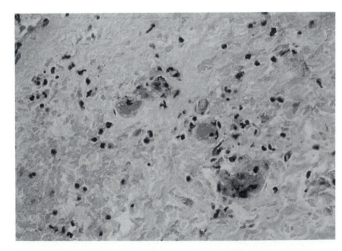

11-4-1 PURPURA FULMINANS: Massive hemorrhage without significant inflammation. (200×)

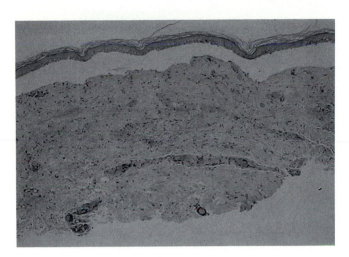

11-4-2 PURPURA FULMINANS: Subepidermal bulla with early epidermal necrosis. (40×)

sels may show platelet and fibrin thrombi and have associated small areas of vessel wall necrosis (Plate 11-4-2). The epidermis and superficial portions of the dermis may also show necrosis, which is on the basis of ischemia. Bulla formation in this condition is not uncommon, with the separation at the dermal-epidermal interface (Figure 11-4-2). The separated epidermis is frequently necrotic. Similar changes may occur in organs other than the skin.

Differential Diagnosis
Anticoagulant necrosis
Disseminated intravascular coagulation
Venomous bite reaction

11-5 ANGIOKERATOMA

CLINICAL DESCRIPTION

Angiokeratomas may occur as isolated or multiple lesions. In the latter instance they may have hereditary patterns and/or associated metabolic defects.

Etiology and Incidence
The etiology of this benign vascular tumor is unknown. It is relatively uncommon in children but is more often seen in adolescents.

Clinical Features
Lesions appear as small (2 to 8 mm), reddish black, sharply circumscribed papules with a verrucous surface (Plate 11-5-1). They often bleed briskly after being traumatized and may subsequently involute. Their appearance may mimic that of malignant melanoma.

Isolated Angiokeratoma
Isolated lesions may occur anywhere on the body. Most commonly, they are present on the extremities.

Angiokeratoma of Mibelli
Multiple angiokeratomas on the dorsa of the digits and over joints (knees and elbows) may be inherited as an autosomal dominant trait in families. In such cases they are often associated with cold intolerance and are known as angiokeratoma of Mibelli.

Angiokeratoma Circumscriptum
Angiokeratomas may rarely present as a group of papules or nodules on an extremity of an infant or young child, forming a plaque. A verrucous surface assists in making the diagnosis of angiokeratoma circumscriptum. Such lesions may increase in size in adolescence.

Fabry's Disease
Large numbers of angiokeratomas arising on the lower abdomen, hips, buttocks, and thighs of a prepubertal child suggest the possibility of Fabry's disease. This X-linked recessive disorder is fully expressed in males who carry the gene on their X chromosome but only partially expressed in females who carry the trait on one of their X chromosomes. In addition to angiokeratomas in large numbers on the body, affected individuals have recurrent fevers, limb pain, flushing of acral sites, paresthesias of their extremities, renal impairment, and corneal opacities.

Differential Diagnosis
Alpha-fucosidase deficiency
Sialidosis

HISTOLOGICAL DESCRIPTION

Angiokeratomas are essentially telangiectasias and not proliferations of new vessels. The features seen are those of widely dilated papillary dermal vessels with associated epidermal hyperplasia that appears to enclose some of the dilated vessels, giving the appearance of an intraepidermal vascular space (Figure 11-5-1). There is associated epidermal hyperkeratosis and there may be focal parakeratosis. The dilated vessels may extend into the midreticular dermis. There is usually no significant associated inflammatory response.

Angiokeratoma circumscriptum shows, in addition to widely dilated papillary dermal vessels, prominent hyperkeratosis and acanthosis, dilated vascular spaces that are similar to those seen in lymphangiomas. Vascular ectasia extends into the lower dermis and subcutaneous tissue. The vessels in this area are the same as those in cavernous hemangioma and may

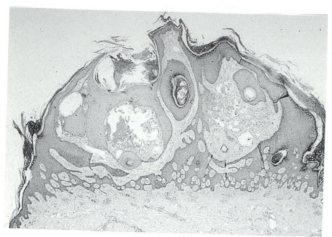

11-5-1 ANGIOKERATOMA: Sharply defined tumor of ectat papillary dermal vessels closely approximating a verrucous epidermis. (20×)

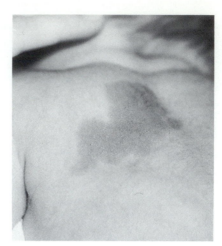

11-6-1 PORT-WINE STAIN: Irregular erythematous plaque on an infant's back.

be filled with red blood cells. There is no associated inflammation. Angiokeratoma circumscriptum is essentially an angiokeratoma with an associated cavernous hemangioma. Vascular thrombi may occur in this condition.

In Fabry's disease, granular lipid deposits can be found in endothelial cells of blood vessels, dermal macrophages, and fibroblasts and are related to a defect of the lysosomal enzyme alpha-galactosidase. This defect causes the accumulation of ceramide trihexoside in these cells as well as in the heart and kidneys.

Differential Diagnosis
Hemangioma

11-6 PORT-WINE STAIN (NEVUS FLAMMEUS)

CLINICAL DESCRIPTION

Etiology and Incidence
Port-wine stains are present at birth. The etiology is unknown.

Clinical Features
Port-wine stains are usually on the face (Figure 11-6-1) but may occur on any body surface. They are varying shades of red and blue in color. The lesion is initially flat, but with time develops angiomatous papules and overgrowth of the underlying tissues.

Differential Diagnosis
Salmon patch

HISTOLOGICAL DESCRIPTION

The histological features of nevus flammeus are ectatic, mature, thin-walled vessels that occur in the upper dermis (Figure 11-6-2). These may be filled with red blood cells. This vascular ectasia may be entirely confined to the papillary dermis. In contrast to capillary hemangioma, there is no endothelial cell proliferation and the dermis appears either somewhat edematous or normal in character.

Differential Diagnosis
Salmon patch
Essential telangiectasias

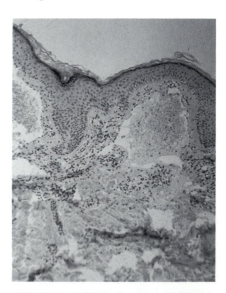

11-6-2 NEVUS FLAMMEUS: Ectatic superficial and middermal vessels lined by endothelial cells and distended by erythrocytes. (40×)

11-7 CAVERNOUS HEMANGIOMA (DEEP HEMANGIOMAS)

CLINICAL DESCRIPTION

Etiology and Incidence

Cavernous hemangioma may be present at birth. Its etiology is unknown.

Clinical Features

Cavernous hemangioma may occur in combinations with strawberry hemangioma (superficial) (Figure 11-7-1). They grow most rapidly in the first six months of life, decelerate the next six months, and complete most of their growth by two years of age. Subsequently 90% involute spontaneously (50% by five years, 70% by seven years, and 90% by nine years).

Differential Diagnosis

Lymphangioma
Lipoma
Pyogenic granuloma
Spitz nevus
Strawberry hemangioma

HISTOLOGICAL DESCRIPTION

On histological study, three types of congenital hemangiomas are usually seen: capillary hemangioma, nevus flammeus, and cavernous hemangioma.

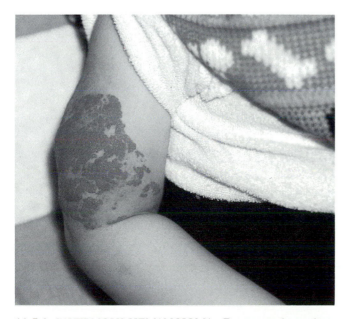

11-7-1 CAVERNOUS HEMANGIOMA: Deep-seated vascular mass, which causes irregularity of the contour of the upper arm. The surface is studded with erythematous papules and confluent plaques.

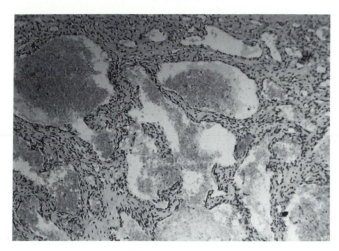

11-7-2 CAVERNOUS HEMANGIOMA: Thick-walled dilated vessels in the mid- to deep dermis, the deep component of a cavernous hemangioma. (40×)

Capillary Hemangioma

The histological feature of capillary hemangioma is a proliferation of small, well-formed vessels with distinct plump endothelial cells. Endothelial cell proliferation may be significant; in many areas there is aggregation of endothelial cells without the presence of vascular lumina. The younger the lesion in terms of development, the more endothelial cell cords and collections of cells without the presence of vascular lumina. As the lesion matures, vascular lumen become more apparent as does the presence of numerous red blood cells. Hemorrhage may be noted within some of these tumors. The stroma may be hyalinized and/or somewhat mucinous. In older lesions that are regressing, capillary walls show thickening and hyalinization. The inflammatory response is variable but is usually lymphocytic. Capillary hemangioma may be impossible to separate from pyogenic granuloma on histological grounds.

Cavernous Hemangioma

Cavernous hemangiomas have widely dilated vascular spaces in the lower dermis, extending into the subcutaneous tissue. The vessels are thin-walled with flattened endothelial cells (Figure 11-7-2). Fibrosis may be noted in the intervening spaces between vessels and there is usually no significant inflammation. Some vessels in the lower dermis may have thicker walls with the presence of a muscularis. Most commonly there is no overlying superficial vascular component.

Differential Diagnosis

Capillary Hemangioma
Pyogenic granuloma

Cavernous Hemangioma
Lymphangioma

11-8 BLUE RUBBER-BLEB NEVUS

CLINICAL DESCRIPTION

Etiology and Incidence

Blue rubber-bleb nevus occurs at birth and in infancy. It is associated with systemic lesions in the gastrointestinal tract.

Clinical Features

These lesions resemble compressible prunes in that they are blue-purple-black in color and raised above the skin surface and have a wrinkled surface. They vary in size from 0.3 to 6 cm. These tumors usually occur in multiples but do occur as single lesions (Plate 11-8-1). They may be tender when palpated.

Differential Diagnosis

Hemangioma
Melanocytic nevus

HISTOLOGICAL DESCRIPTION

Blue Rubber-Bleb Nevus

The histological features of blue rubber-bleb nevus and cavernous hemangioma are similar. Both have large, dilated vascular spaces in the dermis, filled with red blood cells. The vessel walls may be hyalinized and fibrotic. Some vascular spaces may show thrombi. These tumors may have a superficial component of small vessel proliferation (Figures 11-8-1 and 11-8-2).

Differential Diagnosis

Cavernous hemangioma
Glomus

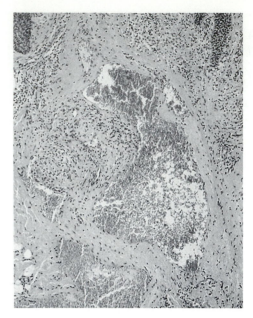

11-8-2 BLUE RUBBER-BLEB NEVUS: The deep dermal component shows thick-walled dilated blood vessels. (100×)

11-9 GENERALIZED ESSENTIAL TELANGIECTASIA

CLINICAL DESCRIPTION

Etiology and Incidence

Generalized essential telangiectasia (GET) occurs in adolescence, usually in females. Its etiology is unknown.

Clinical Features

Telangiectasias begin locally and either spread to involve an extremity or become generalized (Plate 11-9-1). They are asymptomatic and benign but cause a significant cosmetic problem. The lesions rarely regress.

Differential Diagnosis

Hyperestrogenemia
Spider angioma

HISTOLOGICAL DESCRIPTION

The histological features are dilated thin-walled vessels in the upper dermis, which may be engorged with red blood cells. The vessels have a thin endothelial cell lining and do not contain a muscularis. Vessels in this condition show extremely thin, fragile-appearing walls. There is no associated inflammation.

Differential Diagnosis

Hereditary telangiectasia
Spider nevus
Unilateral telangiectasia

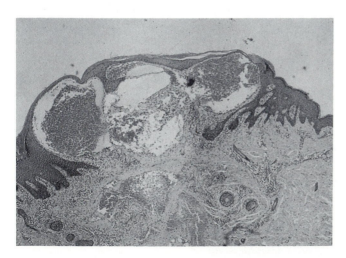

11-8-1 BLUE RUBBER-BLEB NEVUS: Low magnification shows that the vascular arrangement can mimic that of an angiokeratoma. (40×)

11-10 GLOMUS TUMOR

CLINICAL DESCRIPTION

Etiology and Incidence

Multiple glomus tumors are more common in children than in adults. Solitary lesions occur infrequently in children. The condition is dominantly inherited. The etiology is unknown.

Clinical Features

Glomus tumors mainly involve the lower extremities, but other skin surfaces may also be involved. The lesion is a purplish nodule (Plate 11-10-1) very similar to a blue rubber-bleb nevus. It ranges in size from millimeters to several centimeters in diameter. In contrast to solitary glomus tumors, multiple glomus tumors are usually nontender. The distribution differs from the inherited form in that it usually appears on the upper extremities, especially the nailbeds. Solitary glomus tumors are tender lesions and give rise to spontaneous paroxysms of pain.

Differential Diagnosis

Neurofibroma
Dermatofibroma
Melanoma
Blue nevus
Leiomyoma
Blue rubber-bleb nevus

HISTOLOGICAL DESCRIPTION

Single glomus tumors are solitary dermal nodules surrounded by compressed fibrous connective tissue capsule. Within this capsule are numerous small vessels that have a single endothelial lining and are surrounded by a varying number of glomus cells. Glomus cells are characterized by eosinophilic cy-

toplasm, and large, round, uniform-appearing centrally placed nuclei (Figure 11-10-1). Glomus cells can occasionally be confused with nevus cells. The surrounding stroma is fibrocellular and often shows chronic inflammation. Stains with S-100 protein often show numerous small nerve fibers associated with this vascular tumor.

Multiple glomus tumors occur more diffusely in the dermis and are not surrounded by a capsule. Glomus cells are fewer in number than in solitary glomus tumors. Vessels are thin-walled and show a somewhat compressed, thin endothelial cell. S-100 stains show nerve fibers associated with this tumor also.

Differential Diagnosis

Capillary hemangioma

11-11 GRANULOMA PYOGENICUM

CLINICAL DESCRIPTION

Etiology and Incidence

Granuloma pyogenicum is seen throughout childhood. One etiologic hypothesis is that these lesions result from vascular proliferation in response to trauma.

Clinical Features

The lesions occur on exposed skin and skin subjected to trauma (i.e., face and extremities, especially the fingers). The lesions usually occur singularly as red, raised, moist pedunculated nodules that bleed easily (Figure 11-11-1). They arise

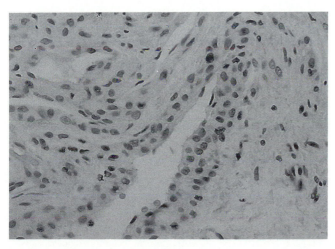

11-10-1 GLOMUS TUMOR: Dilated dermal vessels are surrounded by uniform cuboidal cells. (200×)

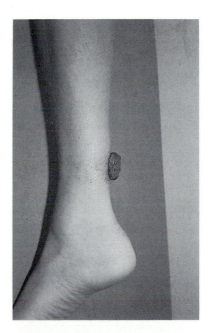

11-11-1 PYOGENIC GRANULOMA: Exophytic erythematous mass that arose after a soccer injury.

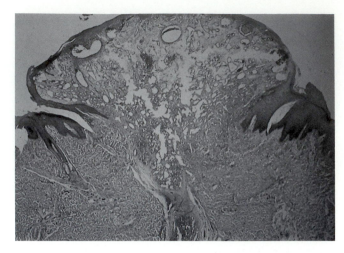

11-11-2 PYOGENIC GRANULOMA: Exophytic nodule surrounded by an epithelial collarette. The stroma contains large numbers of small vessels in a myxoid-appearing matrix. (40×)

rapidly, appearing over several weeks. Spontaneous regression can occur but removal is frequently necessary. Following removal, satellite lesions may develop, especially on the back.

Differential Diagnosis
Capillary hemangioma
Spitz nevus

HISTOLOGICAL DESCRIPTION

The histological features are marked proliferation of small mature vessels in a very edematous stroma. The overlying epidermis is often effaced and there is lateral epidermal acanthosis. This configuration (epidermal collarette formation) is often seen in lesions that show rapid central proliferation of dermal components. There are also cords and groups of endothelial cells without a central lumen (Figures 11-11-2 and

11-11-3). In nonulcerated pyogenic granuloma, there is a mononuclear cell inflammatory infiltrate of lymphocytes and histiocytes. As the thin epidermis ulcerates, secondary change ensue in the form of acute inflammatory cells, hemorrhage, necrosis, and increased ground substance within the stroma. Pyogenic granulomas in their early stage, before secondary change occur, are often difficult or impossible to differentiate from capillary hemangioma.

Differential Diagnosis
Capillary hemangioma
Kaposi's sarcoma

11-12 LYMPHANGIOMAS
CLINICAL DESCRIPTION

Etiology and Incidence
Most lymphangiomas present between birth and two years of age. There are four main types: lymphangioma simplex, cavernous lymphangioma circumscriptum, lymphangioma circumscriptum, and cystic hygroma. Their etiology is unknown.

Clinical Features
Lymphangioma Simplex
Seen during infancy, these lesions are found mainly on the upper half of the body. They are flesh-colored swellings that vary in size.

Cavernous Lymphangioma Circumscriptum
These are larger, less well-defined swellings (Figure 11-12-1), which are difficult to treat and which frequently recur. Their distribution is much the same as that of lymphangioma simplex.

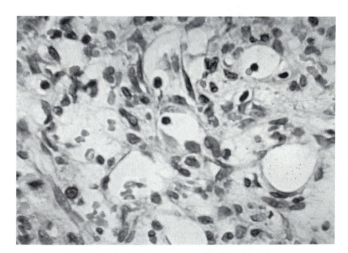

11-11-3 PYOGENIC GRANULOMA: Matrix composed of very edematous stroma surrounding delicate blood vessels. (400×)

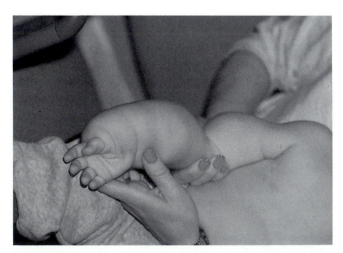

11-12-1 LYMPHANGIOMA: Cavernous lymphangioma, causing gross deformity of the right forearm.

Lymphangioma Circumscriptum

These lesions are found most commonly on the proximal extremities, upper trunk, and lateral chest wall. Patches of translucent vesicles, some blood-filled, sit on normal-appearing or diffusely swollen skin. The vesicles periodically vary in size and color. Recurrences are common if only the superficial lesions are removed.

Cystic Hygroma

These benign lymphatic tumors of the neck frequently increase in size, becoming quite large. Unlike lymphangioma circumscriptum they rarely recur following surgery.

Differential Diagnosis

Cavernous hemangioma

Verruca

Angiokeratoma

HISTOLOGICAL DESCRIPTION

Lymphangioma Simplex

The histological features in lymphangioma simplex are superficial dilated, thin-walled vessels that occupy the papillary dermis. These vessels have flattened, ill-defined endothelial cell lining. Epidermal participation consists of acanthosis and hyper- and parakeratosis. In addition to dilated cystic vascular spaces in the papillomatous portion of the dermis, there are large dilated lymph vessels that extend into the deeper dermis and often into the subcutaneous fat. These large dilated vessels may show a muscularis and may be associated with intervening zones of fibrosis.

Cavernous Lymphangioma Circumscriptum

In the subcutaneous tissue there are large, dilated cystic spaces lined by a thin, flattened layer of endothelium and sometimes filled with an eosinophilic- and/or basophilic-staining amorphous material in which there are few mononuclear cells (mainly lymphocytes). There is often associated fibrosis in the subcutaneous tissue and lower dermis. A muscularis may be associated with these large spaces. There is no overlying superficial component in this type of lymphangioma.

Lymphangioma Circumscriptum

This is the most superficial form of this type of lymphatic tumor, consisting of dilated lymphatic vessels in the papillary dermis (Figure 11-12-2). The epidermis shows hyperkeratosis and may show focal parakeratosis as well as rather marked acanthosis, often with collarette formation. An occasional red blood cell may be seen within the lymph spaces, but usually there are mononuclear cells (lymphocytes) associated with amorphous basophilic-staining material (Figure 11-12-3). There is usually no deep component to this tumor, al-

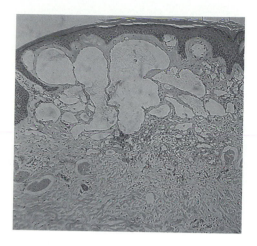

11-12-2 LYMPHANGIOMA CIRCUMSCRIPTUM: The latticelike appearance of the dermis is caused by widely ectatic lymphatics. (40×)

though lymphatic spaces may be seen in the midreticular dermis. Inflammatory changes are minimal.

Cystic Hygroma

The histological features of cystic hygroma are the same as those of cavernous lymphangioma. There are large dilated vascular spaces lined by flattened endothelial cells. There is no associated inflammation (Figure 11-12-4). The stroma is often fibrotic and hyalinized. Muscle fibers and/or bundles can also be found. The location of this tumor on the neck and in the axilla defines cystic hygroma.

Differential Diagnosis

Hemangioma

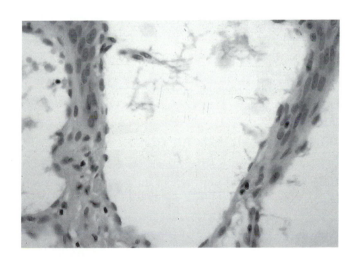

11-12-3 LYMPHANGIOMA CIRCUMSCRIPTUM: Endothelial cells line these vascular spaces. Note the absence of erythrocytes and the presence of proteinaceous material in the lumen. (400×)

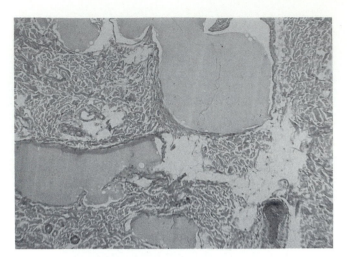

11-12-4 CYSTIC HYGROMA: Abundant proteinaceous material fills vascular lumina in the deep dermis. (200×)

11-13 LIVEDO RETICULARIS

CLINICAL DESCRIPTION

Persistent bluish-red discoloration of the skin that is minimally affected by changes in temperature.

Etiology and Incidence

This disorder may occur at any age. The etiology is unknown. Livedo reticularis is similar to cutis marmorata—the physiologic change produced by exposure to cold temperatures that disappears with rewarming of the skin. In livedo reticularis, however, these skin changes do not clear with rewarming (Plate 11-13-1). This persistent condition symmetrically affects the extremities and trunk of healthy females. When these skin changes occur in an asymmetric patchy distribution the presence of vasculitis (livedo vasculitis) and associated collagen vascular disease must be considered. Children with livedo vasculitis may develop ulcerations and edema.

Differential Diagnosis

Cutis marmorata
Cutis marmorata telangiectaticum congenita
Livedo vasculitis

HISTOLOGICAL DESCRIPTION

The histological features in this condition are variable. There may be only a mild perivascular inflammatory response of lymphocytes. When there is significant vascular involvement (usually blue-purple areas), there are vascular reactions that vary from vascular occlusion (thrombosis) to marked endothelial swelling and proliferation of the endothelium to the point of occlusion. There can be infiltration of the area by inflammatory cells, including lymphocytes, histiocytes, and neutrophils. The end stage of this process is fibrosis.

Differential Diagnosis

Atrophy blanche
Embolic conditions
Vasculitis

REFERENCES

Cryoglobulinemia

Ellis FA: The cutaneous manifestations of cryoglobulinemia. Arch Dermatol 1964; 89:690.

Garcia-Fuentes M, Chantler C, Williams DG: Cryoglobulinaemia in Henoch-Schönlein purpura. Br Med J 1977; 2:163.

Henoch-Schönlein Purpura

Ansell BM: Henoch-Schönlein purpura with particular reference to the prognosis of the renal lesion. Br J Dermatol 1970; 82:211.

Pigmented Purpura

Randal SJ, Kierland RR, Montgomery H: Pigmented purpuric eruptions. Arch Dermatol Syph 1951; 64:177.

Purpura Fulminans

Chu DZJ, Blaisdell FW: Purpura fulminans. Am J Surg 1982; 143:356.

Cram DL, Soley RL: Purpura fulminans. Br J Dermatol 1968; 80:323.

Gurses N, Ozkan A: Neonatal and childhood purpura fulminans: A review of seven cases. Cutis 1988; 41:361.

Petrini P, Segnestam K, Ekelund H, Egberg N: Homozygous protein C deficiency in two siblings. Pediatr Hematol Oncol 1990; 7:165.

Spicer TE, Rau JM: Purpura fulminans. Am J Med 1976; 61:566.

Angiokeratoma

Esterly NB: The skin. In Behrman RE, Kliegman RM, Nelson WE, et al., eds. Textbook of Pediatrics, 14th ed. Philadelphia: W.B. Saunders, 1992.

Fabry J: Uber einen Fall von Angiokeratoma circumscriptum am Oberschenkel. Dermatol Z 1915; 22:1.

Fabry J: Ein Beitrag zur Kenntnis der Purpura haemorrhagica nodularis (Purpura papulosa haemorrhagica) Arch Derm Syph 1898; 43:187.

Goldman L, Gibson SH, Richfield DF: Thrombotic angiokeratoma circumscriptum simulating melanoma. Arch Dermatol 1981; 117:138.

Imperial R, Helwig EB: Angiokeratoma: A clinicopathological study. Arch Dermatol 1967; 95:166.

Hemangioma

Taxy JB, Gray SR: Cellular angiomas of infancy: An ultrastructural study of two cases. Cancer 1979; 43:2322.

Findley JL, Noe JM, Arndt KA, et al.: Port wine stains: Morphologic variations and developmental lesions. Arch Dermatol 1984; 120:1453.

Blue Rubber-Bleb Nevus

Fretzin DF, Potter B: Blue rubber bleb nevus. Arch Intern Med 1965; 116:924.

Generalized Essential Telangiectasia

McGrae JD Jr, Winkelmann RK: Generalized essential telangiectasia: Report of a clinical and histochemical study of 13 patients with acquired cutaneous lesions. JAMA 1963; 185:909.

Glomus Tumor

Tarnowski WM, Hashimoto K: Multiple glomus tumors. J Invest Dermatol 1969; 52:474.

Granuloma Pyogenicum

Warner J, Jones E: Pyogenic granuloma recurring with multiple satellites: A report of 11 cases. Br J Dermatol 1986; 8:627.

Lymphangioma

Flanagan BF, Helwig EB: Cutaneous lymphangioma. Arch Dermatol 1977; 113:24.

Harkins GA, Sabiston DC Jr: Lymphangioma in infancy and childhood. Surgery 1960; 47:811.

Livedo Vasculitis

Bard IW, Winkelmann RK: Livedo vasculitis. Arch Dermatol 1967; 96:489.

12

Cutaneous Manifestations of Systemic Disease

Contents

12-1 ACRODERMATITIS ENTEROPATHICA

CLINICAL DESCRIPTION

Acrodermatitis enteropathica is a recessively inherited disorder characterized by diarrhea, dermatitis, and alopecia.

Etiology and Incidence

The etiology of this entity was unknown until Moynahan, in 1973, demonstrated low serum zinc levels in affected children (< 50 mg/dl). Since that time some individuals with this syndrome have been found to have normal zinc levels. Zinc deficiency states and acrodermatitis enteropathica have also been noted in patients on long-term parenteral hyperalimentation, full-term and premature infants fed breast milk only, patients who have had intestinal bypass procedures and those with diets deficient in zinc.

The onset of this disorder is usually in the first two years of life, with an average age of nine months.

Clinical Features

A vesiculobullous eruption begins in the periorificial skin regions in a symmetrical fashion. Frequently a misdiagnosis of moniliasis is made. The skin areas involved (periorificial and acral) are often eroded, crusted, and sharply marginated (Plate 12-1-1). A psoriasiform diaper eruption is present. The child becomes very irritable and then begins losing hair. Later in the course of the disease, diarrhea is a prominent feature. Other findings include conjunctivitis, stomatitis, paronychia, nail dystrophy, and growth retardation. If left untreated, patients become mentally deficient.

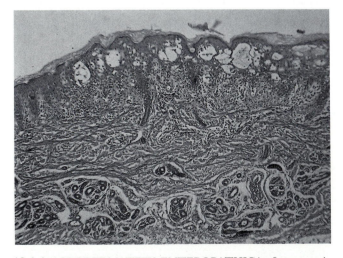

12-1-1 ACRODERMATITIS ENTEROPATHICA: Low magnification shows striking vacuolar degeneration of the epidermis. (20×)

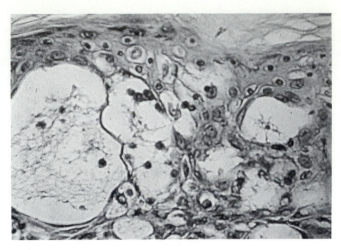

12-1-2 ACRODERMATITIS ENTEROPATHICA: High magnification shows intraepidermal microvesicles secondary to vacuolar degeneration. (400×)

Differential Diagnosis

Chronic mucocutaneous candidiasis
Psoriasis
Essential fatty acid deficiency
Biotin deficiency
Multiple carboxylase deficiency
Acquired immunodeficiency syndrome

HISTOLOGICAL DESCRIPTION

Epidermal vacuolization, clear epidermal cells, and parakeratosis are the striking histological features of this condition. Intraepidermal vesicles can result when vacuolar degeneration in the epidermis is extensive (Figures 12-1-1 and 12-1-2). The primary changes are all epidermal; the dermis shows a sparse lymphohistiocytic inflammatory infiltrate. Because of the superficial epidermal vacuolar change the upper epidermis stains less intensely than the lower portion of the epidermis, resulting in a two-phase staining pattern. Late lesions show mainly parakeratosis and acanthosis, a finding similar to that in chronic dermatoses.

Differential Diagnosis

Necrolytic migratory erythema
Toxic epidermal necrolysis
Burn

12-2 ALLERGIC GRANULOMATOSES (VASCULITIDES)

CLINICAL DESCRIPTION

Under this category are grouped Wegener's granulomatosis, allergic granulomatosis (Churg-Strauss syndrome), and lymphomatoid granulomatosis.

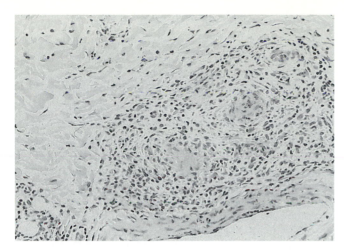

12-2-1 WEGENER'S GRANULOMATOSIS: The infiltrate is composed of lymphocytes, histiocytes, and multinucleated giant cells, which give the infiltrate a granulomatous appearance. (200×)

Etiology and Incidence

These entities are of unknown etiology and very rare in childhood. Necrotizing granulomas induced by vasculitis are a prominent feature in each. Skin findings are seen in 25% to 50% of patients with Wegener's granulomatosis, 66% of patients with allergic granulomatosis, and 45% of those with lymphomatoid granulomatosis.

Clinical Features

Wegener's granulomatosis is characterized by upper and lower respiratory findings of sinusitis, nasal mucosal ulcerations, otitis media, cough, and hemoptysis. Petechiae and purpura can be found on the face, trunk, and limbs. At times these findings suggest Henoch-Schönlein purpura. Papulonodules, subcutaneous nodules, and ulcerations can appear on any part of the body. At times eye abnormalities (e.g., episcleritis, retinal artery thrombosis, and proptosis) are prominent.

Allergic granulomatosis is similar to periarteritis nodosa but has symptoms that suggest an atopic condition (i.e., recurrent wheezing and pneumonitis). A prominent feature of this condition is a marked peripheral eosinophilia. The vasculitic lesions also involve the skin (nodules, ulcers, erythema multiforme-like skin changes), central nervous system, and gastrointestinal tract (abdominal pain, bloody diarrhea).

Lymphomatoid granulomatosis also involves the lungs (cough, chest pain, shortness of breath). Skin changes are often the first sign of this disorder and consist of erythematous macules, papules, nodules, and ulcerations.

Differential Diagnosis

Atopic lung disease
Collagen vascular disease
Other vasculitides
Periarteritis nodosa

HISTOLOGICAL DESCRIPTION

Granulomatous vasculitis includes three clinical syndromes—Wegener's granulomatosis, allergic granulomatosis, and lymphomatoid granulomatosis— share in common vasculitis and granuloma formation. Subtle histological and clinical differences separate them. Lymphomatoid granulomatosis most likely represents cutaneous T cell lymphoma with vasculitis.

Wegener's Granulomatosis

Characteristically, necrotizing vasculitis and necrotizing granulomas are seen (Plate 12-2-1). The vasculitis is of small to medium-sized vessels and shows leukocytoclasis, vessel wall invasion by inflammatory cells, endothelial swelling, and vascular obliteration. Vascular obliteration leads to ulceration. Fibrinoid deposits can be found about vessels. In addition to polymorphonuclear leukocytes, the infiltrate contains lymphocytes, histiocytes, mast cells, and hemorrhage. The granulomas have central necrosis surrounded by an infiltrate of neutrophils, lymphocytes, plasma cells, and multinucleated giant cells (Figure 12-2-1). The central focus of a granuloma may be small vessel destruction with subsequent granuloma formation (Figure 12-2-2). Some biopsy specimens may show only ulceration and the ravages of prior vasculitis and necrotic granulomas.

Allergic Granulomatosis

The histological features in this condition are similar to these in Wegener's granulomatosis, except that in the areas of leukocytoclastic vasculitis many eosinophils are present. Fibrin deposits are alsao found about the involved vessels. The granulomatous changes have central collagen degeneration with degranulated eosinophils. Such areas are surrounded by histiocytes and multinucleated giant cells as well as plasma cells.

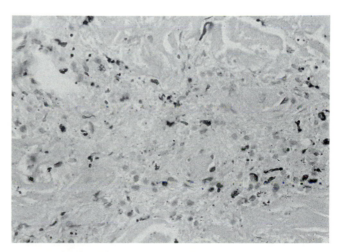

12-2-2 WEGENER'S GRANULOMATOSIS: Zones of dermal necrosis surrounded by remains of ill-defined outlines of blood vessels. (400×)

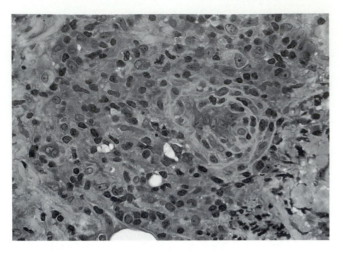

12-2-3 LYMPHOMATOID GRANULOMATOSIS: One-micron sections showing a brisk angiocentric infiltrate about a damaged blood vessel. The infiltrate is composed of pleomorphic mononuclear cells with mitoses. (400×)

The collagen alteration with eosinophils is similar to the flame figures of Well's disease. Eosinophilia is an essential feature of this condition; without it, the diagnosis becomes more tenuous.

Lymphomatoid Granulomatosis
The striking feature of this condition is a perivascular infiltrate of atypical lymphocytes, histiocytes and plasma cells (Figure 12-2-3). This infiltrate is angiocentric and is associated with vasculitis. The vascular destructive changes are usually of lower dermal vessels, where endothelial swelling, fibrin deposits, and leukocytoclasis can be seen.

Differential Diagnosis
Granulomatous inflammation secondary to infection
Collagen vascular diseases

12-3 ANNULAR ERYTHEMAS

CLINICAL DESCRIPTION
The annular erythemas include erythema marginatum, erythema annulare centrifugum, annular erythema of infancy, and erythema chronicum migrans.

Etiology and Incidence
Erythema marginatum is one of the major clinical criteria defined by Jones used in making the diagnosis of rheumatic fever, as it occurs in 10% of patients with rheumatic fever. Streptococcal infections occur most frequently between five and fifteen years of age, also the years when erythema marginatum is seen. Although many antigens and toxins are associated with the streptococcal organism, none has been defin-

itively identified as being directly responsible for rheumatic fever or the rash. Furthermore, when this finding is associated with rheumatic fever, it occurs only following streptococcal infections of the throat, not the skin.

Erythema annulare centrifugum is a skin finding of unknown etiology. The childhood form is theorized to be a hypersensitivity reaction to infection (especially group A beta hemolytic streptococci) or collagen vascular disease.

Annular erythema of infancy is uncommon and of unknown etiology. Erythema chronicum migrans is described in the section on tick bites, Chapter 18.

Clinical Features
Erythema marginatum is characterized by pink macules that gradually enlarge peripherally (while clearing centrally) and connect to form a serpiginous pattern with very sharp margins. The lesions are most commonly found on the trunk (Figure 12-3-1). The eruption may be recurrent over a period of several months, but each episode lasts only two to three weeks.

Erythema annulare centrifugum is similar to erythema marginatum but is distinguished by its raised wide border and smaller ring. Lesions are singular or multiple and located mainly on the trunk (Plate 12-3-1). The lesions begin as erythematous, asymptomatic papules and slowly expand while clearing centrally. New lesions may form within formed rings.

Annular erythema of infancy begins in the first several months of life as erythematous papules. The papules develop into short-lived (two-plus days) annular and arcuate lesions. Cyclical eruptions occur every five to six weeks in this self-limited disorder. The lesions are asymptomatic and disappear

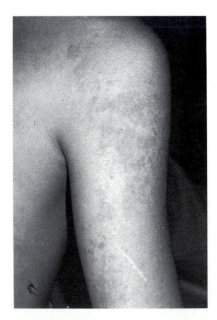

12-3-1 ANNULAR ERYTHEMAS (erythema marginatum): Erythematous macules and small plaques on the arm and trunk of a child with rheumatic fever.

without leaving postinflammatory changes. No systemic problems have been associated with this benign disorder.

Differential Diagnosis
Neonatal lupus erythematosus
Tinea corporis
Granuloma annulare
Pityriasis rosea
Erythema multiforme
Erythema chronicum migrans
Urticaria
Familial annular erythema

HISTOLOGICAL DESCRIPTION

Erythema Marginatum
The epidermis may show spongiosis without epidermal cell injury, although there can be increased epidermal pigmentation. There is dermal edema and a dense infiltrate of lymphocytes about dermal vessels. Collections of neutrophils may be present in dermal papillae. Although nuclear debris may surround blood vessels, there is an absence of fibrin deposition in and around vessel walls and absence of dermal hemorrhage. These features distinguish erythema marginatum from leukocytoclastic vasculitis with focal hemorrhage and a surrounding lymphohistiocytic inflammatory infiltrate.

Erythema Annulare Centrifugum
The striking histological feature in this condition is a dense sheathing of dermal vessels by lymphocytes without vasculitis (Figures 12-3-2 and 12-3-3). The epidermis shows minimal involvement with slight spongiosis and discrete parakeratosis overlying the areas of spongiosis.

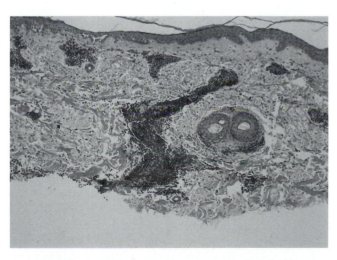

12-3-2 ERYTHEMA ANNULARE CENTRIFUGUM: Tightly cuffed infiltrates surrounding dermal blood vessels with a typical "coat-sleeved" distribution. (20×)

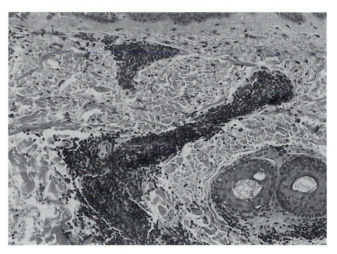

12-3-3 ERYTHEMA ANNULARE CENTRIFUGUM: The infiltrate is composed almost entirely of lymphocytes. (200×)

Annular Erythema of Infancy
Biopsy specimens show a dense perivascular infiltrate of lymphocytes, histiocytes, and occasional plasma cells admixed with variable numbers of eosinophils.

Differential Diagnosis
Secondary syphilis
Urticaria
Collagen vascular disease

12-4 BASAL CELL NEVUS SYNDROME

CLINICAL DESCRIPTION
The major skin finding in this syndrome is a nevoid basal cell tumor that is associated with multiple defects.

Etiology and Incidence
This autosomal dominant disorder is of unknown cause. Basal cell epitheliomas usually first appear at puberty.

Clinical Features
The major skin findings in basal cell nevus syndrome are multiple basal cell epitheliomas. Their appearance can be uncharacteristic because they are flesh-colored or brown, dome-shaped papules without rolled borders and telangiectasia. The main skin areas involved are the neck and upper trunk (Figure 12-4-1). The lesions ulcerate. Palmoplantar pits with a red base are common. Other findings include milia, cysts, lipomas, and comedones.

Other involved systems include the skeletal (mandibular cysts, broad nasal root, frontal bossing, scoliosis, syndactyly), central nervous (calcification of the falx, mental retardation, hydrocephalus, deafness, agenesis of the corpus

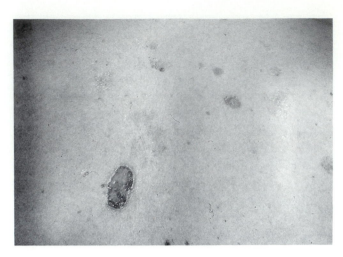

12-4-1 BASAL CELL NEVUS SYNDROME: Basal cell epitheliomas.

callosum), and endocrine (hypogonadism, ovarian cyst, pelvic calcification) systems.

Differential Diagnosis
None

HISTOLOGICAL DESCRIPTION

The histological features of tumors of basal cell nevus syndrome are the same as those of photo-induced basal cell carcinomas. There are islands of basaloid nodules in the dermis, which show peripheral palisading with a central core of cells showing cytological atypia with mitoses (Plate 12-4-1). Often there is a retraction space between the tumor and the stroma. The stroma is fibromyxoid and has a varying inflammatory cell response, usually lymphocytic in character. Basal cell tumors may be derived from the epidermis or the follicular adnexa.

The palmar pits seen in this syndrome show focal loss of the stratum corneum, a thin granular layer, and superficial basal cell tumors at the dermal-epidermal interface. The inflammation in palmar pits is sparse and lymphocytic.

Differential Diagnosis
Cylindroma
Trichoepithelioma

12-5 DERMATOMYOSITIS

CLINICAL DESCRIPTION

Juvenile dermatomyositis is a multisystem inflammatory disorder that involves the skin and muscles.

Etiology and Incidence

Dermatomyositis is the least common of the collagen vascular diseases and rarely begins before the second year of life. The cause of this disorder is unknown. Most believe dermatomyositis is an immunologically mediated disorder. Both cellular and humoral (immune deposits in the vessel walls and increased circulating immune complexes) mechanisms have been described. In contrast to the adult disease, vasculitis is a major pathologic finding in childhood dermatomyositis. HLA-B8 antigen is present in more than 70% of children in some studies.

Clinical Features

The dermatologic features are characteristic in most cases. Heliotrope rash (violaceous discoloration of the upper eyelids and periorbital skin with edema) is quite common and is the presenting sign in 75% of cases. Scaling and erythema of the knuckles are frequent findings (Figure 12-5-1). Following resolution of the inflammatory phase, flat-topped violaceous papules and atrophic scars appear on the interphalangeal joints (Gottron papules). Erythema and scaling are also present on the elbows, knees, and malleoli. Calcification of the skin frequently (20% to 60% of cases) complicates the course of the disease (Plate 12-5-1). Calcinosis cutis can lead to breakdown of the skin and ulcerations. Other skin findings include facial edema, butterfly rash, ulcerations of the fingertips, photosensitivity, violaceous changes over the upper trunk and upper extremities, periungual erythema, and telangiectasias. Postinflammatory hypo- and/or hyperpigmentation may be prominent. The skin may have a shiny appearance and feel edematous (nonpitting).

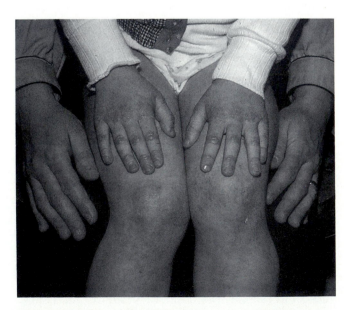

12-5-1 DERMATOMYOSITIS: Erythema and scaling of a child's knuckles and knees.

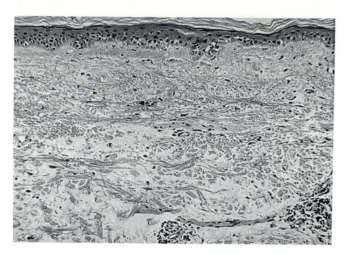

12-5-2 DERMATOMYOSITIS: Partial effacement of the rete ridge pattern, subepidermal vacuolation, and prominent separation of collagen bundles by mucin. (40×)

In contrast to adults, children with dermatomyositis have a greater incidence of atrophy, contractures, calcifications, and gastrointestinal involvement (dysphagia, malabsorption). Children rarely have Raynaud's phenomenon and associated malignancies. Systems involved in addition to the skeletal system are the pulmonary (restrictive) and cardiac (myocarditis, arrhythmias) systems.

Differential Diagnosis
Systemic lupus erythematosus
Scleroderma
Mixed connective tissue disease
Other vasculitides

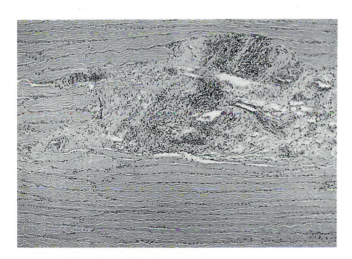

12-5-3 DERMATOMYOSITIS: Inflammation of skeletal muscle, causing fragmentation and degeneration of muscle bundles. (40×)

HISTOLOGICAL DESCRIPTION

The histological features in dermatomyositis vary from a non-specific perivascular inflammation and dermal edema to epidermal atrophy with discrete liquefaction degeneration of the basal cells and increased ground substance (mucin) in the dermis (Figure 12-5-2). Fibrinoid deposition can occur in droplet form as well as being linear at the basement membrane. Inflammatory change gives way to epidermal atrophy; lichenoid inflammation is manifested clinically by poikiloderma. Essentially the changes seen in the skin in dermatomyositis are similar to those seen in other collagen vascular diseases, in particular lupus erythematosus. The papular lesions of the extremities (Gottron papules) show changes similar to those described above with epidermal hyperplasia.

Muscle changes vary, as in the skin, from sparse to severe inflammation with fragmentation and degeneration of muscle bundles. Hyperplasia of the skeletal muscle nuclei, altered staining of muscle bundles, loss of muscle striations, and a perivascular lymphohistiocytic inflammatory infiltrate (Figure 12-5-3) can be seen. Muscle biopsies are best performed on symptomatic muscles. Currently, magnetic resonance imaging studies are used in some centers to localize inflammatory changes and target areas best to biopsy. Sampling for histologic studies should be performed before electromyographic studies to avoid artifactual alterations in tissue.

12-6 DYSKERATOSIS CONGENITA

CLINICAL DESCRIPTION

This genetic disorder is seen infrequently. The major findings are reticular skin pigmentation, nail dystrophy, and leukokeratosis.

Etiology and Incidence
Less than sixty cases of dyskeratosis congenita have been reported in the literature. This genetic disorder is inherited via an autosomal recessive mode. There is some question as to whether transmission is X-linked because of the predominance of males with this disorder. The classic changes generally appear in the first decade of life.

Clinical Features
A reticular gray-brown pattern very similar to poikiloderma appears on the face, neck, and trunk. The nails fail to reach the distal margin of the digits and are dystrophic. White patches appear on the buccal mucosa (leukokeratosis). Erosions and blisters may appear. Hyperkeratosis of the palms and soles is also found. About 50% of patients develop an

aplasticlike pancytopenia. Some patients present with thrombocytopenia as the first finding in this disease.

Differential Diagnosis
Fanconi's syndrome
Pachyonychia congenita

HISTOLOGICAL DESCRIPTION

The histological changes in dyskeratosis congenita vary depending on the lesion studied. Atrophic lesions show epidermal atrophy with basal layer liquefaction degeneration, dermal melanophage pigmentation, and a perivascular infiltrate of lymphocytes about dermal vessels. The retiform areas of hyperpigmentation show pigment laden melanophages with lymphocytic inflammation and superficial telangiectasia.

Differential Diagnosis
Postinflammatory hyperpigmentation
Fixed drug eruption

12-7 EPIDERMAL NEVUS AND NEVUS SEBACEUS SYNDROMES

CLINICAL DESCRIPTION

Epidermal nevus syndrome and nevus sebaceus syndrome are grouped together because of their great similarity. Both involve nevi (generally extensive) that are associated with skeletal and central nervous system abnormalities.

Etiology and Incidence
The exact incidence of these disorders is unknown, but it is unlikely that they occur with great frequency. Their etiology has not been defined.

Clinical Features
In the epidermal nevus syndrome, a major feature is a verrucous, pigmented lesion of varying size and distribution. The nevus may be unilateral and extensive or systematized (streaming over the entire body). Some lesions are whorled. Almost any portion of the skin surface may be involved (Figure 12-7-1). The skin lesions may be present at birth or develop and extend at any time after birth.

In the nevus sebaceus syndrome there are velvety or verrucous lesions that frequently involve the scalp and/or face. These lesions are present at birth and are flat, hairless skin areas of varying size (generally large) that are yellow to orange in color. Often the lesion involves the midline of the face in a linear fashion. Secondary tumors (including basal cell epitheliomas) may develop within the nevus during puberty in 10% to 15% of children. A lipodermoid of the conjunctiva may be associated.

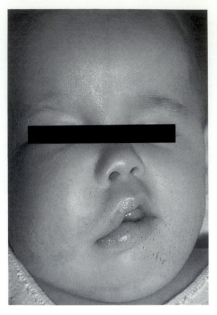

12-7-1 EPIDERMAL NEVUS SYNDROME: Raised tan epidermal nevus on left side of face of child with hemihypertrophy and seizures.

Both types of nevi are associated with skeletal (e.g., kyphoscoliosis, vertebral defects, short limbs) and central nervous system (brain tumors, especially astrocytomas, hydrocephaly, mental retardation, seizures) abnormalities.

Differential Diagnosis
Linear inflammatory epidermal nevus
Ichthyosis hystrix
Lichen striatus
Linear lichen planus
Linear psoriasis
Aplasia cutis congenita
Alopecia areata

HISTOLOGICAL DESCRIPTION

Epidermal Nevus
The histological features of localized and systemic epidermal nevis are orthohyperkeratosis, acanthosis, papillomatosis, and lymphohistiocytic inflammatory infiltrate about dermal vessels. The features may resemble those of the seborrheic keratosis and are frequently diagnosed as such when there is no clinical history. Unlike seborrheic keratosis, however, this condition does not show significant keratin tunnels or cysts. Epithelial alterations in epidermal nevi include dyskeratotic cells, corps rounds, and grains; and/or include epidermolytic hyperkeratosis.

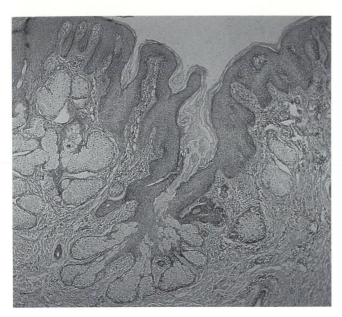

12-7-2 NEVUS SEBACEUS: Prominent papillomatosis and moderate acanthosis of the epidermis associated with large numbers of sebaceous lobules in the subjacent dermis. Note aberrant opening of sebaceous ducts directly onto the surface. (40×)

Nevus Sebaceus

The histological features of nevus sebaceus depend on the time in the patient's life it was biopsied. The usual features are (1) the presence of large mature sebaceous glands and sebaceous follicles; (2) epidermal hyperplasia (Figure 12-7-2); (3) papillomatosis, with the papillary dermis showing a less fibrillar pattern; (4) rudimentary hair germ structures; (5) dilated apocrine glands in the lower dermis; and (6) sometimes an associated syringocystadenoma papilliferum and/or basal cell carcinoma.

In newborns, features one through four will be present. In childhood through the prepubertal years, features one through four will have diminished and the histological features will not be characteristic. In the postpubertal years, all of the features will have developed, with feature six being the variable.

Differential Diagnosis

Epidermal Nevus
Darier's disease
Congenital ichthyosiform erythroderma
Papilloma
Verruca
Seborrheic keratosis

Nevus Sebaceus
Epithelial nevus
Sebaceous hyperplasia

12-8 JUVENILE RHEUMATOID ARTHRITIS

CLINICAL DESCRIPTION

Dermatologic findings are generally associated with the systemic form of juvenile rheumatoid arthritis, which is categorized as one of the connective tissue diseases.

Etiology and Incidence

Estimates are that 250,000 children in the United States have juvenile rheumatoid arthritis. Five percent of all cases begin in childhood, usually after two years of age, with two peaks, the first between two and four years of age and the second at adolescence (in females).

Although the etiology of juvenile rheumatoid arthritis is unknown, it is thought to be immunologically mediated. The trigger for this immune mechanism may be an infectious agent as yet unidentified.

Clinical Features

The dermatologic features include an evanescent rash (in up to 50% of patients), subcutaneous nodules (up to 10%), and cuticular telangiectasias (15%). The skin eruption is seen most commonly during a fever spike. The small macules or papules are salmon-colored. Frequently there is central clearing and circumferential pallor (Figure 12-8-1). The rash is found mostly on the trunk and proximal extremities, but any body surface, including the palms and soles, may be involved.

Subcutaneous nodules vary in size from a few millimeters to several centimeters. They are subcutaneous and found

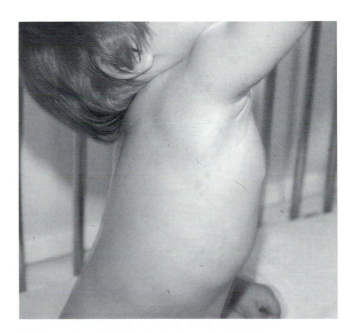

12-8-1 JUVENILE RHEUMATOID ARTHRITIS: Evanescent truncal eruption (erythematous macules with central clearing).

mostly on extensor surfaces (e.g., forearm, near the elbow, back of the hands, knees). They are asymptomatic.

Under magnification tortuous capillaries can be identified in the cuticles. These changes are the same as those seen in other collagen vascular disorders.

Differential Diagnosis
Viral exanthem
Drug reaction
Other collagen vascular diseases
Traumatically induced subcutaneous nodule

HISTOLOGICAL DESCRIPTION

Erythematous Eruption
The histological features of erythematous eruption (rheumatoid neutrophilic dermatitis) are perivascular lymphocytic infiltration with a sparse reaction about the follicular structures (Plate 12-8-1). The infiltrate consists of lymphocytes with fragmented neutrophils (Figure 12-8-2). There is distinct papillary dermal edema. Later in the evolution of this process there is exocytosis of lymphocytes into spongiotic foci of the epidermis associated with the formation of overlying parakeratosis.

Rheumatoid Nodules
The striking histological feature in rheumatoid nodules is a deep-seated zone of fibrinoid (eosinophilic) necrosis in the dermis. A palisaded array of histiocytes and lymphocytes surrounds such areas, outlining them in tissue (Figure 12-8-3). Rheumatoid nodules differ from deep-seated granuloma annulare in the extent of the necrosis and the absence of eosinophils, which can often be found in deep granuloma annulare.

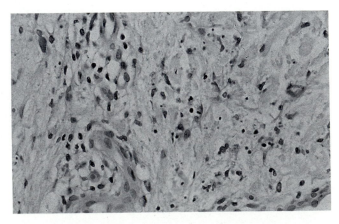

12-8-2 JUVENILE RHEUMATOID ARTHRITIS: The infiltrate is composed of lymphocytes and fragmented neutrophils. (400×)

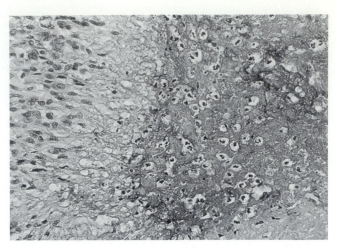

12-8-3 JUVENILE RHEUMATOID ARTHRITIS: A radial array of histiocytes surrounds a zone of fibrinoid necrosis. (100×)

Differential Diagnosis
Persistent erythema
Deep granuloma annulare
Necrobiosis lipoidica
Beryllium granuloma

12-9 LUPUS ERYTHEMATOSUS

CLINICAL DESCRIPTION

Neonatal, discoid, subacute, and systemic lupus erythematosus are discussed here.

Etiology and Incidence
Systemic lupus erythematosus (SLE) in pediatric patients is not uncommon. Twenty percent of patients have the onset of SLE in childhood, generally in adolescence. The other lupus subtypes occur less frequently. A female predominance exists for all types.

There is a genetic predisposition to lupus, but the etiology has not been ascertained. An autoimmune basis is presumed. Drugs (e.g., Dilantin, sulfonamides) have been known to precipitate a lupuslike syndrome without renal manifestations. Neonatal lupus is passively transferred from women who test positive for the antinuclear anti-Ro (SSA) or anti-La (SSB) antibodies.

Clinical Features
Eighty percent of patients with SLE eventually have skin manifestations. These dermatologic changes are numerous and in most cases represent the effects of vasculitides. Twenty-five percent present with one of these skin findings. More than thirty percent of patients have malar erythema and scaling (butterfly rash) (Plate 12-9-1). Interphalangeal

erythema and scaling, periungual erythema and telangiectases, and macular erythema of the palms and soles are all common findings. Local infarcts and ulcerations of the skin can occur. Photosensitivity, Raynaud's phenomenon, livedo vasculitis, and numerous membrane ulcerations all occur. Violaceous plaques, individual urticarial lesions lasting more than twenty-four hours, and scarring alopecia are seen. Thinning of hair has also been described.

Discoid lesions are well-demarcated plaques that vary in color from red to purple and have adherent scales. Areas of atrophy, telangiectasia, and dilated plugged follicular pores are present.

Subacute lupus is very rarely seen in childhood. The findings are much the same as in adults: photosensitivity, erythematous, scaling lesions similar to those seen in psoriasis (in a photodistribution), and annular polycyclic coalescent lesions on sun-exposed surfaces (extensor).

Two-thirds of neonatal lupus patients are born with skin changes, which may be macules, macular erythematous patches, or rings. The lesions display atrophy (80%), scaling (60%), telangiectasis (33%), follicular plugging (15%), and hypo- and hyperpigmentation (20%). Skin changes are distributed on the face (around the eyes), scalp, neck, and upper chest and are only rarely generalized. The lesions fade by the time the infant is six to twelve months of age.

Differential Diagnosis

Any collagen vascular disease
Rheumatic fever
Neonatal lupus:
   Bloom's syndrome
   Rothmund-Thomson syndrome
   Cockayne's syndrome

HISTOLOGICAL DESCRIPTION

The histological findings in all varieties of lupus erythematosus have common features, varying in severity.

Discoid Lupus Erythematosus

Discoid lupus erythematosus has distinct features of hyperkeratosis, follicular hyperkeratosis (follicular plugging), epidermal atrophy, and liquefaction degeneration of basal cells (Plate 12-9-2). In persistent/long standing lesions the basement membrane is thickened and tortuous. The papillary dermis is edematous and there is almost always an increase in ground substance (hyaluronic acid) in the reticular dermis (Figure 12-9-1). There is always a perivascular lymphocytic infiltrate. The adnexal structures show a variable degree of inflammation, often found about the dermal sweat gland coils. The features seen in discoid lupus erythematosus vary; not all features are seen in all cases. However, the increased ground substance and perivascular inflammation are consistent find-

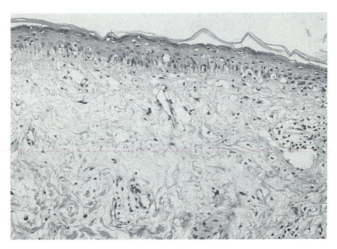

12-9-1 DISCOID LUPUS ERYTHEMATOSUS: Prominent effacement of the rete ridge pattern and interstitial mucin deposition. These changes are seen after inflammation subsides. (100×)

ings. Neonatal lupus shows histologic findings similar to those of discoid or subacute cutaneous lupus erythematosus, but they may be much more subtle. In such cases direct immunofluorescence studies may be helpful since they show positive band test findings in lesional skin in approximately fifty percent of patients.

Subacute Lupus Erythematosus

Subacute lupus erythematosus often shows more epidermal involvement than discoid and has features more in common with systemic lupus erythematosus. As in discoid lupus, there are ground substance changes in the reticular dermis and a perivascular lymphocytic inflammatory infiltrate. Hyperkeratosis and follicular hyperkeratosis are not prominent features in subacute lupus. There is marked necrosis of basilar keratinocyte and loss of the normal rete ridge pattern. Because of the marked vacuolar degeneration in subacute lupus, dermalepidermal separation often occurs on sections, and this change can be confused with bullous dermatoses. Colloid bodies are also commonly found in subacute lupus. Adnexal involvement is variable but less than that seen in discoid lupus erythematosus.

Systemic Lupus Erythematosus

Systemic lupus erythematosus shows minimal histological features early on, including edema of the papillary dermis, rare necrotic epidermal cells, and sparse to rare vacuolar degeneration of the basal cell layer. This change resembles alterations in graft versus host disease. Dermal vessels may show a sparse perivascular infiltrate of lymphocytes. In systemic lupus erythematosus fibrinoid can sometimes be found deposited between collagen bundles, staining distinctly eosinophilic and periodic acid-Schiff-positive. There can be an

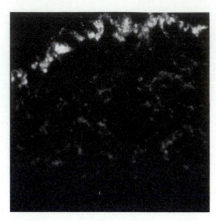

12-9-2 LUPUS ERYTHEMATOSUS: Positive lupus band test: variably sized granular deposits of IgG along the epidermal-dermal junction. (100×)

inflammatory infiltrate at the dermal subcutaneous junction, with a significant increase in hyaluronic acid in this area. This change is similar to that seen in lupus profundus but is less severe.

Immunofluorescence Findings

In involved skin, granular IgG, IgM, IgA, and C_3 can be seen at the dermal-epidermal junction as well as about dermal vessels. In systemic lupus immunoreactant deposits can be found in clinically uninvolved (non-lesional) skin in up to 80% of cases (Figure 12-9-2).

Differential Diagnosis

Graft versus host disease
Lichen planus
Erythema multiforme
Polymorphous light eruption

12-10 MIXED CONNECTIVE TISSUE DISEASE

CLINICAL DESCRIPTION

This collagen vascular disorder seems to be a combination of systemic lupus erythematosus, dermatomyositis, scleroderma, and juvenile rheumatoid arthritis.

Etiology and Incidence

Mixed connective tissue disease is very rare in childhood and is seen almost exclusively in adolescence. Its cause is unknown.

Clinical Features

The clinical features are described in the individual sections describing the other collagen vascular diseases (see dermato-

myositis, scleroderma, SLE). The diagnosis is made serologically by finding an anti-RNP titer greater than 1:1,000.

Differential Diagnosis

Any of the collagen vascular diseases

HISTOLOGICAL DESCRIPTION

The histological findings in mixed connective tissue disease depend on the clinical manifestation of the condition. If the changes seen are mainly those of scleroderma, the histological features of that condition are manifested. If the clinical manifestations are mainly those of lupus erythematosus, the histological features will be those of lupus erythematosus. The histological features of these entities are described under each condition.

Differential Diagnosis

Any of the collagen vascular diseases

12-11 MUCOSAL NEUROMA SYNDROME

CLINICAL DESCRIPTION

Etiology and Incidence

Mucosal neuroma syndrome (multiple adenomatosis syndrome; MEA 2B) is an autosomal-dominant disorder that is rare in childhood. Its cause is unknown.

Clinical Features

Affected individuals have unusual appearing facies with protuberant fleshy lips (upper greater than lower) and a marfanoid habitus. Pedunculated, pink nodules are present early in life (at times in newborns) on the tip and anterior half of the tongue. Patients have intestinal ganglioneuromatosis, medullary thyroid cancer, parathyroid adenomas, and pheochromocytomas.

Differential Diagnosis

Other multiple endocrine adenomatosis syndromes

HISTOLOGICAL DESCRIPTION

The cutaneous neuromas in this condition show in the dermis large bundles of cutaneous nerves without a capsule. There is no associated inflammatory infiltrate. The histological findings of large bundles of nerves within a somewhat fibrocellular dermis are similar to those in traumatic neuromas and accessory digits. Usually the epidermis reflects the site of the biopsy; that is, those on the mucosa show mucosal epithilium and those on the extremities show extremity skin. Thus, bundles of cutaneous nerves are found in various anatomic locations in mucosal neuroma syndrome.

Differential Diagnosis
Accessory digit
Traumatic neuroma
Idiopathic neuroma

12-12 NECROBIOSIS LIPOIDICA DIABETICORUM

CLINICAL DESCRIPTION

Although this skin finding is found in association with diabetes mellitus, at times it can be an isolated skin change.

Etiology and Incidence
Necrobiosis lipoidica diabeticorum is seen in childhood. It occurs in less than 0.5% of all patients with diabetes. There is a predilection for females.

Vascular occlusion seems to be associated with the dermal changes seen in this disorder. Its exact etiology is unknown, but some association with trauma is suspected.

Clinical Features
Necrobiosis lipoidica diabeticorum begins with erythematous macules that enlarge into plaques. There is gradual discoloration and atrophy of the skin (Plate 12-12-1). The expanding border remains violaceous. The end result is a waxy, red-yellow, translucent atrophic plaque with vessels traversing its surface. These lesions are susceptible to breakdown and ulceration. The skin changes occur over the pretibial area in most instances, but any skin surface maybe involved.

Differential Diagnosis
Amyloidosis
Scleroderma
Morphea
Pretibial myxedema
Acrodermatitis atrophicans chronica

HISTOLOGICAL DESCRIPTION

Necrobiosis lipoidica diabeticorum shows a zone of necrobiosis in the reticular dermis that extends to the subcutaneous junction and is often broad-based and diffuse. The zones of collagen alteration often take on a "layer cake" appearance as seen with low magnification. The intervening collagen bundles are often sclerotic and thickened and extend into the areas of necrobiosis (Plate 12-2-2). Necrosis can occur but is not a consistent feature. At the margins of the necrobiotic area are palisades of histiocytes and lymphocytes as well as plasma cells (Figure 12-12-1).

Often, the epidermis is thinned and effaced and the papillary dermis is edematous with vascular prominence. The palisade of inflammatory cells in this condition may be

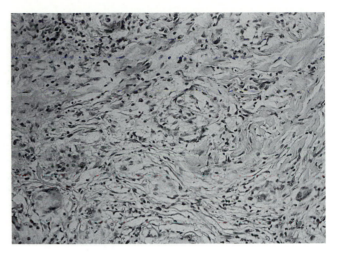

12-12-1 NECROBIOSIS LIPOIDICA DIABETICORUM: Infiltrate composed of lymphocytes, plasma cells, and lipidized histiocytes, some of which are multinucleated. (200×)

marked, with the presence of many histiocytes and multinucleated giant cells. This reaction can be so prominent as to almost obscure the areas of necrobiosis. This has been called a granulomatous stage of necrobiosis lipoidica and may represent a later stage in the evolution of this process.

Differential Diagnosis
Rheumatoid nodule
Deep granuloma annulare
Foreign body with granuloma formation

12-13 NEVUS ACHROMICUS

CLINICAL DESCRIPTION

This lesion represents a nevoid type of hypopigmentation.

Etiology and Incidence
The exact etiology and incidence have not been determined.

Clinical Features
At birth there are fixed areas of hypopigmentation (Figure 12-13-1). The area of involvement varies from small patches to large segments. Involvement is frequently truncal and unilateral but may be bilateral or swirling. Due to its association with mental retardation and hemihypertrophy, this lesion may be confused with Ito's hypomelanosis.

Differential Diagnosis
Incontinentia pigmenti
Nevus anemicus
Vitiligo
Piebaldism

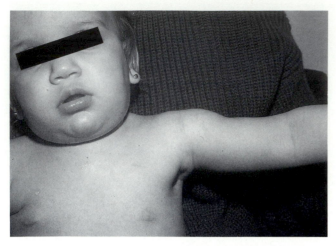

12-13-1 NEVUS ACHROMICUS: Depigmented area on a child's shoulder and chest. Erythema and edema secondary to scratching (triple response of Lewis) differentiates achromic nevus from nevus anemicus (negative response).

Waardenburg syndrome
Albinism

HISTOLOGICAL DESCRIPTION

On a single biopsy specimen without comparative normal skin, a diagnosis of nevus achromicus is difficult if not impossible to make. Only sparse inflammation about dermal vessels and the absence of pigment in the basal cell zone suggest the diagnosis, although pigment granules can be seen in some keratinocytes. Fresh dopa-stained tissue shows a diminution or absence of functional melanocytes in the epidermis when compared to uninvolved skin.

Differential Diagnosis
Vitiligo

12-14 PEUTZ-JEGHERS SYNDROME

CLINICAL DESCRIPTION

The skin findings in Peutz-Jeghers (lentigines) are a marker of systemic disease (intestinal polyps).

Etiology and Incidence
This syndrome is inherited via autosomal dominant transmission. Ninety-six percent of polyps occur in the small intestine. Two to 6% are malignant.

Clinical Features
Lentigines are noted by two years of age. They are found on the lips (Plate 12-14-1), perioral and periorbital skin, buccal mucosa, perianal and labial skin, dorsum of the fingers or toes,

and, rarely, the tongue. Lentigines on the tongue in black patients must be distinguished from the normal pigmentation of the papillae. When examining relatives it is best to look at the mucous membranes for pigmented lesions because the lentigines on the lips and skin may disappear following puberty.

Polyps may be found in any gastrointestinal location but are most numerous in the small intestine. Children frequently present with abdominal pain and/or intussusception.

Differential Diagnosis
LEOPARD syndrome
Normal lentigines
Normal tongue pigmentation in black patients

HISTOLOGICAL DESCRIPTION

The histological findings are epidermal hyperplasia with elongated rete in which there is striking basal layer pigmentation (Plate 12-14-2). The papillary dermis may show melanophage pigmentation without significant inflammation. There is no increase in the number of melanocytes in this condition, only that of increased function, as confirmed by dopa-stained fresh tissue.

Differential Diagnosis
Lentigo of other causes
Freckles

12-15 PYODERMA GANGRENOSUM

CLINICAL DIAGNOSIS

In pyoderma gangrenosum there are painful ulcerations of unknown cause that have a characteristic appearance.

Etiology and Incidence
This finding is rare in childhood and is mainly seen during adolescence. Its etiology is unknown but it is thought to be immunologically mediated, at times associated with a vasculitis. It is frequently associated with ulcerative colitis, granulomatous colitis, leukemia, chronic active hepatitis, rheumatoid arthritis, systemic lupus erythematosus, and various paraproteinemias.

Clinical Features
The lesions begin as an erythematous tender papule with surrounding erythema. Enlargement and ulceration ensue. The ulcers have red-purple borders that are raised and tender (Figure 12-15-1). The ulcer base is red, granular, and covered by a purulent exudate. Scarring of involved skin is common. Although the lesions may involve any part of the skin surface, the lower legs are most commonly involved.

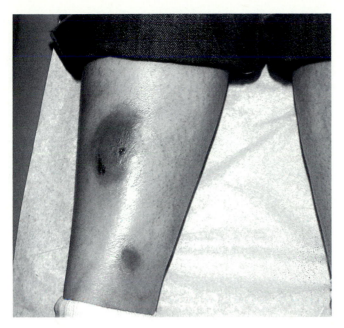

12-15-1 PYODERMA GANGRENOSUM: Child with inflammatory bowel disease.

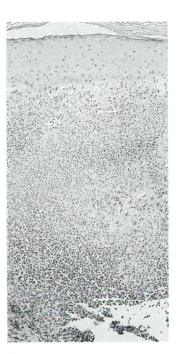

A   B

12-15-2 PYODERMA GANGRENOSUM: (A) Low power shows a deep ulcer. (20×) (B) Higher magnification shows the infiltrate adjacent to the ulcer. The infiltrate is composed entirely of neutrophils. (100×)

Differential Diagnosis

Deep fungal infection
Atypical mycobacterial infection
Cryptococcosis
Amebiasis
Syphilis
Collagen vascular disease
Wegener's granulomatosis

HISTOLOGICAL DESCRIPTION

Pyoderma gangrenosum shows varying histological features, depending on the time of the biopsy within the evolution of this lesion. Early pyoderma gangrenosum may show histological features similar to those of Sweet's syndrome: dermal edema, a diffuse infiltration of neutrophils, and marked perivascular inflammation to the point of leukocytoclastic vasculitis. Other early lesions may show only a lymphocytic perivascular reaction. As the lesion progresses toward ulceration, the vascular changes are more pronounced, with fibrinoid necrosis of vessel walls, thrombosis, and vascular occlusion occurring superficially within the dermis. Ulceration shows all of the changes associated with an ulcer, including inflammation, hemorrhage, and a mixed inflammatory infiltrate. Abscess formation in this condition can occur prior to ulceration. At the base of the ulcer there is fibrosis and inflammation, which may extend to the subcutaneous fat (Figure 12-15-2).

Differential Diagnosis

Sweet's syndrome
Vasculitis
Infectious diseases

12-16 SARCOIDOSIS

CLINICAL DESCRIPTION

This chronic disorder affects many systems and seems to have two different modes of presentation.

Etiology and Incidence

Sarcoidosis occurs infrequently in childhood. Its exact incidence and prevalence is unknown. Most cases occur during adolescence, but a special form is found in children less than four years of age. Sarcoidosis is more common in blacks (75%) than whites (20%). However, affected children who are younger than four years are almost exclusively white. Most cases occur in the southeastern United States.

The geographic distribution of cases suggests that environmental factors are involved in the etiology. An immune dysfunction has also been hypothesized.

Clinical Features

Sarcoidosis involves the lungs, lymph nodes, and eyes in children older than four years and the skin (76%), eyes (58%), and joints (58%) in those younger than four years. Lung disease occurs much less frequently (22%) in the younger age group.

A wide variety of skin lesions may be found, therefore biopsy is very helpful in making the diagnosis. These lesions range from an erythematous scaling macular eruption to yellow-brown, flat-topped papules (Plate 12-16-1). There may be hypopigmented macules, hypertrophic scars, nodules, and infiltrated plaques. The face and extremities (Plate 12-16-2) are frequently involved, as are the neck and trunk.

Fifty percent or more of patients present with fever, weight loss, cough, abdominal pain, and rash. Those younger than four years of age most frequently present with rash, arthritis (simulating rheumatoid arthritis), and uveitis.

Differential Diagnosis
Blau syndrome (arthritis, uveitis, rash, synovial cysts)
Rheumatoid arthritis
Tuberculosis
Other granulomatous diseases

HISTOLOGICAL DESCRIPTION

Sarcoidosis has the same histological features in children as in adults. The classic features are epithelioid cell granulomas in the dermis with a variable infiltrate of lymphocytes (Figures 12-16-1 and 12-16-2). There appears to be a correlation between the age of the lesion and the amount of lymphocytic infiltrate (i.e., earlier lesions show the most pronounced amount of lymphocytic infiltrate about and within the epithelioid nodules). Older lesions show less inflammation, increased numbers of giant cells, and dermal fibrosis. Caseation of the epithelioid nodules is rare but can occur. Epithelioid nodules are of varying size, usually rounded, and found randomly distributed in the dermis, in contrast to granulomas of leprosy, which follow the neurovascular bundles and are more elongated in appearance.

Differential Diagnosis
Infectious granulomas
Tuberculoid leprosy

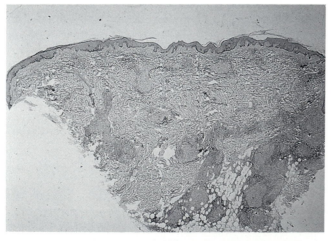

12-16-1 SARCOIDOSIS: Prominent perivascular granulomas in the superficial and deep reticular dermis, as in adipose tissue. (40×)

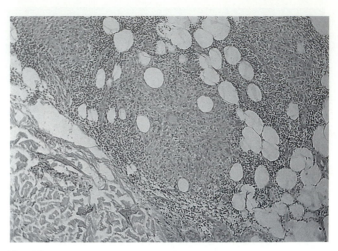

12-16-2 SARCOIDOSIS: The infiltrate is composed of collections of epithelioid histiocytes surrounded by variable numbers of lymphocytes. (200×)

Beryllium granuloma
Lupus vulgaris
Foreign body granuloma

12-17 SCLERODERMA

CLINICAL DESCRIPTION

There are two forms of scleroderma: localized or linear (morphea) and systemic.

Etiology and Incidence
Scleroderma is uncommon in childhood. As in the adult disease, females predominate in the childhood forms. This collagen vascular disease is of unknown etiology. Genetic, vascular, and immunologic mechanisms have been hypothesized.

Clinical Features
The localized form is generally benign and resolves spontaneously. When skin over joints is involved, contractures must be prevented. The earliest changes include erythematous or violaceous plaques that gradually enlarge. The central portion of the lesion becomes firm, yellow-white to white, waxy, and indurated (Plate 12-17-1A). The border remains violaceous as it expands. Lesions vary in size and shape (guttate, plaque, generalized, and linear). Linear lesions can involve the limbs and scalp (coup de sabre). Progression to facial hemiatrophy (Parry-Romberg syndrome) (Plate 12-17-1B) can occur. In the latter syndrome the ipsilateral tongue atrophies as well (Plate 12-17-1C).

The presenting signs of systemic scleroderma include induration of the skin, subcutaneous calcifications, Raynaud's

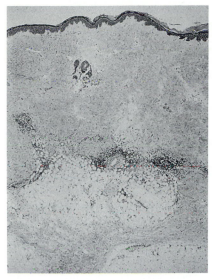

A

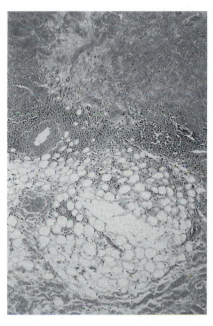

B

12-17-1 MORPHEA: (A) Low magnification shows mononuclear inflammatory infiltrate at the dermal subcutaneous interface. (20×) (B) The inflammatory infiltrate is composed of lymphocytes and plasma cells. There is swollen, homogenous eosinophilic collagen. (200×)

phenomenon, contractures, joint complaints, dysphagia, dyspnea, and muscle weakness. The most common finding is waxy, nonpliable thickening of the skin of the trunk, which extends to the extremities (Plates 12-17-1D and 12-17-1E). The skin on the face becomes tight and smooth. Pinched nose, pursed lips, and a stare leads to a fixed facial expression. The skin on the hands becomes smooth and the fingers contracted. Other findings include ulceration of the fingertips,

subcutaneous calcifications, hypo- and hyperpigmentation, and telangiectasias (cuticular, hands and feet, generalized at times).

Although Raynaud's phenomenon is uncommon in childhood, children with systemic scleroderma frequently present with this condition.

Differential Diagnosis

Vitiligo
Macular atrophy
Lichen sclerosis et atrophicus
Atrophoderma of Pasini and Pierini
Dermatomyositis
Eosinophilic fascitis
Scleredema
Stiff-skin syndrome
Myositis ossificans progressiva

HISTOLOGICAL DESCRIPTION

Scleroderma and morphea have similar histological features and are described as one condition. The inflammatory stage of both shows, at the dermal subcutaneous junction, an infiltrate of lymphocytes that extends into the subcutaneous fat. The septae of the panniculus are thickened and contain a similar inflammatory infiltrate, mainly lymphocytes, although plasma cells can be seen (Figure 12-17-1). New collagen formation occurs at the lower reticular dermis and replaces the fat. The reticular dermis in the inflammatory stage also shows a brisk perivascular lymphocytic infiltrate. As the condition progresses the inflammatory stage passes into the sclerotic stage. The inflammatory infiltrate disappears. Collagen bundles are less cellular and less fibrillar. Follicular structures are absent or present only as remnants. Eccrine gland coils are located high in the dermis, are atrophic and are surrounded by less adipose tissue than is usual. The adipose tissue is replaced to a great extent by new collagen.

Differential Diagnosis

Late radiation change

12-18 SINUS HISTIOCYTOSIS WITH MASSIVE LYMPHADENOPATHY

CLINICAL DESCRIPTION

When sinus histiocytosis with massive lymphadenopathy is seen in children, dermatological findings are likely to be present.

Etiology and Incidence

This rare disorder has no known etiology. An infectious or immunologic disturbance has been hypothesized. Blacks seem more susceptible, especially those in Africa and the West Indies. The course is benign and self-limited.

Clinical Features

Bilateral, painless, massive cervical lymphadenopathy is the most striking feature of this disorder. One study reported skin findings in seven of ten affected children. Singular or multiple papules or nodules (some as large as 4 cm in diameter) having a xanthomatous appearance may be found on any skin surface.

Other findings include fever, leukocytosis, polyclonal hypergammaglobulinemia, and elevated sedimentation rate. Any of the other lymph node chains may be involved. It is rare to have only skin findings.

Differential Diagnosis

Malignant lymphoma
Hodgkin's disease
Malignant reticuloendotheliosis
Dermatofibroma
Juvenile xanthogranuloma
Other xanthomatous disorder

HISTOLOGICAL DESCRIPTION

The epidermal changes vary from thinning and atrophy to acanthosis to parakeratosis. The skin nodules have a well-circumscribed dense infiltrate of cells, which can involve the entire thickness of the dermis. The cellular infiltrate is composed of inflammatory cells, the striking cell being a large histiocyte with abundant cytoplasm and a large vesicular nucleus. Some histiocytes may be multinucleated and exhibit the features of Touton giant cells. Within the infiltrate there are, in varying numbers, eosinophils, plasma cells, and neutrophils. The presence of these latter inflammatory cells within the infiltrate is not consistent and their numbers are variable. Lymphocytophagocytosis and plasmacytophagocytosis occur in this condition.

Differential Diagnosis

Xanthogranuloma
Xanthoma
Dermatofibroma (histiocytic type)
Histiocytosis X
Reticulohistiocytic granuloma

12-19 SWEET'S SYNDROME

CLINICAL DESCRIPTION

Sweet's syndrome (acute febrile neutrophilic dermatosis) is a reactive phenomenon that has been reported infrequently in the pediatric age group. It may indicate the presence of another serious systemic disorder.

Etiology and Incidence

Sweet's syndrome has been reported only rarely in childhood. One patient reported was three months of age. Most speculate that the skin changes associated with this disorder represent a reactive phenomenon to infection or a malignant or premalignant condition.

Clinical Features

The major skin changes are tender, painful erythematous or violaceous plaques or nodules. The plaques may be studded with vesicles or pustules. Frequently, the plaques have raised annular margins with a semitranslucent appearance (Plate 12-19-1). At times there is central clearing or crusting. The lesions vary in size (up to 4 cm in diameter) and may coalesce as they expand. The face, neck, and forearms are most heavily involved, but any skin surface can be affected.

Associated findings include fever, arthralgias, conjunctivitis, leukocytosis (at times, 24,000/mm^3 or more), and elevated sedimentation rate. The disorder is frequently preceded by an infection or fever.

Differential Diagnosis

Erythema multiforme
Erythema annulare centrifugum
Erythema nodosum
Erythema elevatum diutinum
Granuloma faciale

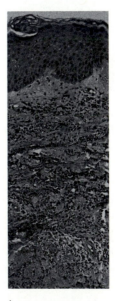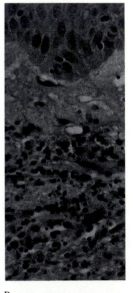

A   B

12-19-1 SWEET'S SYNDROME: (A) Papillary dermal edema and a brisk dermal inflammatory infiltrate. (20×) (B) The infiltrate is composed almost entirely of neutrophils. Note that the blood vessels appear intact. (200×)

Bromoderma
Bowel bypass syndrome

HISTOLOGICAL DESCRIPTION

This is a neutrophilic dermal reaction. The primary infiltrating cell is the neutrophil, although lymphocytes and histiocytes are present. The papillary dermis is markedly edematous, in many instances to the point of dermal-epidermal separation. Neutrophils are found diffusely in this edematous dermis and the infiltrate extends to the dermal-subcutaneous junction. Neutrophils are often fragmented (leukocytoclasia), although there is no vasculitis in this condition (Figure 12-19-1).

Differential Diagnosis

Early pyoderma gangrenosum
Erythema elevatum diutinum
Leukocytoclastic vasculitis

12-20 TOXIC SHOCK SYNDROME

CLINICAL DESCRIPTION

Toxic shock syndrome (TSS) is characterized by shock and a scarlatiniform eruption caused by toxins produced by *Staphylococcus aureus* or group A beta-hemolytic streptococci.

Etiology and Incidence

The exact incidence of this disorder in children is unknown, but 15% of cases are not related to menstruation and tampon use. The incidence in menstruating women is 6.2 per 100,000. Those cases not associated with tampon use usually result from colonization by a phage group-1 toxin-producing staphylococcal strain (e.g., abscesses, cellulitis, emphysema, osteomyelitis, wound infections, nasal packs for nosebleeds, rhinoplasty). Strains of *S. aureus* that cause TSS produce a marker protein (toxic shock toxin-1) responsible for nausea, vomiting, fever, rash, and desquamation. Group A beta-hemolytic streptococci produce pyrogenic toxins, (A, B, and C) which cause similar symptoms.

Clinical Features

Toxic shock syndrome begins suddenly with high fever, vomiting, and diarrhea. The patient complains of a sore throat, headache, and myalgias. A rash develops and within forty-eight hours the patient goes into shock.

Shortly after the onset of illness the patient develops a diffuse, erythematous maculopapular eruption (scarlatiniform) (Plate 12-20-1). Hyperemia of the mucous membranes (with or without strawberry tongue) follows in two to three days. Petechiae may appear toward the end of the first week. Desquamation of the hands and feet completes the dermatologic progression of events at one to two weeks.

Other findings include an elevated white cell count with a shift to the left, thrombocytopenia, disseminated intravascular coagulation, and elevated prothrombin time (PT) and partial thromboplastin time (PTT). Additional abnormalities include elevated blood urea nitrogen (BUN), creatinine, creatine kinase (CPK), serum glutamine oxaloacetic transaminase (SGOT), and serum glutamic pyruvic transaminase (SGPT). The serum calcium and phosphate may be decreased. Group A beta-hemolytic streptococci may be grown from blood cultures or soft tissue infections when this organism, rather than *S. aureus*, is involved.

Differential Diagnosis

Measles
Rocky Mountain spotted fever
Leptospirosis
Scarlet fever
Staphylococcal scalded skin syndrome
Erythema multiforme
Kawasaki's disease

HISTOLOGICAL DESCRIPTION

The histological features in toxic shock syndrome vary from a perivascular infiltrate of lymphocytes and papillary dermal edema to an infiltrate about blood vessels that consists of neutrophils and eosinophils as well as lymphocytes. There is exocytosis of neutrophils with the formation of spongiotic microvesicles in which neutrophils are seen within the foci of spongiosis, somewhat similar to the spongiform pustule. There can be marked papillary dermal edema in this condition, with the production of subepidermal bullae.

Differential Diagnosis

Sweet's syndrome
Erythema multiforme
Infection
Psoriasiform dermatoses

12-21 URTICARIA

CLINICAL DESCRIPTION

The clinical diagnosis of urticaria is generally easy, but determining the underlying etiology for this common disorder is time-consuming and frustrating.

Etiology and Incidence

Approximately 15% of individuals will experience at least one episode of urticaria during their lives. Exact figures for children are not available.

Basically, urticaria is due to vasodilation and transudation of fluid from small cutaneous vessels. This process may be mediated by immunologic or nonimmunologic factors.

The release of histamine from the mast cell can be triggered in either situation. Immunologically, type 1 reactions occur most frequently, followed by type III reactions. In general, immunologic mechanisms are involved more often in acute than in chronic urticaria. Nonimmunologic factors include chemical histamine liberators, direct effects of physical agents, and cholinergic effects.

Chronic urticaria in children is undiagnosed in 90% of cases but fortunately most improve without discovery of a serious underlying disorder. In one study that described an etiology for fifteen of ninety-four chronic urticaria patients, cold urticaria was most common, followed by infections, collagen vascular disease, food allergies, and a complement defect. The primary diagnostic tool continues to be a detailed history, with emphasis on precipitating events.

Clinical Features

Urticaria appears as white, edematous papules with a halo of erythema, both of varying size (Figure 12-21-1). Frequently the lesions have serpiginous borders, which enlarge and coalesce with other lesions, forming quite interesting patterns.

Urticaria may be acute (less than six weeks duration) or chonic (greater than six weeks duration). About one-third of cases are acute. Individual lesions rarely last longer than twelve to twenty-four hours. Lesions lasting more than twenty-four hours are generally due to the presence of an underlying vasculitis.

Differential Diagnosis

Table 12-21-1 lists the various causes of urticaria and some distinguishing characteristics.

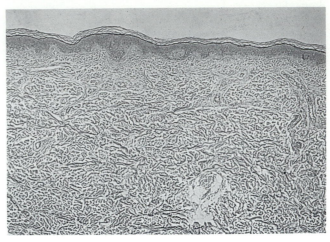

12-21-2 URTICARIA: Low-power view shows essentially normal epidermis and dermis. (20×)

HISTOLOGICAL DESCRIPTION

The histological features of urticaria are not specific. There is a perivascular inflammatory infiltrate of lymphocytes associated with dermal edema (Figure 12-21-2). Eosinophilia within the infiltrate is variable and not always present. The epidermis is usually uninvolved. In persistent urticarial plaques—those urticarial lesions that persist longer than twenty-four hours—neutrophils may be found in the inflammatory infiltrate about dermal vessels. There is also some endothelial swelling without a true vasculitis (Figure 12-21-3).

Differential Diagnosis

Chronic dermatoses

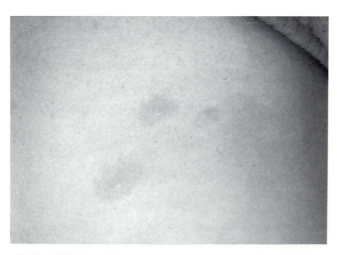

12-21-1 URTICARIA: Slightly raised erythematous plaques on the trunk.

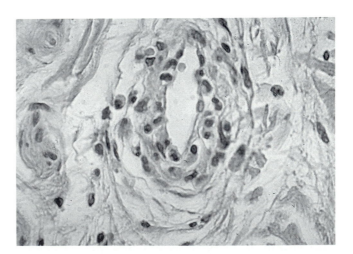

12-21-3 URTICARIA: Closer examination of venules shows migration of neutrophils across vessel walls. Note perivascular edema and eosinophils. (400×)

12-21-1 Causes of Urticaria

Condition	Facts to Consider
Drugs (ingested or injected)	Most common cause of recognized acute urticaria (e.g., penicillin); mediated by type I, type III, or directed degranulation of mast cells (e.g., morphine or codeine)
Foods	More important agent in acute urticaria; food additives frequently involved; skin test usually not helpful
Inhalant allergens	Usually occurs in atopics; IgE-mediated
Infections	Probably secondary to immunologic reactions to antigens introduced by organisms, parasites, viral hepatitis, etc.
Arthropod bites and stings	IgE-mediated
Penetrants and contactants	Not allergic contact dermatitis (e.g., aquagenic urticaria)
Internal diseases	Urticaria pigmentosa; urticaria may herald JRA, SLE (7–23% of cases)
Psychogenic factors	Can exacerbate urticaria but probably not cause it
Genetic abnormalities, hereditary angioedema	Accounts for less than 2% of all causes of angioedema; rarely these patients have urticaria; deficiency of C-1 esterase inhibitor; onset before 10 y, mottling of skin first sign; abdominal pain prominent; 25% have laryngeal obstruction; low levels of C_4 and C_2 at times; C_2 may be normal between attacks
Familial cold urticaria	Autosomal dominant; onset at 4–5 y; burning, nonpruritic urticaria; 0.5–3 h after cold exposure; leukocytosis
Physical agents	All last 30–60 min only
Dermographism	Most common of physical urticarias (8%); some cases IgE-mediated
Pressure urticaria	Frequently delayed in onset (4–6 h after pressure applied)
Cold urticaria	May be associated with cryoglobulins, cold hemolysins, etc.; frequently find purpura, livedo reticularis, and acral cyanosis
Heat urticaria	Immediate (minutes) or delayed (4–6 h) responses rare
Cholinergic urticaria	5–7% of all urticaria induced by heat, emotional states, or exercise; 1–3 mm wheals with large surrounding flares
Solar urticaria	Seen several minutes after exposure to sunlight; lasts 15–30 min.

REFERENCES

Acrodermatitis Enteropathica

Ackerman AB: Acrodermatitis enteropathica. In: Histologic diagnosis of inflammatory skin disease. Philadelphia: Lea & Febiger, 1978:512.

Gonzalez JR, Botet MV, Sanchez JL: The histopathology of acrodermatitis enteropathica. Am J Dermatopathol 1982; 4:303.

Moynahan EJ: Acrodermatitis enteropathica: A lethal inherited human zinc-deficiency disorder. Lancet 1974; 2:399.

Allergic Granulomatoses (Vasculitides)

Chumbley LC, Harrison EG Jr, Deremee RA: Allergic granulomatosis and angiitis (Churg-Strauss syndrome): Report and analysis of 30 cases. Mayo Clin Proc 1977; 52:477.

Chyu JYH, Hagstrow WJ, Soltani K, et al.: Wegener's granulomatosis in childhood: Cutaneous manifestations as the presenting sign. J Am Acad Dermatol 1984; 10:341.

Cupps TR, Favir AS: Wegener's granulomatosis. Int J Dermatol 1980; 19:76.

Finan MC, Winkelman RK: The cutaneous extravascular necrotizing granuloma (Churg-Strauss granuloma) and systemic disease: A review of 27 cases. Medicine (Baltimore) 1983; 62:142.

Jambrosie J, Frome L, Assano D, et al.: Lymphomatoid granulomatosis J Am Acad Dermatol 1987; 17:621.

James WD, Odom RB, Katzenstein ALA: Cutaneous manifestations of lymphomatoid granulomatosis. Arch Dermatol 1981; 117:196.

Annular Erythemas

Bressler GS, Jones RE Jr: Erythema annulare centrifugum. J Am Acad Dermatol 1981; 4:597.

Burla JB: Erythema marginatum. Arch Dis Child 1955; 30:359.

Hebert AA, Esterly NB: Annular erythema of infancy. J Am Acad Dermatol. 1986; 14:339.

Jones criteria (revised) for guidance in the diagnosis of rheumatic fever. Circulation 1965; 32:664.

Peterson AQ Jr, Jarratt M: Annular erythema of infancy. Arch Dermatol 1981; 117:142.

Troyer C, Grossman ME, Silvers DN: Erythema marginatum in rheumatic fever: Early diagnosis by skin biopsy. J Am Acad Dermatol 1983; 8:724.

Basal Cell Nevus Syndrome

Gutierrez MM, Mora RG: Nevoid basal cell carcinoma syndrome: A review and case report of a patient with unilateral basal cell nevus syndrome. J Am Acad Dermatol 1986; 15:1023.

Mason JK, Helwig EB, Graham JH: Pathology of the nevoid basal cell carcinoma syndrome. Arch Pathol 1965; 79:401.

Peck GL, Gross EG, Butkus D, DiGiovanna JJ: Chemoprevention of basal cell carcinoma with isotretinoin. J Am Acad Dermatol 1982; 6:815.

Dermatomyositis

Christianson HB, Brunsting LA, Perry HO: Dermatomyositis. Arch Dermatol 1956; 74:581.

Hanno R, Callen JP: Histopathology of Gottron's papules. J Cutan Pathol 1985; 12:389.

Janis JF, Winkelman RK: Histopathology of the skin in dermatomyositis. Arch Dermatol 1968; 97:640.

Taieb A, Guichard C, Salamon R, et al.: Prognosis in juvenile dermatopolymyositis: A cooperative retrospective study of 70 cases. Pediatr Dermatol 1985; 2:275.

Dyskeratosis Congenita

Sirinavin C, Trawbridge AA: Dyskeratosis congenita: Clinical features and genetic aspects—Report of a family and review of the literature. J Med Genet 1975; 12:339.

Tchou PK, Kohn T: Dyskeratosis congenita: An autosomal dominant disorder. J Am Acad Dermatol 1982; 6:1034.

Epidermal Nevus and Nevus Sebaceus Syndrome

Clancy RR, Kartz MB, Baker D, et al.: Neurologic manifestations of the organoid nevus syndrome. Arch Neurol 1985; 42:236.

Domingo J, Helwig EB: Malignant neoplasms associated with nevus sebaceous of Jadassohn. J Am Acad Dermatol 1979; 1:545.

Lentz CL, Altman J, Mopper C: Nevus sebaceus of Jadassohn. Arch Dermatol 1968; 97:294.

Moskowitz R, Honig PJ: Nevus sebaceous in association with an intracranial mass. J Am Acad Dermatol 1982; 6:1078.

Su WPD: Histopathologic varieties of epidermal nevus. Am J Dermatopathol 1982; 4:161.

Juvenile Rheumatoid Arthritis

Lowney ED, Simons HM: Rheumatoid nodules of the skin. Arch Dermatol 1963; 88:853.

Schaller J, Wedgwood RJ: Juvenile rheumatoid arthritis: A review. Pediatrics 1972; 50:940.

Lupus Erythematosus

Brangert JL, Freeman RG, Sontheimer RD, et al.: Subacute cutaneous lupus erythematosus and discoid lupus erythematosus: Comparative histopathologic findings. Arch Dermatol 1984; 120:332.

Fox RJ, McCusition CH, Schoch EP Jr: Systemic lupus erythematosus: Association with previous neonatal lupus erythematosus. Arch Dermatol 1979; 115:340.

Glidden RS, Mantzouranis EC, Borel Y: Systemic lupus erythematosus in childhood: Clinical manifestations and improved survival in fifty-five patients. Clin Immunol Immunopathol 1983; 29:196.

Provost TT: The relationship between discoid lupus erythematosus and systemic lupus erythematosus. Am J Dermatopathol 1979; 1:181.

Tani M, Shimizu R, Ban M, et al.: Systemic lupus erythematosus with vesiculobullous lesions. Arch Dermatol 1984; 120:1497.

Mixed Connective Tissue Disease

Singsen BH, Bernstein BH, Kornresch HK, et al.: Mixed connective tissue disease in childhood: A clinical and serological survey. J Pediatr 1977; 90:893.

Tiddens HAWM, Van der Net JJ, de Graeff-Meeder ER, et al.: Juvenile-onset mixed connective tissue disease: Longitudinal follow-up. J Pediatr 1993; 122:191.

Mucosal Neuroma Syndrome

Gorlin RJ, Sedano HO, Vickers RA, et al.: Multiple mucosal neuromas, pheochromocytoma, and medullary carcinoma of the thyroid: A syndrome. Cancer 1968; 22:293.

Necrobiosis Lipoidica Diabeticorum

Boulton AJM, Cuffield AM, Abouganem D, et al.: Necrobiosis lipoidica diabeticorum: A clinicopathologic study. J Am Acad Dermatol 1988; 18:530.

Gray HR, Gorshem JH, Johnson WS: Necrobiosis lipoidica: A histopathological and histochemical study. J Invest Dermatol 1965; 44:369.

Nevus Achromicus

Solomon LM, Esterly NB: Pigmentary abnormalities, nevus achromicus. In: Neonatal dermatology. Philadelphia: W.B. Saunders, 1973; 106.

Sugarman GI, Reed WB: Two unusual neurocutaneous disorders with facial cutaneous signs. Arch Neurol 1969; 21:242.

Peutz-Jeghers Syndrome

Utsunomiga J, Gocho H, Miyanaga T, et al.: Peutz-Jeghers syndrome: Its natural course and management. Johns Hopkins Med J 1975; 136:71.

Yamadak K, Matsukawa A, Havi Y, et al.: Ultrastructural studies on pigmented macules of Peutz-Jeghers syndrome. J Dermatol (Tokyo) 1981; 8:367.

Pyoderma Gangrenosum

Barnes L, Lucky AW, Bucuvalas JC, et al.: Pustular pyoderma gangrenosum associated with ulcerative colitis in childhood: Report of two cases and review of the literature. J Am Acad Dermatol 1986; 15:608.

Su WPD, Schroeter DL, Perry HO, et al.: Histopathologic and immunopathologic study of pyoderma gangrenosum. J Cutan Pathol 1986; 13:323.

Sarcoidosis

Barrie HJ, Bogoch A: The natural history of the sarcoid granuloma. Am J Pathol 1953; 29:451.

Blau EB: Familial granulomatous arthritis, iritis and rash. J Pediatr 1985; 107:689.

Hetherington S: Sarcoidosis in young children. Am J Dis Child 1982; 136:13.

Scleroderma

Fleischmayer R, Nedwich A: Generalized morphea: 1. Histology of the dermis and subcutaneous tissue. Arch Dermatol 1972; 106:509.

Goel KM, Shanks RA: Scleroderma in childhood. Arch Dis Child 1974; 49:861.

Sinus Histiocytosis with Massive Lymphadenopathy

Foucar E, Rosai J, Dorfman R: Sinus histiocytosis with massive lymphadenopathy: An analysis of 14 deaths occurring in a patient registry. Cancer 1984; 54:1834.

Thawerani H, Sanchez RI, Rosai J, et al.: The cutaneous manifestations of sinus histiocytosis with massive lymphadenopathy. Arch Dermatol 1978; 114:191.

Sweet's Syndrome

Crow RD, Kendal-Vegas F, Rook A: Acute febrile neutrophilic dermatosis: Sweet's syndrome. Dermatologica 1969; 139:123.

Levin DL, Esterly NS, Herman JJ, et al: The Sweet syndrome in children. J Pediatr 1981; 99:73.

Toxic Shock Syndrome

Abdul-Karim FW, Lederman MM, Carter JR, et al.: Toxic shock syndrome. Hum Pathol 1981; 12:16.

Cone LA, Woodard DR, Schlievert PM, et al.: Clinical and bacteriologic observations of a toxic shock-like syndrome due to Streptococcus pyogenes. N Engl J Med 1987; 317:146.

Wesenthal AM, Todd JK: Toxic shock syndrome in children aged 10 years or less. Pediatrics 1984; 74:112.

Urticaria

Russell Jones R, Bhogal, Dash A, et al.: Urticaria and vasculitis: A continuum of histological and immunopathological changes. Br J Dermatol 1983; 108:695.

Sofer NA: Acute and chronic urticaria and angioedema. J Am Acad Dermatol 1991; 25:146.

13

Metabolic Diseases

Contents

13-1 ANGIOKERATOMA CORPORIS DIFFUSUM

CLINICAL DESCRIPTION

In 1898, Anderson in England and Fabry in Germany independently described angiokeratoma corporis diffusum. This is the cardinal cutaneous manifestation of Fabry's disease, a storage disorder which involves the skin, eyes, kidneys, and nervous system.

Etiology and Incidence

The disorder is inherited as a sex-linked trait. It is caused by the absence of or a defect in the enzyme ceramide trihexosidase (alpha-galactosidase A). Over 400 cases have been reported with an estimated incidence of about 1 in 40,000. The gene maps to the long arm of the X chromosome (Xq 21.33 → q 22) and has been cloned. Clinical signs reflect progressive deposition of globotriaosylceramide in vascular endothelium.

Clinical Features

The earliest cutaneous finding is clusters of telangiectasia that usually begins in childhood or adolescence. Angiokeratomas increase in number with age and become elevated (Plate 13-1-1). These blood-filled macules or papules are dark red to blue-black and vary from less than 1 to 3 mm. They do not blanche with pressure and may be hyperkeratotic. The lesions are most dense between the umbilicus and knees, involving all intervening structures and are often bilaterally symmetric. Involvement of the oral mucosa and conjunctiva is common, as well as other mucosal areas. The tongue, face, ears, nails, and scalp are spared. In addition to these vascular lesions, hypohidrosis or anhidrosis is an early and almost universal finding. Patients and heterozygous females develop spokelike posterior capsular cataracts and conjunctival and retinal vascular lesions. Another early manifestation of Fabry's disease is periodic crises, severe burning or shooting pains in the lower extremities, ("Fabry crises") as well as acroparesthesias, which may be extremely debilitative. The terminal event is usually renal failure in the fourth decade of life or death due to cardiac or cerebrovascular disease.

Differential Diagnosis:

Fucosidosis type 3 (absence of alpha-L-fucosidase)
Sialidosis (absent neuraminidase)
Normal individuals
Aspartylglucosaminuria
Adult type β-galactosidase deficiency (GMI gangliosidosis)

HISTOLOGICAL DESCRIPTION

The skin lesions are telangiectasias or small superficial angiomas; the larger, older, acral lesions may have overlying hyperkeratosis.

As with most of the lipid storage diseases, the histological features are not revealing on routine hematoxylin and eosin sections. There may be epidermal hyperplasia with hyperkeratosis. There may also be an associated lymphocytic perivascular infiltrate. Vascular ectasia may be present within the papillary dermis (see Figure 11-6-2). The striking features are seen on fresh frozen or formalin-fixed frozen tissue. Polariscopic examination of such tissue shows doubly refractile lipid stored in the endothelial cells of dermal vessels as well as in the arrector pili muscles. Sections predigested with diastase and stained with periodic acid-Schiff reveal glycolipid in the same locations. These reactions can also be demonstrated using Sudan black B. Fucosidosis is a storage disease similar to Fabry's disease that presents a similar, if not identical, histological picture. The lipid in this condition stains equally well with oil red O or Sudan black B.

In Fabry's disease, atrophic or scarce sweat and sebaceous glands have been reported.

Differential Diagnosis

Fucosidosis
Other storage diseases

13-2 CALCINOSIS CUTIS

CLINICAL DESCRIPTION

There are two forms of calcinosis cutis: dystrophic and metastatic. Forms with unknown causes also exist.

Etiology and Incidence

The most common form of calcinosis cutis (dystrophic) occurs in damaged skin and may be localized (calcinosis circumscripta) or widespread (calcinosis universalis). Patients have connective tissue diseases (e.g., dermatomyositis, scleroderma, CREST syndrome, SLE), subcutaneous fat necrosis of the newborn, pseudoxanthoma elasticum, Albright's hereditary osteodystrophy, and Ehlers-Danlos disease. These children usually have normal serum levels of calcium and phosphorus.

Metastatic calcinosis cutis occurs less commonly in childhood and is seen with bone destruction and/or elevated levels of calcium, phosphorus, or both. Examples of disorders associated with this entity include hyperparathyroidism, pseudohyperparathyroidism, hypervitaminosis D, sarcoidosis, osteomyelititis, chronic renal disease, and other diseases associated with bone destruction (leukemia, Paget's disease, metastatic carcinoma). Solitary nodular calcifications occur without explanation and are usually observed on the scalp or face of children. A familial disease of tumoral calcinosis with large subcutaneous masses of calcium overlying pressure areas and joints has also been described.

Clinical Features

Dystrophic calcification is characterized by firm papules, plaques, or tumors that are skin-colored to violaceous (Plate 13-2-1). Although they may appear on any part of the body, they occur most frequently on the upper extremities near the joints. They may perforate through the skin.

Metastatic calcification consists of firm, white papules measuring 1 to 4 mm in size. These lesions are frequently symmetrical and arranged linearly in the popliteal spaces and posterior axillary folds, and on the iliac crests.

Differential Diagnosis

Limited
Traumatic calcinosis cutis (associated with exposure to
calcium chloride)

HISTOLOGICAL DIAGNOSIS

Calcinosis can be recognized on hematocylin and eosin-stained sections as purple, blue, or black particulate matter often surrounded by granulomatous inflammation. Calcium can be demonstrated using von Kossa stain, which stains calcium black. The epidermis may be thinned, acanthotic, or ulcerated, but most commonly, is unaffected. Calcium is distributed in granular form and may be found surrounded by epithelioid histiocytes, multinucleated giant cells, plasma cells, and lymphocytes (Figures 13-2-1 and 13-2-2). In lesions of longer duration, calcium is found in a more amorphous form, less granular and devoid of any inflammation. In systemic lupus erythematosus, dermatomyositis, scleroderma, and fat necrosis, other histological features of these conditions in addition to the presence of cutaneous calcium can be demonstrated. Cutaneous calcification, whether metastatic, dys-

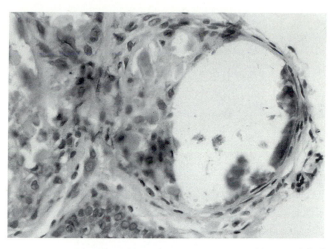

13-2-2 CALCINOSIS CUTIS: Amorphous basophilic material of variable size particles of calcium deposits. (200×)

trophic, or idiopathic, shows almost identical histological features and the etiology cannot be determined by histological observations alone.

Differential Diagnosis

Tattoo
Osteoma cutis

13-3 ECZEMATOUS ERUPTIONS

CLINICAL DESCRIPTION

There are many metabolic disorders associated with a rash similar in appearance to atopic eczema (Figure 13-3-1): phenylketonuria, acrodermatitis enteropathica, histidinemia,

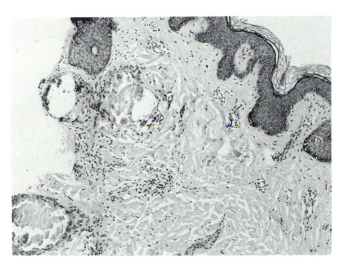

13-2-1 CALCINOSIS CUTIS: Dermal collections of amorphous basophilic material surrounded by a sparse inflammatory infiltrate. (40×)

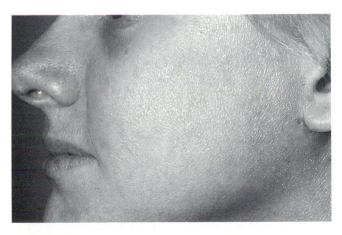

13-3-1 ECZEMATOUS ERUPTIONS: Adolescent with phenylketonuria, showing erythematous scaling papules and excoriations of the face.

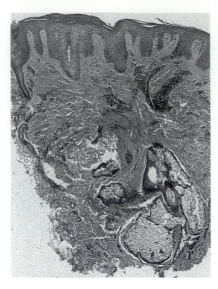

13-3-2 ECZEMATOUS ERUPTIONS: Changes of subacute eczematous process, including those associated with metabolic disorders: irregular acanthosis, spongiosis, collections of serum in the scale, and superficial dermal perivascular inflammatory infiltrates. (100×)

gluten-sensitive enteropathy, Hartnup syndrome, and Hurler's syndrome, biotinidase deficiency, multiple carboxylase deficiency, essential fatty acid deficiency, and hyper IgE syndrome.

HISTOLOGICAL DESCRIPTION

The histological features are the same as those of eczema (Chapter 5). Overall, the changes are those of epidermal and dermal inflammation and edema (Figure 13-3-2).

13-4 GAUCHER'S DISEASE

CLINICAL DESCRIPTION

This storage disease was first described in 1882.

Etiology and Incidence

This autosomal recessive disease is characterized by the deposition of glucocerebroside in histiocytes (the Gaucher cell), resulting in visceromegaly and/or neurologic disease. Accumulation occurs because of the lack of the enzyme glucocerebrosidase. This uncommon disorder occurs mostly (two-thirds of cases) in Ashkenazi Jews with an estimated carrier rate in this population of 1:25. The gene has been cloned and maps to chromosome 1 q 21. There are several clinical subtypes of the disease.

Clinical Features

Brownish yellow pigmentation is seen on the face, neck, hands or shins. Some areas of pigmentation are wedge-shaped. Furuncles, easy bruising, and hemorrhagic folliculitis occur on the extremities due to bone marrow involvement. Pingueculae are seen in the conjunctivae. These skin changes occur in the chronic Type I (nonneuropathic) type, which is two times more common than the infantile or acute form. The skin findings may not appear until after adolescence.

Differential Diagnosis

Other storage diseases

HISTOLOGICAL DESCRIPTION

The histological feature in this condition is epidermal basal layer hyperpigmentation. The epidermis may be thickened, with overlying hyperkeratosis. The dermis contains a mixture of cells, including lymphocytes, histiocytes, and larger histiocytic forms (Gaucher cells), which can be as large as 120 μm. The latter are multinucleated and their cytoplasms appear striped like wrinkled tissue paper or crumpled silk. They stain positively with acid phosphatase and may be PAS+. The folliculitis shows perifollicular and intrafollicular infiltration with acute inflammatory cells, including neutrophils and lymphocytes. Hemorrhage is found within the stroma around the inflamed follicles; in these acutely inflamed areas Gaucher cells are less apparent (Plate 13-4-1).

Differential Diagnosis

Reticulohistiocytosis
Other storage diseases
Leukemias
Thalassemia
Congenital dyserythropoletic anemia

13-5 JUVENILE XANTHOGRANULOMA

CLINICAL DESCRIPTION

This entity is in most instances a benign, self-limiting disorder. However, extensive involvement can cause significant cosmetic deformity.

Etiology and Incidence

The disease has no known cause. Serum lipids are normal. The lesions are present at birth in 20% of patients and appear within the first year of life in the remainder of patients. Only rarely has this entity been reported with adult onset. Lesions increase in number and then spontaneously disappear in 90% of cases in 3-6 years.

Clinical Features

Lesions seem to concentrate on the head, upper chest, and proximal extremities. They occasionally involve the mucous membranes or mucocutaneous junctions. Rarely the eyes, lungs, testes, pericardium, spleen, or liver are involved. Uncommonly, there is an association with neurofibromatosis and with chronic juvenile myeloid leukemia. Spontaneous hyphemas are seen, but infrequently. The lesions are usually yellow or reddish brown papules that vary in size (Plate 13-5-1). At times the lesions coalesce to form large plaques.

Differential Diagnosis

Xanthoma
Pyogenic granuloma

HISTOLOGICAL DESCRIPTION

The classic feature of xanthogranuloma is an infiltrate that fills the dermis and is composed of lipidized histiocytes, Touton giant cells (multinucleated foam cells), eosinophils, lymphocytes, and nonlipidized histiocytes (Figure 13-5-1). Foreign body giant cells can also be found in this infiltrate. The epidermis is often effaced and there is exocytosis of inflammatory cells and histiocytic cells. Some sections show only dense collections of histiocytes without the infiltration of eosinophils and without Touton giant cells. Fibrosis and fewer cells in the infiltrate represent the end stage of these conditions. Although this condition is called juvenile xanthogranuloma, similar lesions occur in adults.

Differential Diagnosis

Histiocytosis X
Reticulohistiocytic granuloma
Xanthoma disseminatum

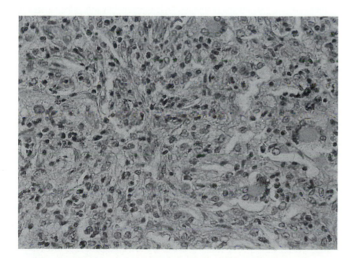

13-5-1 JUVENILE XANTHOGRANULOMA: Dense dermal infiltrates of lipidized histiocytes, Touton giant cells, and eosinophils. (100 ×)

13-6 MYXEDEMA

CLINICAL DESCRIPTION

Myxedema in childhood indicates the presence of hypothyroidism.

Etiology and Incidence

Myxedema is a late clinical sign of severe hypothyroidism. Pretibial changes are seen in adolescence, on rare occasions and are also associated with hyperthyroidism. The skin changes are due to an increase of dermal mucin. The edema is due to the affinity of mucin for water.

Clinical Features

There is generalized puffiness without pitting and a palpable infiltration of the skin. Diffuse hair loss may be seen, particularly loss of the outer third of the eyebrows. The skin is pale, dry, and somewhat waxy in appearance. Yellow waxy papules localized to the anterior portion of the lower extremities represent pretibial myxedema. Hypohidrosis and hyperpigmentation are also associated findings.

In congenital hypothyroidism (cretinism), children have short stature, dysmorphic facies (hypertelorism, thick lips, macroglossia) and pale mottled edematous skin. They are also mentally retarded. Pigmentation may be decreased. These changes may be at least partially prevented if therapeutic replacement is given early on, within the first few weeks of life.

Differential Diagnosis

Hypopituitarism
Hypothalamic hypothyroidism
Edema secondary to any cause

HISTOLOGICAL DESCRIPTION

On hematoxylin and eosin-stained sections there is fragmentation and separation of dermal collagen. Within the spaces in the dermis there is dermal mucin, manifested by basophilic staining of somewhat stringy granular material (Figure 13-6-1). This change may extend to the lower reticular dermis. There is a sparse lymphocytic perivascular infiltrate. The epidermis is usually effaced and thinned and separated from these changes by a zone of papillary dermal sparing (Grenz zone). Stains with colloidal iron are positive (Plate 13-6-1). Sections predigested with hyaluronidase will not stain with the colloidal iron reaction, indicating that the material in the dermis in this condition is hyaluronic acid. The end stage of this process is fibrosis.

Differential Diagnosis

Lupus erythematosus
Focal cutaneous mucinosis

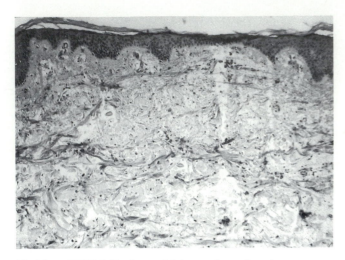

13-6-1 MYXEDEMA: In pretibial myxedema there is a separation of dermal collagen bundles by mucin. (40×)

Lichen myxedematosis
Plaquelike cutaneous mucinosis
Acral papular mucinosis

13-7 LIPODYSTROPHY

CLINICAL DESCRIPTION

Lipodystrophy—the loss of subcutaneous fat—exists in three forms: congenital generalized (lipoatrophic diabetes, Betardinelli syndrome), acquired generalized, and partial.

Etiology and Incidence

The pathogenesis of this rare group of disorders is unknown. The congenital form consists of generalized loss of body fat, an increased rate of skeletal growth, acanthosis nigricans, enlarged external genitalia, hepatomegaly, and insulin-resistant diabetes; the inheritance pattern is autosomal recessive. The onset of partial lipodystrophy is usually between five and fifteen years of age, but may be earlier. The female to male ratio is 4:1 and this disorder is sporadic. The generalized forms are congenital or acquired, with a female to male ratio of 2:1. Affected individuals appear muscular and initially tall. Males have phallic enlargement, but the androgens and gonadotropins are not elevated. Mental retardation has been noted in about 50% of children with the congenital form.

Clinical Features

Children with partial lipodystrophy have loss of subcutaneous fat from the face and sometimes the rest of the upper trunk. The lower extremities are spared. The progress may be slow. Renal disease (with progression to chronic sclerosing glomerulonephritis), neurologic abnormalities, an enlarged liver, hy-

perlipemia (especially of the triglycerides), and nonketotic insulin-resistant diabetes and hyperglucagonemia can be associated with this disorder.

The major dermatologic findings in generalized lipodystrophy (congenital or acquired) other than loss of subcutaneous fat (Figure 13-7-1) include hypertrichosis, hyperpigmentation, acanthosis nigricans, curly scalp hair, and systemic cystic angiomatosis. Also associated are prominent muscles, large hands and feet, hepatomegaly, phallic enlargement, advanced bone age and height, neurologic abnormalities, cardiomegaly, insulin resistance, and hyperlipemia. Fatal cirrhosis with esophageal varices may occur.

Differential Diagnosis

Leprechaunism
Dunnigan syndrome
X-linked dominant partial lipodystrophy
SHORT syndrome
Progeria
Werner syndrome
Diencephalic syndrome

HISTOLOGICAL DESCRIPTION

Fat cells (adipocytes) in lipodystrophy, in contrast to normal fat cells, are smaller in size, fewer in number, and irregular in shape. The total volume of fat is reduced. Early in the process there is an inflammatory infiltrate in the fat lobules that is composed almost entirely of lymphocytes. The fat in lipodystrophy resembles fetal fat (Figure 13-7-2).

Differential Diagnosis

Sclerema neonatorum
Panniculitis

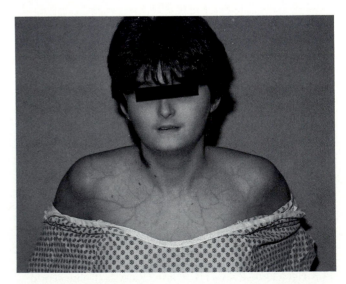

13-7-1 LIPODYSTROPHY: Chest wall veins are easily visualized because of the absence of fat.

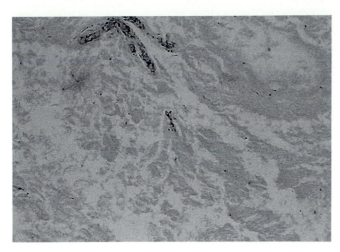

13-7-2 LIPODYSTROPHY: Immature fat with fibrous tissue. (100×)

13-8 NIEMANN-PICK DISEASE

CLINICAL DESCRIPTION

This is an autosomal recessive group of disorders, all of which are characterized by hepatosplenomegaly, foam cells in bone marrow, and variably increased amounts of cholesterol, glycolipid or bis(monoacyl glycero) phosphate in the spleen and liver.

Several forms are associated with marked central nervous system involvement, but some subtypes have little or no neurologic changes associated.

Etiology and Incidence

This rare disorder is due to a deficiency of sphingomyelinase (type I disease) or is due to uncertain primary defects (type II disease). Acute and subacute forms of type I are more frequently seen in Ashkenazi Jews.

Clinical Features

The skin change seen is the presence of yellow, pink, or orange xanthomas. The lesions are concentrated on the face, hands, extremities, and shoulders.

Differential Diagnosis

Xanthoma

HISTOLOGICAL DESCRIPTION

Niemann-Pick disease is a member of the histiocytic storage diseases in which sphingomyelins are stored in a variety of cells. Altered cells can be found in the dermis and are similar to those seen in Gaucher's disease. Cells are large—greater than 100 μm in diameter—and contain cytoplasmic vacuoles that stain with Sudan black. The pigmentary change is due to basal layer hyperpigmentation. The other lesions seen in

these patients, eruptive xanthomas, show foamy histiocytes in the dermis with lymphocytes, histiocytes, neutrophils, and occasional eosinophils. Touton giant cells can be seen in the later stages of this process.

Differential Diagnosis

Other xanthomas
Xanthogranuloma
Gaucher's disease

13-9 PERIORIFICIAL DERMATITIS

CLINICAL DESCRIPTION

Periorificial dermatitis has many different causes, including metabolic derangement such as acrodermatitis enteropathica and carboxylase deficiencies.

Etiology and Incidence

Acrodermatitis enteropathica is a hereditary disorder (autosomal recessive) that produces a defect in the absorption of zinc, leading to zinc deficiency. It has also been seen in patients receiving hyperalimentation with inadequate zinc supplements, with zinc-deficient (frequently vegetarian) diets, and with intestinal bypass surgery and in premature infants fed breast milk.

Essential fatty acid deficiency caused by prolonged parenteral nutrition may cause a similar periorificial dermatitis. An inherited (autosomal recessive) defect in holocarboxylase synthase results in decreased amounts of three carboxylase enzymes: 3-methyl crotonyl-CoA carboxylase, pyruvic acid carboxylase, and propionyl-CoA carboxylase, and results in severe lactic acidosis of neonatal onset. Inherited deficiency of another enzyme, biotinidase, results in an infantile form of the disease with variable manifestations (ataxia, seizures, acidosis, recurrent infection, sparse hair, and periorificial dermatitis) and is readily treated with biotin supplementation.

Clinical Features

All of these conditions demonstrate a periorificial dermatitis (erythematous, maculopapular to vesicular eruption similar to moniliasis and or psoriasis [Chapter 12]). Those with acrodermatitis enteropathica also demonstrate diarrhea and alopecia. Many fail to grow and are very irritable. The biotin disorders are associated with anorexia, lassitude, acidosis, seizures, ataxia, hypotonia, smooth tongue, glossitis, alopecia, keratoconjunctivitis, and anemia.

Differential Diagnosis

Mucocutaneous candidiasis
Glucagonoma syndrome

Zinc deficiency
Biotin deficiency
Biotinidase deficiency
Multiple decarboxylase deficiency
Essential fatty acid deficiency
Psoriasis
Neonatal citrullinemia

HISTOLOGICAL DESCRIPTION

Acrodermatitis enteropathica (Chapter 12) serves as a proto-type for all conditions that produce the clinical syndrome of periorificial dermatitis. The histological findings are not in themselves specific. The primary eruption in acrodermatitis enteropathica is vesiculobullous, symmetrical, and grouped. Later, crusts form and the epidermis shows focal or diffuse parakeratosis. There is psoriasiform epidermal hyperplasia with dyskeratosis and keratinocyte vacuolar alterations. In the dermis there is a perivascular infiltrate of lymphocytes and histiocytes. If there is significant involvement with yeast organisms, neutrophils can be seen in the infiltrate.

Differential Diagnosis

Psoriasis
Contact dermatitis
Candida dermatitis
Epidermolysis bullosa

13-10 MULTICENTRIC RETICULOHISTIOCYTOSIS

CLINICAL DESCRIPTION

This disorder affects the skin, joints, and other organ systems.

Etiology and Incidence

Multicentric reticulohistiocytosis is a rare disorder of unknown etiology. Eighty-five percent of those affected are Caucasians. Onset may be during adolescence. The female to male ratio is 3:1.

Clinical Features

Fifty percent of patients present with a papulonodular skin eruption and 50% with arthritis. If the arthritis precedes the skin changes, it does so by months to years. There is also an association (in up to 24% of adult patients) with carcinomas.

The skin lesions are flesh-colored to red-brown and vary in size (mm to cm). They may coalesce into a cobblestone-appearing plaque (Figure 13-10-1). They are distributed on the head, hands, periarticular skin, neck, and trunk. When on the nailfolds they are closely arranged, giving a beaded appearance (Plate 13-10-1). Fifty percent of patients have nodules involving the oral mucous membranes. The lesions may wax

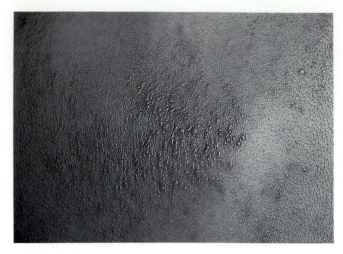

13-10-1 MULTICENTRIC RETICULOHISTIOCYTOSIS: Grouped, cobblestone-appearing papules on the dorsum of a patient's hand.

and wane in any of the locations. Nail changes include atrophy, longitudinal ridging, and hyperpigmentation. One-third of patients have xanthelasma.

Differential Diagnosis

Rheumatoid arthritis
Sarcoidosis
Xanthoma disseminatum
Congenital self-healing reticulohistiocytosis
Generalized eruptive histiocytoma
Familial histiocytic dermatoarthritis
Lepromatous leprosy
Fibroxanthoma
Lipoid proteinosis
Disseminated lipogranulomatosis

HISTOLOGICAL DESCRIPTION

This condition shares histological features with reticulohistiocytic granuloma. The epidermis is effaced and may be atrophic with a moderate keratin scale (Figure 13-10-2). The striking feature is the presence of large (40 to 110 μm) giant cells with multiple small nuclei. There are also large cells of a similar nature without multiple nuclei. These cells have smooth-appearing (ground glass) amphophilic cytoplasm with fine granules and small vacuoles (Plate 13-10-2). By electron microscopy, 40% of the histiocytic cells contain pleomorphic cytoplasmic inclusions. The number of these cells within the inflammatory infiltrate is variable. Other cells in the infiltrate are lymphocytes, eosinophils, plasma cells, and histiocytes in varying numbers. As the lesions evolve there is increasing fibrosis. Later there may be only a few giant cells embedded in the dense fibrocellular dermis.

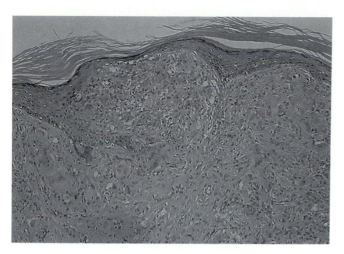

13-10-2 MULTICENTRIC RETICULOHISTIOCYTOSIS: Collections of multinucleated giant cells and lymphocytes efface the contour of the overlying epidermis. (100×)

Differential Diagnosis
Xanthoma
Dermatofibroma with monster cells

13-11 XANTHOMA DISSEMINATUM

CLINICAL DESCRIPTION
The name of this disorder describes its major feature.

Etiology and Incidence
This rare disorder is of unknown etiology. Thirty percent of cases begin before puberty. Diabetes insipidus is present in

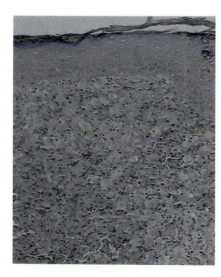

13-11-1 XANTHOMA DISSEMINATUM: Large numbers of histiocytes with variable lipidization are surrounded by lymphocytes. (40×)

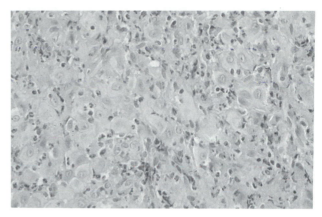

13-11-2 XANTHOMA DISSEMINATUM: Higher magnification of the infiltrate shows histiocytes with peripherally foamy cytoplasm and lymphocytes. (200×)

40% of cases; serum lipoproteins are normal. The disease appears mostly in young men.

Clinical Features
The lesions are distributed on the face, neck, antecubital fossae, periumbilical area, genitalia, and perineum. The conjunctivae may also be affected. They are yellow-orange, yellow-brown, or purpuric papules, nodules, or plaques (Plate 13-11-1). The epiglottis, larynx, and trachea are involved in 40% of cases.

Differential Diagnosis
Hand-Schüller-Christian disease
Multicentric reticulohistiocytosis
Xanthoma
Juvenile xanthogranuloma

HISTOLOGICAL DESCRIPTION
Xanthoma disseminatum show an infiltrate of histiocytes, foamy histiocytes, lymphocytes, eosinophils, neutrophils, and Touton giant cells (Figures 13-11-1 and 13-11-2). These form a dermal nodule with the overlying epidermis being effaced and atrophic. The infiltrate may extend into the dermal subcutaneous junction.

Differential Diagnosis
Other xanthomas
Reticulohistiocytic granuloma
Histiocytosis X
Juvenile xanthogranuloma

REFERENCES

Angiokeratoma Corporis Diffusum
Calhoun DH, Bishop DF, Bernstein HS, Quinn M, Hantzopoulos P, Desnick RJ: Fabry disease: Isolation of a

CDNA clone encoding human α-galactosidase A Proc Natl Acad Sci USA 1985; 82:7364.

Frost P, Spaeth GL, Tanaka Y: Fabry's disease: Glycosidic lipidosis. Arch Intern Med 1966;117:440.

Pyeritz RE, Bender WL, Lipford EH III: Anderson-Fabry disease. Johns Hopkins Med J 1982;150:181.

Calcinosis Cutis

Llainer SS, Andres ME, Jorizzo JL: Metastatic calcinosis cutis. Cutis 1983;32:463.

Tezoka T: Cutaneous calculus: Its pathogenesis. Dermatologica. 1980;161:191.

Gaucher's Disease

Barranger JA, Murray GJ, Ginns El: Genetic heterogeneic of Gaucher's disease. In Barranger HA, Brady RO, eds: Molecular basis of lysosomal storage disorders. New York: Academic Press, 1984:311.

Zimran A, et al.: Prediction of severity of Gaucher's disease by identification of mutations at DNA level. Lancet 1989;II:349.

Lee Robinson DR, Glen RH: Gaucher's disease: A modern enzymatic and anatomic methods of diagnosis. Arch Pathol 1981;105:102.

Xanthogranuloma

Chen BA, Hood A: Xanthogranuloma: Report on clinical and histologic findings in 64 patients. Pediatr Dermatol 1989;6:262.

Cooper PH, et al.: Association of juvenile xanthogranuloma with juvenile myeloid leukemia. Arch Dermatol 1984;120:371.

Gianotti F, Caputo R. Histicytic syndromes: A review. J Am Acad Dermatol 1985;13:383.

Makino K, Noainoue T, Shimeo S: Lipodystrophia centrifugalis abdominalis infantilis. Arch Dermatol 1972;106:899.

Renick SO, Woosley J, Azaizkham RG: Giant juvenile xanthogranulomas: Exophytic and endophytic varieties. Pediatr Dermatol 1990;7:185.

Senior B, Sellis SS: The syndrome of total lipodystrophy and partial lipodystrophy. Pediatrics 1964;33:593.

Mucinoses

Heyman WR: Cutaneous manifestation of thyroid disease. J Am Acad Dermatol 1992;26:885.

Schermer DR: Cutaneous myxedematosus (mucoid) states. Cutis 1968;4:939.

Tiuban AP, Roenizk HH: The cutaneous mucinosis. J Am Acad Dermatol 1986;14:1.

Lipogranuloma

Schmoeckel G, Hohlfed M: A specific ultrastructural marker for disseminated lipogranulomata (Farber). Arch Dermatol Res 1979;266:187.

Reticulohistiocytoses

Cotterall MD, et al.: Multicentric reticulohistiocytosis and malignant disease. Br J Dermatol 1978, 98:221.

Lesher JA Jr, Allen BS: Multicentric reticulohistiocytosis. J Am Acad Dermatol 1984; 11:713.

Raphael S, Cawdery SL, Faerber EN, et al.: Multicentric reticulohistocytosis in a child. J Pediatr 1989;114:266.

Periorificial Dermatitis

Moynuhan EJ: Acrodermatitis enteropathenia: A lethal inherited human zinc-deficiency disorder. Lancet 2; 1974;399.

Nyhan WL: Inborn error of metabolism. Arch Dermatol 1987;123:1696.

Wells BT, Wrinkelman RK: Acrodermatitis enteropathica: Report of 6 cases. Arch Dermatol 1961;84:40.

Williams ML, Packman S, Cowan MJ: Alopecia and periorificial dermatitis in biotin responsive multiple carboxylase deficiency. Arch Dermatol 1987;123:1696.

Xanthoma Disseminatum

Altman J, Wilkelmann RK: Xanthoma disseminatum. Arch Dermatol 1962;86:582.

Mishkell MA, Cockshott WP, Nazir DJ, et al.: Xanthoma disseminatum: Clinical metabolic pathologic and radiologic aspects. Arch Dermatol 1977;113:1094.

Niemann-Pick Disease

Crocker AC, Faber S: Niemann-Pick disease. A review of 18 patients. Medicine 1958;37:1.

Spence MW, Callahan JW: Sphingomyelin-cholesterol lipidoses: The Niemann-Pick group of diseases. In Scriver CR, Beaudet AL, Sly WS, Valle D (eds). The Metabolic Basis of Inherited Disease. New York, McGraw Hill, 1989, pp. 1655.

14

Inflammatory Diseases
of Sebaceous
and Sweat Glands

Contents

14-1 ACNE

CLINICAL DESCRIPTION

Acne is a folliculosebaceous inflammatory disorder that may occur in various clinical settings. Because most forms of acne share common histological features, they are discussed collectively in this section.

Etiology and Incidence

Clinical and experimental observations suggest that androgens are prerequisite for the development of acne, although their exact etiologic role has not been defined. Speculation exists with regard to the possible role(s) of microorganisms (*Propionibacterium acnes*), emotional stress, and diet in the genesis and persistence of acne. Certain drugs (steroids, diphenylhydantoin, phenobarbital) and topical agents that may result in follicular occlusion (pomade) may also produce acne.

The most common form of acne, acne vulgaris, affects well over 30 million individuals in the United States alone and accounts for the vast majority of dermatologic problems in children during adolescence. Certain forms of acne may occur or persist at any time during life, including the neonatal period (0.04% of newborns) and early adulthood to middle age (2% to 8% affected). Acne vulgaris has well-established hereditary and genotypic associations, although a precise inheritance pattern has not been established.

Clinical Features

The salient clinical characteristics of acne are (1) open comedones (blackheads) that appear as follicular ostia expanded by black keratotic and sebaceous material; (2) closed comedones (whiteheads)—small, pale to white noninflammatory papules that may progress to form open comedones or inflammatory

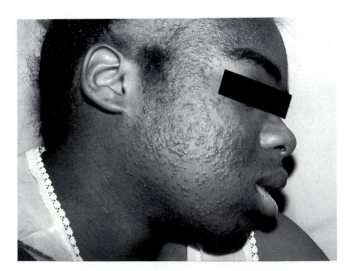

14-1-1 DRUG-INDUCED ACNE: Monomorphous-appearing erythematous papules on the face and neck of an adolescent receiving systemic corticosteroids.

lesions; (3) erythematous papulopustules; (4) deep, painful nodules, abscesses, and sinus tracts; and, with healing, (5) raised or depressed scars. Differences in the morphology and distribution exist concerning the various forms of acne that may affect the pediatric population (Table 14-1-1).

Neonatal Acne

Neonatal acne presents at birth or in early infancy, more often in males than in females. Most often comedones are present on the cheeks. Erythematous papules or pustules may also be present. Although the chin and forehead may be affected, the back and trunk are spared (see Chapter 3 for clinical and histological photographs).

The cause of neonatal acne is thought to be stimulation of neonatal sebaceous glands by maternal androgens received through the placenta. This form of acne spontaneously involutes within a few months.

Infantile Acne

Acne occurring after three to four months of life is known as infantile acne (Plate 14-1-1). In contrast to neonatal acne, it can persist for several years. Inflammatory papules and pustules are more common than nodules, and the cheeks are most commonly affected.

A child affected with this form of acne who has a family history of acne may be subject to more severe acne in puberty. A source of androgen excess should be sought if the acne is severe and refractory to therapy.

Drug-Induced Acne

A wide array of drugs can cause acneiform eruptions. Topically applied or systemically administered corticosteroids (Figure 14-1-1) or adrenocorticotrophic hormone (ACTH) produce a widespread monomorphous eruption of erythematous papulopustules. Antidepressants (lithium carbonate), antiepileptic agents (diphenylhydantoin, trimethadione, phenobarbital), and vitamins [B12] are known to produce similar eruptions.

Pomade Acne

Application of oily substances to the face or scalp causes the formation of large numbers of closed comedones in or adjacent to the application site. This is most commonly seen on the foreheads of black children in whom an oily lubricant has been applied to the scalp (Figure 14-1-2).

Acne Vulgaris

In acne vulgaris, lesions are generally distributed on the face and trunk and demonstrate a wide range of morphologic appearances, from open and closed comedones to pustules. It commonly arises in puberty but has been reported in children

14-1-1 Differential Diagnosis of Pediatric Acne

	Neonatal Acne	Infantile Acne	Drug-Induced Acne	Pomade Acne	Acne Vulgaris	Acne Conglobata
Age	20% of newborns	3–4 mo to 3 y	Variable	Childhood and adolescence	Adolescence	Late adolescence and young adulthood
Distribution	Face (cheeks > chin and forehead)	Face > trunk	Widespread	Forehead and temples	Face and trunk	Head, neck, trunk, arms
Morphology	Comedones > papulopustules	Comedones to pustules	Monomorphous, pustular	Closed comedones	Comedones (open and closed), pustules, some cysts	Inflammatory cysts, abscesses, and sinuses
Etiology	Transplacental androgenic stimulation of sebaceous glands	Unknown	Steroids, lithium, diphenylhydantoin, phenobarbital, trimethadione, vitamin B12	Oil-based face and scalp preparations	Androgen-related and genetic factors	XYY genotype, S. aureus, β-hemolytic streptococci
Microscopic	Prominent sebaceous glands with plugging; lymphoid response	See acne vulgaris	Acute folliculitis and pustule formation	Follicular plugging; lymphoid response	Keratotic follicular plugs, perifollicular lymphocytes, follicular rupture, microabscesses	Follicular rupture, abscesses
Clinical differential diagnosis	Drug-related acne	Drug-related or contact	Other forms of acne	Characteristic location and appearance	Acne of other causes	Bacterial pyoderma
Microscopic differential diagnosis			Pustular phase of acne vulgaris		Folliculitis (acute and chronic); perforating folliculitis	Cellulitis, pyoderma

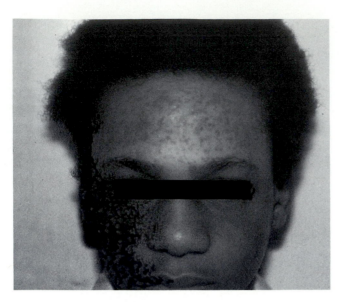

14-1-2 POMADE ACNE: Comedones and rare papulopustules localized to the forehead of this adolescent secondary to the application of oils to the hair.

younger than ten years. Males are more often and more severely affected than females. Although acne generally resolves in the third decade, in a small percentage of patients it persists into the fourth and fifth decades.

Acne Conglobata

A disfiguring variant of acne is acne conglobata. It is characterized by nodules, cysts, and abscesses. Often sinus tracts form and indicate persistence of this process. Males in their late teens or older are most commonly afflicted and display lesions on the face, trunk, and upper arms. A relationship to the XYY phenotype and coagulase-positive staphylococcal or group A beta-hemolytic streptococcal colonization is postulated.

Differential Diagnosis

Various subtypes of acne listed above
Adenoma sebaceum
Eruptive vellous hair cysts

HISTOLOGICAL DESCRIPTION

Open comedones, or blackheads, are histologically superficial dermal cysts lined by stratified squamous epithelium that contain keratin and lipid. They have widely ectatic orifices that connect to the surface of the skin (Figure 3-1-4). Melanin and oxidized keratinous material give these cyst contents a black color.

Closed comedones are histologically similar to open comedones but have a narrow orifice that connects them to the surface. As they become distended with keratin and lipid material the wall becomes thinned and ruptures. Neutrophils

may collect in the center of the comedone, forming a small abscess, and may surround a portion of the epithelial wall as well (Figures 3-1-2 and 3-1-3).

Nodules and cysts are similar inflammatory lesions that arise from follicles but are deeper-seated than comedones. Depending on their depth and degree of accompanying inflammation, variable scar formation occurs. In acne conglobata, epithelial-lined sinus tracts are surrounded by variable acute and chronic inflammatory infiltrates and dermal fibrosis.

Differential Diagnosis

Cutaneous infections
Perforating folliculitis

14-2 FOX-FORDYCE DISEASE

CLINICAL DESCRIPTION

Another name for this disorder is apocrine miliaria.

Etiology and Incidence

The cause of this disorder is thought to be occlusion of apocrine ducts. It occurs almost exclusively in females, postpubertal more often than prepubertal.

Clinical Features

Pruritic follicular papules in the axillary (Figure 14-2-1), areolar, and pubic region characterize this disorder. Pruritus is intermittent and frequently exacerbated by stress.

Differential Diagnosis

Folliculitis
Perforating folliculitis

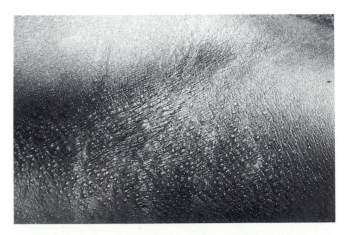

14-2-1 FOX-FORDYCE DISEASE: Characteristic hyperpigmented perifollicular papules of the axilla.

HISTOLOGICAL DESCRIPTION

When a keratotic plug obstructs the infundibular portion of a hair follicle, retention of apocrine secretions occurs at the junction of the apocrine duct with follicular epithelium. At this site a vesicle forms and the apocrine duct ruptures. An inflammatory infiltrate may surround this area and extend about the affected portion of the hair follicle. Multiple histological sections may be necessary to find these subtle histological findings.

Differential Diagnosis

Folliculitis
Follicular eczema

14-3 HIDRADENITIS SUPPURATIVA

CLINICAL DESCRIPTION

Hidradenitis suppurativa is a chronic inflammatory and scarring process affecting axillary, inguinal, and perianal skin.

Etiology and Incidence

The exact cause of hidradenitis is unknown. Some believe it represents inflammation of apocrine glands, while others believe it is part of the follicular occlusion triad (dissecting cellulitis of the scalp, acne, and hidradenitis suppurativa) in which apocrine and eccrine glands are secondarily involved. The disease may be triggered by occlusion of apocrine gland ducts by keratinous follicular contents, resulting in ductal rupture and inflammation. As in Fox-Fordyce disease, hidradenitis is rare before puberty. It affects both sexes.

Clinical Features

Hidradenitis suppurativa presents as solitary or multiple deep-seated erythematous nodules and abscesses in the axillary, inguinal, and perianal areas. As acute lesions increase in size they may discharge seropurulent material by perforating overlying skin. Deep scars form as affected areas heal (Figure 14-3-1). Old lesions heal while new ones continue to form. With chronicity sinus tracts and fistulae may develop.

Differential Diagnosis

Ruptured epidermal inclusion cyst

HISTOLOGICAL DESCRIPTION

The histological features vary with the stage of evolution of lesions. Early lesions show occlusion of apocrine ducts and associated hair follicles with keratin. As epithelial structures become dilated and rupture, they become surrounded by neutrophilic inflammatory infiltrates. Over time, lympho-

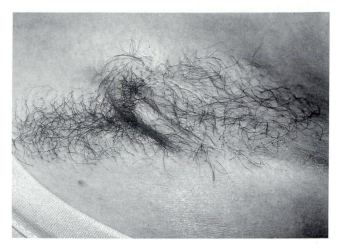

14-3-1 HIDRADENITIS SUPPURATIVA: Axillary vault of an adolescent demonstrating a deep-seated erythematous nodule and puckering of skin due to scarring in hidradenitis suppurativa.

cytes, histiocytes, multinucleated giant cells, and plasma cells are attracted to sites of rupture and the dermal stroma is replaced by granulation tissue. As fibrosis ensues, normal adnexal structures (hair follicles, apocrine, and eccrine glands) are lost. In late stages, sinus tracts may be evident as epithelium-lined channels within fibrotic stroma.

Differential Diagnosis

Ruptured cyst
Cutaneous infection (bacterial, mycobacterial, fungal)

REFERENCES

Acne

Berge T, Gunderson J: Acne conglobata. Acta Derm Venereol 1967;47:41.

Henry MCY: Lithium carbonate toxicity: Acneiform eruptions and other manifestations. Arch Dermatol 1982;118:246.

Hitch JM: Acneiform eruptions induced by drugs and chemicals. JAMA 1969;200:879.

Latif R, Laude TA: Steroid acne in a 14 month old boy. Cutis 1982;29:3133.

Voorhees JJ, Wilkins JW, Hayes E, et al.: Nodulocystic acne as a phenotype feature of XYY genotype. Arch Dermatol 1972;105:913.

Winston MH, Shalita AR: Acne vulgaris: Pathogenesis and treatment. Pediatr Clin North Am 1991;38:889.

Fox-Fordyce Disease

Mevorah B, Duboff GS, Wass RW: Fox-Fordyce disease in pre-pubescent girls. Dermatologica 1968;136:43.

Shelley WB, Levy EJ: Apocrine sweat retention in man. II. Fox-Fordyce disease (apocrine miliaria). Arch Dermatol 1956;73:38.

Hyland CH, Kheir SM: Follicular occlusion disease with elimination of abnormal elastic tissue. Arch Dermatol 1980;116:925.

Hidradenitis Suppurativa

Brunsting HA: Hidradenitis suppurativa: Abscess of the apocrine sweat glands. Arch Dermatol Syph 1939;39:108.

15

Hair and Nails

Contents

15-1 TRICHORRHEXIS INVAGINATA

CLINICAL DESCRIPTION

This hair defect appears in infancy and may affect all body hair to varying degrees.

Etiology and Incidence

This rare defect is found in patients affected with Netherton's syndrome, an ectodermal genodermatosis possibly transmitted in an autosomal recessive manner and characterized by defective keratinization.

Clinical Features

Patients with trichorrhexis invaginata have lusterless, short hair. Abnormal invaginations along the length of the shaft give hair the appearance of bamboo (Figure 15-1-1). These invaginations also cause hair to be extremely fragile and thus unable to attain significant length. This is particularly problematic in areas subject to friction. If the problem improves by adulthood, characteristic hair shaft changes may be discerned only in the eyebrows or on the extremities.

Patients with trichorrhexis invaginata and the autosomal recessive papulosquamous disorder of ichthyosis linearis circumflexa have Netherton's syndrome. They also usually have an atopic background, which may include a personal or family history of asthma, allergic rhinitis, urticaria, angioneurotic edema, anaphylactoid reactions, or flexural eczema. Their ichthyosiform skin alterations are characterized by polycyclic scaling lesions with a double-edged scale, known as ichthyosis linearis circumflexa. Other ectodermal structures (e.g., teeth, nails, palms, or soles) are rarely affected.

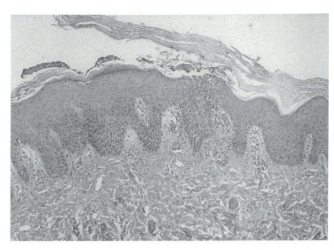

15-1-2 NETHERTON'S SYNDROME: There is regular epidermal hyperplasia associated with the formation of hyperorthokeratotic scale. A pulse of exocytosis with spongiosis and a focus of mild eosinophilic degeneration are also seen. (100×)

Differential Diagnosis

Other hair shaft abnormalities

HISTOLOGICAL DESCRIPTION

Microscopy (light and scanning electron microscopy) shows characteristic nodes along the hair shaft. These nodes have a ball-and-socket arrangement, with the socket defect located proximally and the ball located distally (Figure 15-1-1). There is no distinct periodicity to this defect, nor does it grossly affect all hairs. Other associated abnormalities include twisted hair shafts, variable caliber of shafts, and strictures. Ultrastructural studies have confirmed defective keratinization to be the cause of this problem. Skin biopsy of a figurate lesion of ichthyosis linearis circumflexa may show eosinophilic degeneration of the Malpighian layer (Figure 15-1-2).

Differential Diagnosis

Trichorrhexis nodosa
Other hair shaft abnormalities

15-2 TRICHORRHEXIS NODOSA

CLINICAL DESCRIPTION

Trichorrhexis nodosa is the most common hair shaft defect. Roughly translated, it means ruptured hair with nodelike changes.

Etiology and Incidence

Trichorrhexis nodosa may be acquired or congenital. The acquired form is common, while the congenital form is rare. The latter can be sporadic or familial and has rarely been

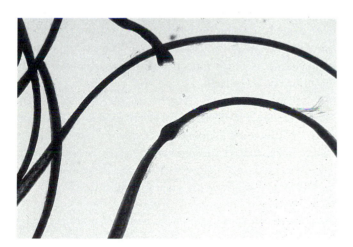

15-1-1 TRICHORRHEXIS NODOSA: A hair mount, showing invaginations along the hair shaft, giving it a bamboolike appearance. (20×)

associated with tooth and nail abnormalities as well as other hair shaft defects.

Clinical Features

The acquired form occurs in patients of all ages and both sexes. Affected individuals usually note that their hair breaks off a short distance from the scalp. Hair may have a somewhat beaded appearance on the scalp (Plate 15-2-1). There is no zone of complete hair loss. This form of the disorder occurs when harsh physical and/or chemical grooming techniques are employed. In black patients, it commonly affects the proximal hair shafts, while in Caucasians and Asians it affects the distal hair shafts. The problem usually abates or resolves over time if the poor grooming techniques are discontinued and hair is cared for in a gentle manner.

The congenital form may or may not affect hair other than scalp hair. It may be accompanied by other ectodermal defects. Trichorrhexis nodosa may manifest itself a few months after birth as broken hairs of variable length.

In infants and children this hair shaft abnormality may be associated with mental retardation and argininosuccinic aciduria. The inborn error of metabolism stems from an abnormality of argininosuccinate lyase, an enzyme which splits argininosuccinic acid to arginine and fumaric acid. As a result, argininosuccinic acid levels are elevated in blood, urine, and cerebrospinal fluid. Associated clinical manifestations range from seizures to physical and mental retardation. Since damage from argininosuccinic aciduria can be prevented or halted with dietary manipulation, it is imperative to recognize trichorrhexis nodosa as a possible clue to an underlying metabolic disorder.

Differential Diagnosis

Other hair shaft defects
Hair shaft defects associated with mental retardation

HISTOLOGICAL DESCRIPTION

Under low magnification the fracture site may resemble a node. Higher magnification (Figure 15-2-1) and scanning electron microscopy show a characteristic fracture in which the hair cortex is splayed. The change mimics the appearance of bristles of two brushes being pushed into each other. These changes are located along the length of the shaft and differ from fraying of the distal end, which occurs with weathering. The defect is thought to occur from weakness of the cortex and/or cuticle.

Differential Diagnosis

Trichoschisis (complete fracture of shafts)
Other hair shaft defects

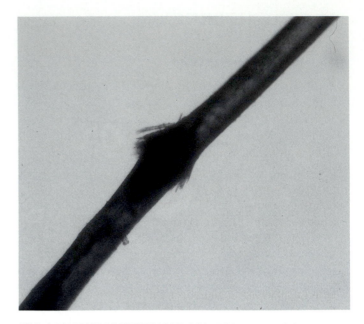

15-2-1 TRICHORRHEXIS NODOSA: Hair mount of the patient in Plate 15-2-1. Along the length of hair shafts are multiple zones of outward splaying of cortex, mimicking bristles of two brushes being pushed together. (40×)

15-3 PILI TORTI

CLINICAL DESCRIPTION

This hair shaft defect is the one most frequently misdiagnosed. It is also known as twisted hair.

Etiology and Incidence

Pili torti is a rare disorder and its cause is unknown. Congenital and acquired forms exist.

Clinical Features

Although hair may be normal or abnormal at birth, by two years of age it is noticeably fragile, brittle, and short because of breakage. It appears frizzy and unruly. The twisted configuration of the hair shaft reflects light irregularly and gives the hair a spangled appearance.

In its classic form (Ronchese), pili torti occurs more often in females than males and is inherited in an autosomal pattern. Affected individuals are frequently blond and have short, broken hair. In this form pili torti may be accompanied by other ectodermal defects (ichthyosis, sensorineural hearing defects, corneal opacities, nail dystrophy, keratosis pilaris, dental defects). The association of cochlear-type hearing loss in association with pili torti (Bjornstad's syndrome) should prompt auditory testing of children with this hair defect.

A second form, probably transmitted in an autosomal dominant fashion, is the late-onset type (Beare). As its name implies, the changes are noted later than in the classic form,

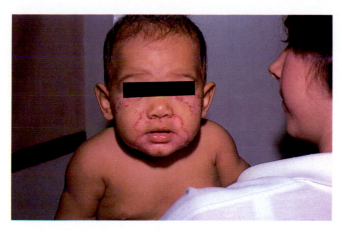

Plate 12-1-1 ACRODERMATITIS ENTEROPATHICA: Crusted, sharply marginated skin eruption around eyes and mouth of child with zinc deficiency.

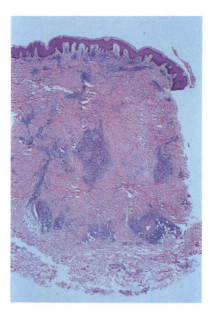

Plate 12-2-1 WEGENER'S GRANULOMATOSIS: Low power shows a deep-seated dermal inflammatory infiltrate surrounding an ill-defined zone of dermal necrosis. There is also prominent papillary dermal edema. (20×)

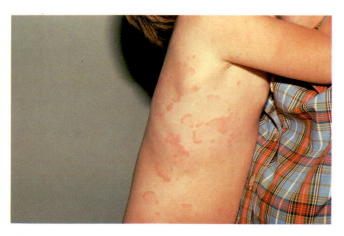

Plate 12-3-1 ANNULAR ERYTHEMAS: Arcuate rings on trunk of child with erythema annulare centrifugum.

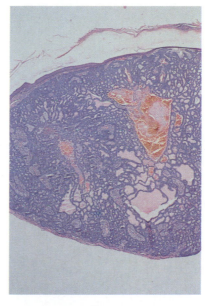

Plate 12-4-1 BASAL CELL NEVUS SYNDROME: Nodular tumor composed of basaloid cells arranged in cords with peripheral palisading, a typical feature. (40×)

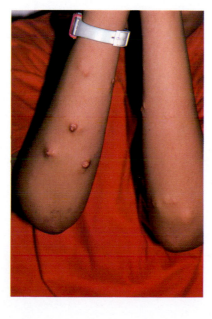

Plate 12-5-1 DERMATOMYOSITIS: Calcium deposits (calcinosis cutis) in an adolescent's skin.

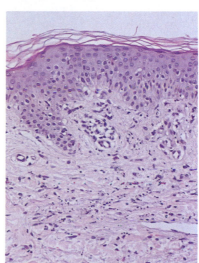

Plate 12-8-1 JUVENILE RHEUMATOID ARTHRITIS: Sparse perivascular and interstitial inflammation of rheumatoid neutrophilic dermatitis. (100×)

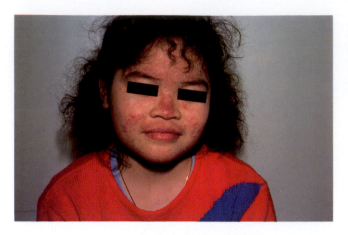

Plate 12-9-1 LUPUS ERYTHEMATOSUS: Butterfly rash in child with systemic lupus erythematosus.

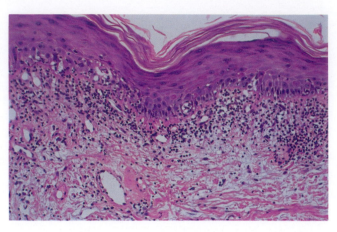

Plate 12-9-2 DISCOID LUPUS ERYTHEMATOSUS: Inflammatory lesion, showing a bandlike infiltrate of lymphocytes approximating the epidermal-dermal junction and associated with subepidermal vacuolization and early basilar keratinocyte necrosis. (100×)

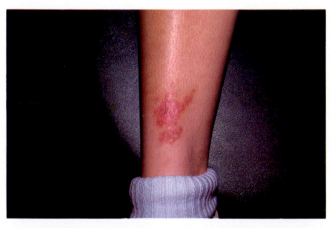

Plate 12-12-1 NECROBIOSIS LIPOIDICA DIABETICORUM: Early atrophy.

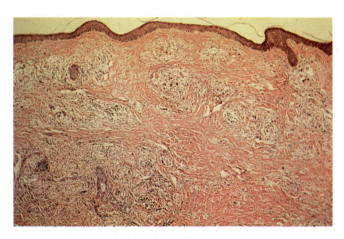

Plate 12-12-2 NECROBIOSIS LIPOIDICA DIABETICORUM: Multiple foci of granulomatous inflammation beneath an atrophic epidermis. (20×)

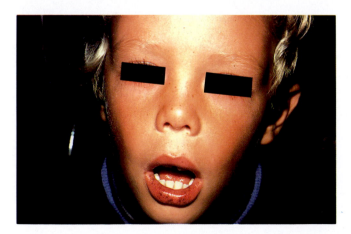

Plate 12-14-1 PEUTZ-JEGHERS SYNDROME: A child with characteristic lentigenes of oral mucosa.

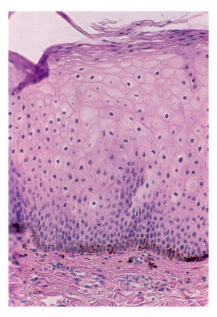

Plate 12-14-2 PEUTZ-JEGHERS SYNDROME: Mucosal epithelium with basalar hyperpigmentation. (20×)

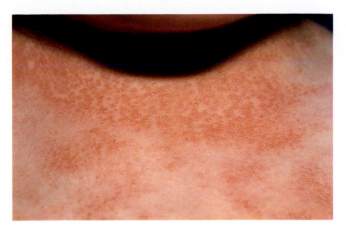

Plate 12-16-1 SARCOIDOSIS: Yellow-brown flat-topped papules on chest of child younger than one year old.

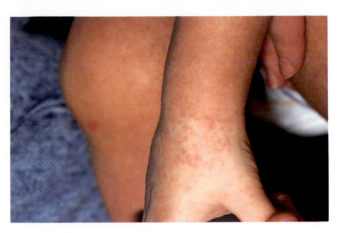

Plate 12-16-2 SARCOIDOSIS: Lesions similar to those in Figure 12-5-2 and synovial thickening of wrist.

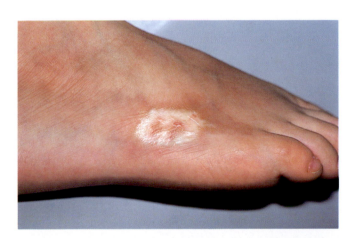

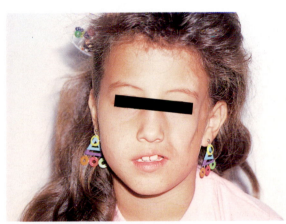

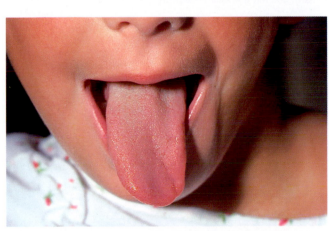

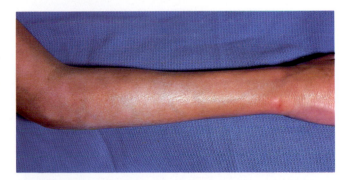

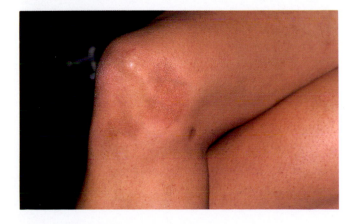

Plate 12-17-1 LINEAR SCLERODERMA (MORPHEA): A (top left) Hard, white central area of morphea surrounded by hyperpigmentation. **B** (top right) Child with facial hemiatrophy (Parry-Romberg disease). **C** (above left) Atrophy of tongue on ipsilateral side. **D** (above right) Note tight atrophic shiny skin on arm of child with systemic scleroderma. **E** (right) Large atrophic grainy patches of atrophoderma of Pasini and Pierini.

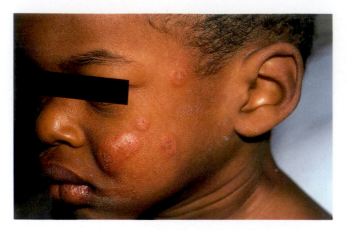

Plate 12-19-1 SWEET'S SYNDROME: Multiple round juicy lesions on a child's face.

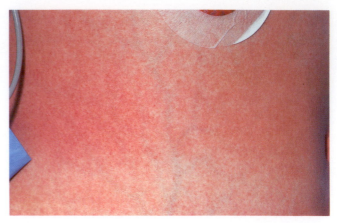

Plate 12-20-1 TOXIC SHOCK SYNDROME: Truncal rash that looks very much like scarlet fever.

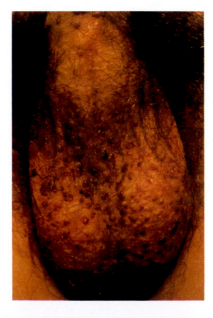

Plate 13-1-1
ANGIOKERATOMA
CORPORIS
DIFFUSION: Multiple
raised violaceous
papules on an adoles-
cent's scrotum.

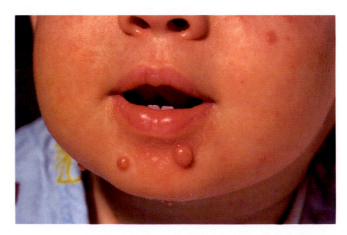

Plate 13-2-1 CALCINOSIS CUTIS: Dystrophic calcification on forearm of child who had infiltrated IV.

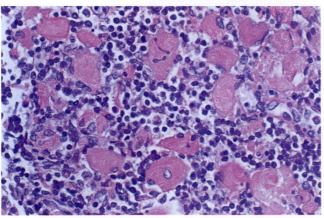

Plate 13-4-1 GAUCHER'S DISEASE: Histiocytes containing periodic acid-Schiff-positive mucopolysaccharides. (400 ×) (Courtesy of Lawrence Kenyon, M.D., Ph.D., resident in pathology, University of Pennsylvania School of Medicine.)

Plate 13-5-1 JUVENILE XANTHOGRANULOMA: Characteristic multiple sharply circumscribed yellowish papules.

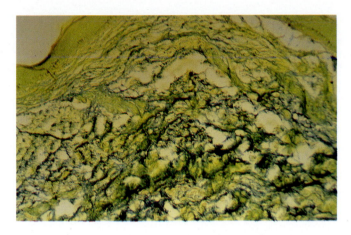

Plate 13-6-1 MYXEDEMA: Special stains, such as colloidal iron stain, highlight the presence of dermal mucin in the dermis. (100×)

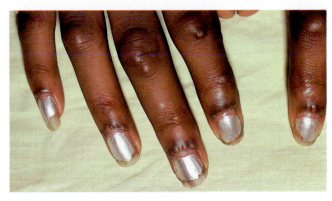

Plate 13-10-1 MULTICENTRIC RETICULOHISTIOCYTOSIS: Hyperpigmented papulonodules on the knuckles and at the posterior nailfolds.

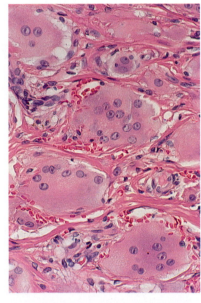

Plate 13-10-2 MULTICENTRIC RETICULOHISTIO- CYTOSIS: The multi- nucleated cells of reticulohistiocytosis characteristically have "ground glass" or "muddy rose" cyto- plasm. (200×)

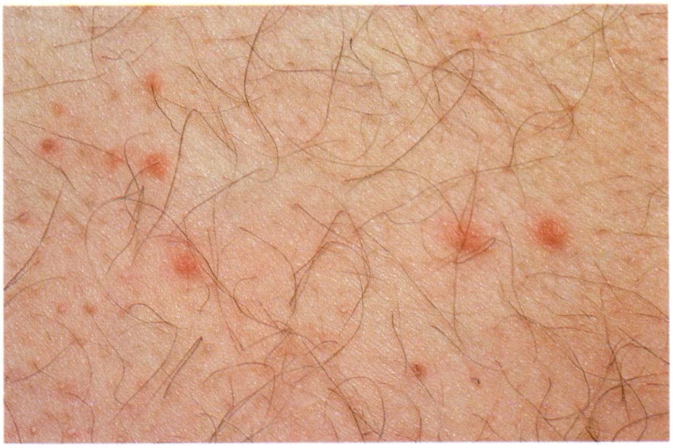

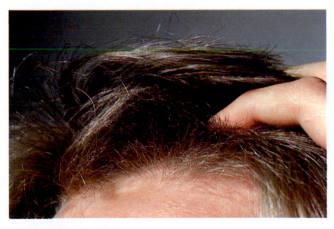

Plate 13-11-1 XANTHOMA DISSEMINATUM: Multiple discrete yellow papules on the trunk.

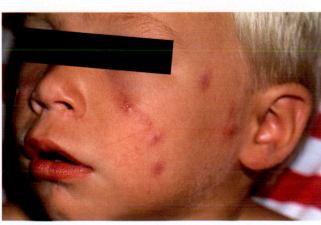

Plate 14-1-1 INFANTILE ACNE: Deep-seated erythematous nodules on the cheek and temple of this toddler.

Plate 15-2-1 TRICHORRHEXIS NODOSA: The hair has a some- what glistening, beaded appearance.

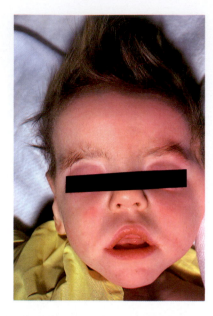

Plate 15-6-1 MENKES' KINKY HAIR SYNDROME: Note peculiar hair, twisted eyebrows, and pallor of the skin in this young boy.

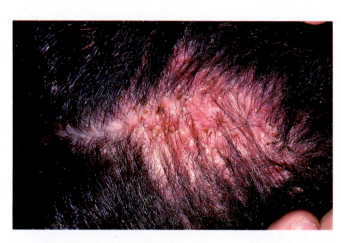

Plate 15-6-2 MENKES' KINKY HAIR SYNDROME: Polariscopy of monilethrix, showing multiple hourglass configurations connected in a chain. (20 ×)

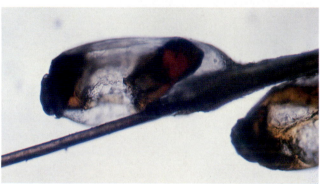

Plate 15-10-1 PEDICULOSIS CAPITIS: Hair mount, showing an adherent nit containing a louse. (200 ×)

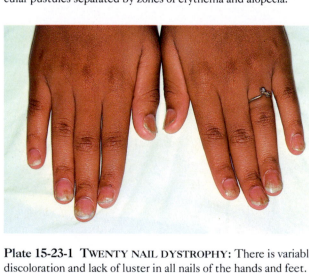

Plate 15-11-1 FOLLICULITIS DECALVANS: There are perifollicular pustules separated by zones of erythema and alopecia.

Plate 15-11-2 FUNGAL FOLLICULITIS: High magnification shows the presence of fungal spores within a hair shaft located in the deep dermis. Special stains were not necessary in this case to identify the organism. (400 ×)

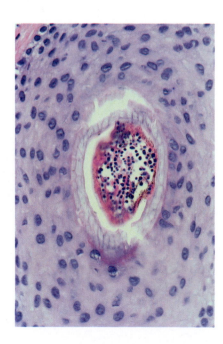

Plate 15-23-1 TWENTY NAIL DYSTROPHY: There is variable discoloration and lack of luster in all nails of the hands and feet.

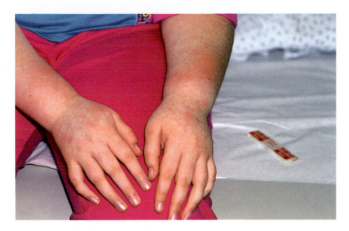

Plate 16-1-1 HISTIOCYTIC CYTOPHAGIC PANNICULITIS: A ten-year-old girl with T cell lymphoma involving the subcutis.

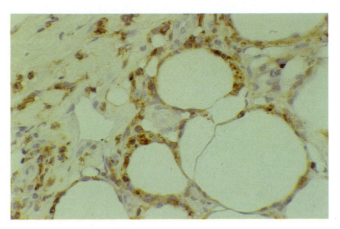

Plate 16-1-2 HISTIOCYTIC CYTOPHAGIC PANNICULITIS: Monoclonal antibody stains for T cells (UCHL-1) show the pleomorphic extracellular and the intrahistiocytic cells to stain as T lymphocytes. This case was associated with T cell lymphoma. (200×)

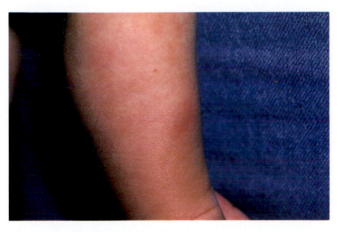

Plate 16-2-1 WEBER-CHRISTIAN PANNICULITIS: The erythematous nodular plaque seen on this fourteen-month-old child's leg was proven to be Weber-Christian panniculitis on biopsy.

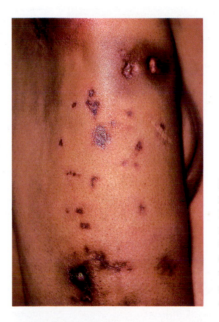

Plate 16-3-1 LUPUS PANNICULITIS: Erythematous subcutaneous plaques on upper arm of an adolescent. Note resolution with hyperpigmented scars and soft tissue depressions.

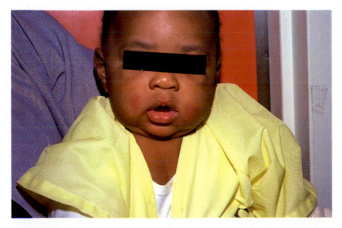

Plate 16-5-1 COLD PANNICULITIS: This eight-month-old child was taken outside in subzero weather. Two days later he presented with hard red plaques on both cheeks.

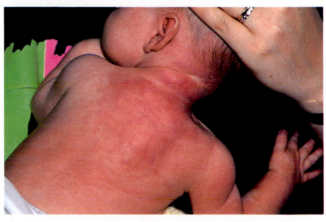

Plate 16-7-1 SUBCUTANEOUS FAT NECROSIS OF THE NEWBORN: Indurated erythematous to violaceous lobulated plaque on an infant's upper back.

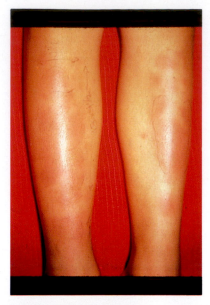

Plate 16-9-1
ERYTHEMA
NODOSUM:
Erythematous nodules
on the shins of an
adolescent female.

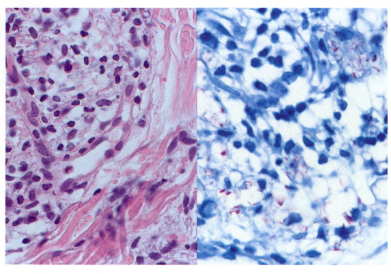

Plate 16-10-1 EOSINOPHILIC FASCIITIS: Individual adipo-cytes are outlined by eosinophils and lymphocytes. (400 ×)

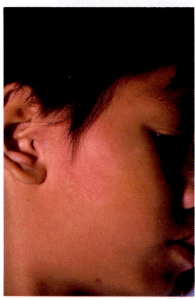

Plate 17-1-2 LEPROMATOUS LEPROSY: (left) The infiltrate surrounds and permeates small nerves. (right) Acid-fast stains reveal several foamy histiocytes containing Mycobacterium leprae. (400 ×)

Plate 17-1-1 LEPROSY: A hypopig-mented anesthetic plaque on the face of a twelve-year-old Cambodian child.

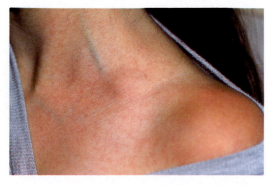

Plate 17-2-1 CAT-SCRATCH DISEASE: The same patient as in Figure 17-2-1 with a supraclavicular node on the same side as the papule.

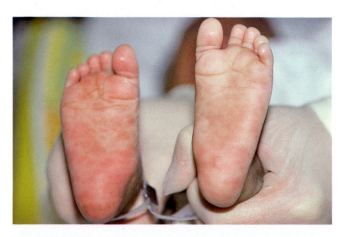

Plate 17-3-1 CONGENITAL SYPHILIS: Ham-colored plantar macules.

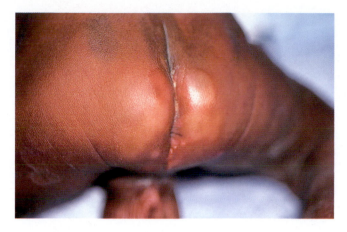

Plate 17-3-2 CONGENITAL SYPHILIS: Anal involvement.

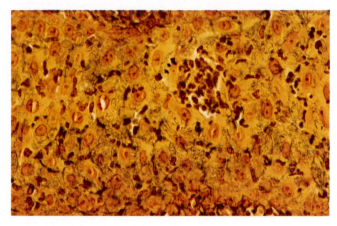

Plate 17-3-3 SYPHILIS: Special stains (Steinert) disclose the presence of numerous fine, threadlike organisms with corkscrew configuration. (400×)

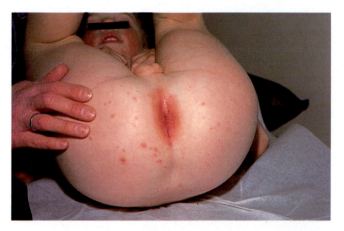

Plate 17-4-1 STREPTOCOCCAL DISEASE: Intense perianal erythema, indicating the presence of streptococcal disease.

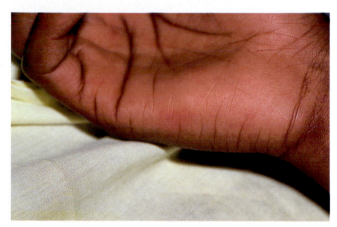

Plate 17-4-2 DERMATITIS-ARTHRITIS: Erythematous papule with beginning area of central duskiness indicative of dermatitis arthritis secondary to *N. gonorrhea*.

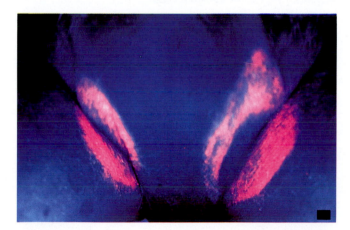

Plate 17-4-3 ERYTHRASMA: Wood's light examination of a patient with erythrasma shows coral red fluoresence of an axillary plaque.

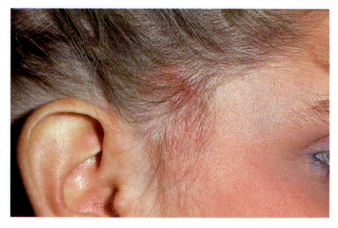

Plate 17-5-1 LEISHMANIASIS: A pigmented depressed scar of cutaneous leishmaniasis within the hairline.

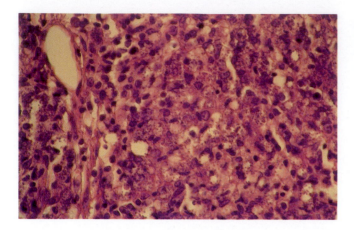

Plate 17-5-2 LEISHMANIASIS: High magnification shows parasitized histiocytes. (200 ×)

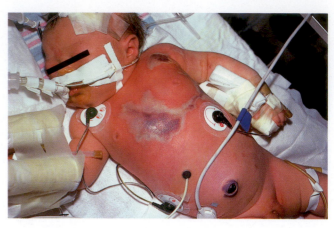

Plate 17-6-1 NECROTIZING FASCIITIS: Areas of gangrene and pallor developing in inflamed skin of an infant.

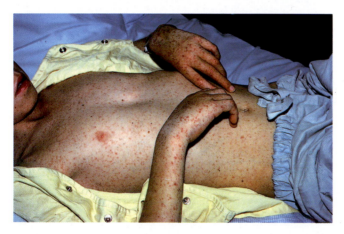

Plate 17-7-1 ROCKY MOUNTAIN SPOTTED FEVER: Vasculitic lesions.

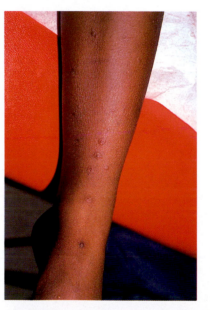

Plate 17-7-2 RICKETTSIALPOX: Papules surmounted with vesicles in a child.

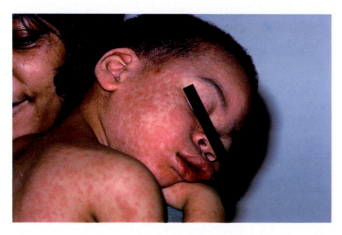

Plate 17-9-1 RUBEOLA: Morbilliform eruption.

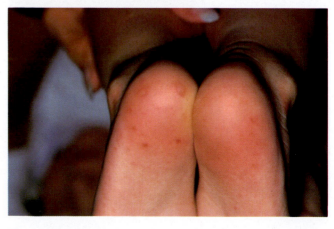

Plate 17-9-2 HAND-FOOT-MOUTH DISEASE: Vesicles secondary to Coxsackievirus A16 on the bottom of a child's foot.

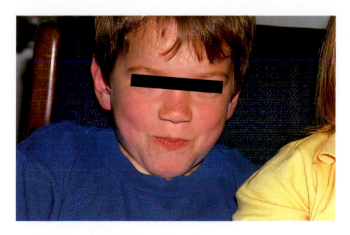

Plate 17-9-3 ERYTHEMA INFECTIOSUM: "Slapped cheeks."

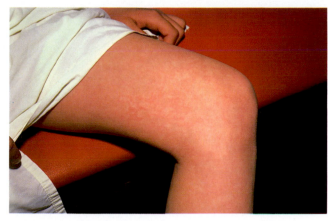

Plate 17-9-4 ERYTHEMA INFECTIOSUM: Reticulated, lacy eruption.

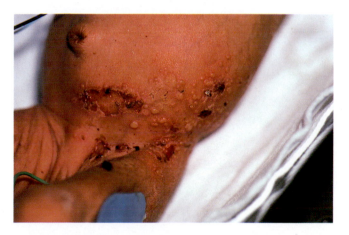

Plate 17-9-5 HERPES SIMPLEX: Newborn with blisters secondary to HSV II in a zosteriform distribution.

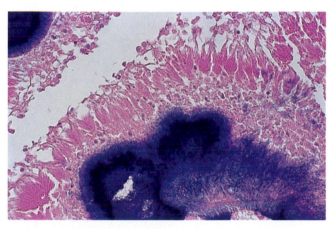

Plate 17-10-1 ACTINOMYCOSIS: Large basophilic granule surrounded by eosinophilic thin filaments with clubbed ends. (200 ×)

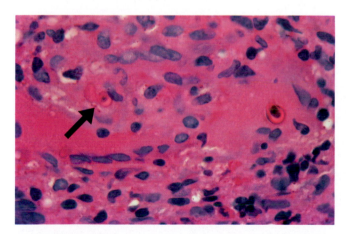

Plate 17-10-2 NORTH AMERICAN BLASTOMYCOSIS: Periodic acid-Schiff stain shows characteristic PAS-positive organisms with broad-based buds. (400 ×) (Courtesy of Clay Cockerell, M.D.)

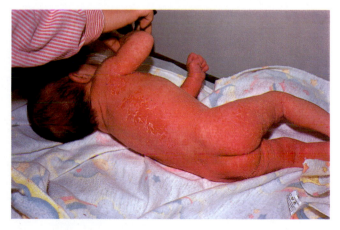

Plate 17-10-3 CANDIDIASIS: Diffuse scaling and erythema in congenital cutaneous candidiasis.

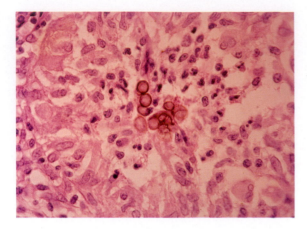

Plate 17-10-4 CHROMOBLASTOMYCOSIS: Round brown organisms ("copper pennies") of chromoblastomycosis surrounded by histiocytes, multinucleated giant cells, and lymphocytes. (100×)

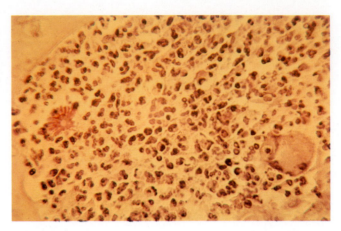

Plate 17-10-5 SPOROTRICHOSIS: Periodic acid-Schiff stain shows a large spore with radiating elongations. Brisk neutrophilic infiltrates are also seen. (200×)

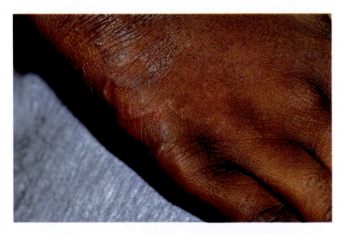

Plate 18-2-1 CUTANEOUS LARVA MIGRANS: Patient presented with erythematous serpiginous line on back of hand after visiting the Southeastern U.S. shore.

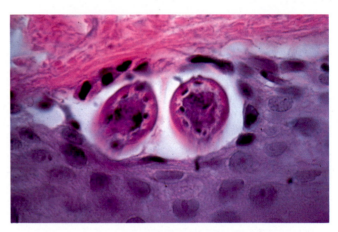

Plate 18-2-2 CUTANEOUS LARVA MIGRANS: The larva of Ancylostoma in cross section, within the superficial epidermis. (100×) Periodic acid Schiff stain.

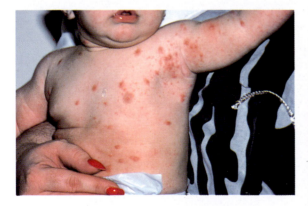

Plate 18-7-1 SCABIES: Erythematous nodules in the axilla of an infant with scabies.

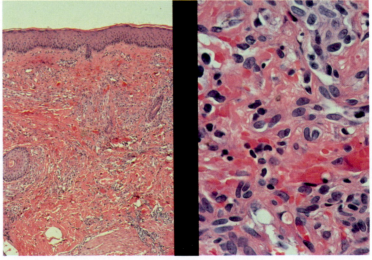

Plate 19-1-1 KAPOSI'S SARCOMA: A plaque-type lesion. (left) Increased cellularity to the dermal stroma on a background of hemorrhage. (40×) (right) High magnification of the spindle cells proliferating in the dermal stroma surrounding extravasated erythrocytes and forming slitlike spaces. (200×)

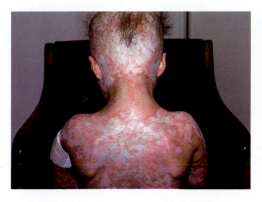

Plate 19-2-1 GRAFT VERSUS HOST DISEASE: Indurated, sclerodermoid, hypopigmented plaques on a young boy. There is significant associated hair loss.

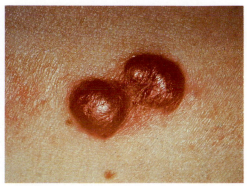

Plate 19-3-1 LYMPHOCYTOMA CUTIS: Red-brown nodules.

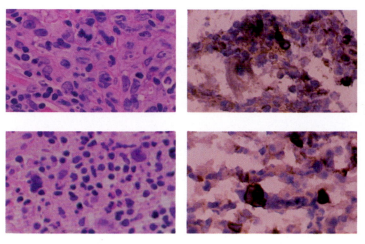

Plate 19-4-1 LYMPHOMATOID PAPULOSIS: (upper left) Atypical mitoses within a lesion of lymphomatoid papulosis. (lower left) Large mononuclear cells reminiscent of Reed-Sternberg cells of Hodgkin's disease. (upper right) Immunohistochemical reactivity of the infiltrate with the interleukin-2 receptor (TAC). (lower right) The immunohistochemical reactivity pattern of the large mononuclear cells with Ki-1. (400×)

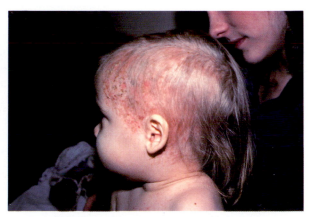

Plate 19-5-1 HISTIOCYTOSIS X/ LETTERER-SIWE DISEASE: Crusted and focally eroded lesions in the scalp (seborrheic distribution) of an eighteen-month-old child.

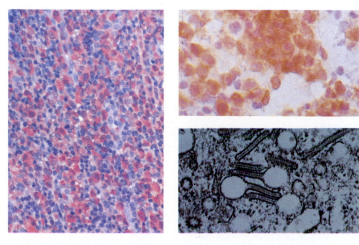

Plate 19-5-2 HISTIOCYTOSIS X: (left) S-100 positivity of infiltrating cells. (100×) (upper right) CD1 positivity of infiltrating cells. (400×) (lower right) Electron microscopy shows Birbeck granules in cell cytoplasms. (33,000×)

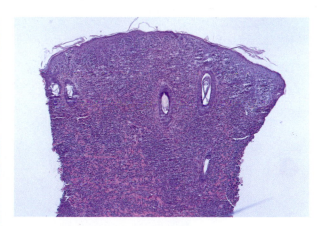

Plate 19-6-1 BENIGN CEPHALIC HISTIOCYTOSIS: Low-power view of the lesion shown in Figure 19-6-2. The dermis is diffusely permeated by an inflammatory infiltrate. (20×)

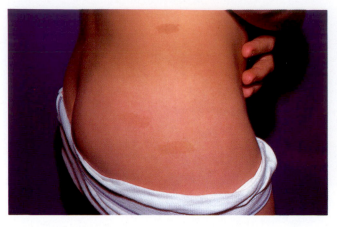

Plate 20-2-1 CAFÉ-AU-LAIT SPOTS: Macules on the trunk of a child with neurofibromatosis.

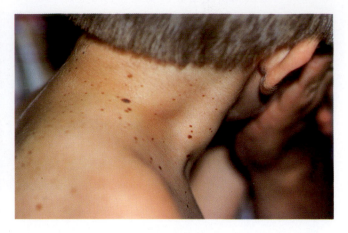

Plate 20-2-2 LENTIGINES SYNDROME: The neck of a child with cardiomyopathy and LEOPARD syndrome.

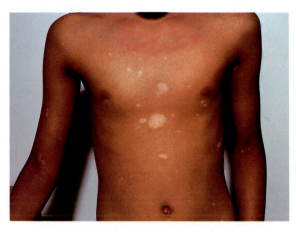

Plate 20-7-1 VITILIGO: Sharply circumscribed patches of depigmentation on a child's chest.

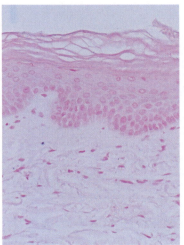

Plate 20-7-2 VITILIGO: Melanin stains show loss of melanin in basilar keratinocytes (left) as compared with normal skin (right). (200×)

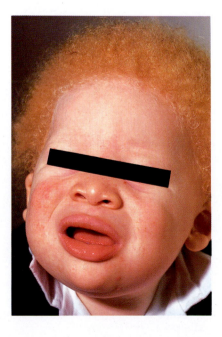

Plate 20-8-1 ALBINISM: Straw-colored hair in a black child.

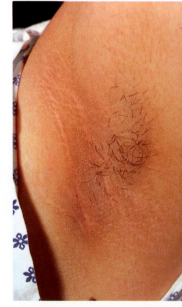

Plate 21-1-1 ACANTHOSIS NIGRICANS: Increased pigmentation and texture of an adolescent's axilla.

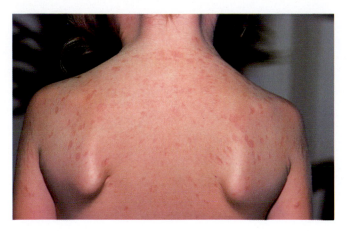

Plate 21-2-1 ANETODERMA: Erythematous atrophic lesions of anetoderma.

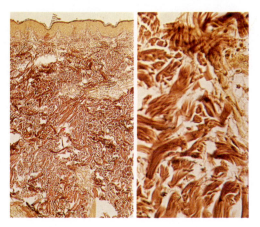

Plate 21-2-2 ANETODERMA: Elastic tissue stains of anetoderma with loss of middermal elastic fibers (Vierhoff-van Gieson) (left, 100 ×; right, 200 ×)

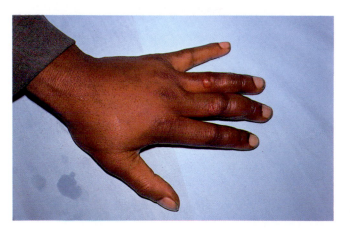

Plate 21-4-1 CUTANEOUS REACTIONS TO COLD: Prominent swelling of the hands and blister formation secondary to frostbite.

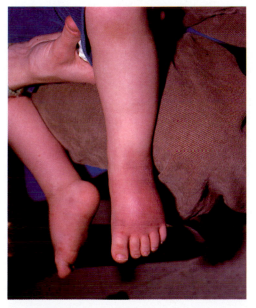

Plate 21-4-2 CUTANEOUS REACTIONS TO COLD: Edema and erythema secondary to wearing wet sneakers in cold weather, producing pernio.

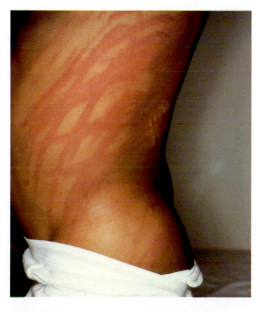

Plate 21-5-1 CHILD BATTERING: Note the whip marks on this child's torso.

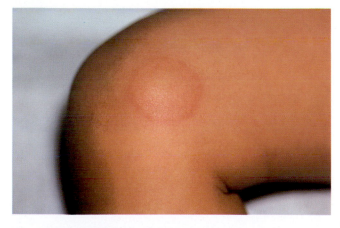

Plate 21-7-1 GRANULOMA ANNULARE: Annular indurated ring. Note central clearing.

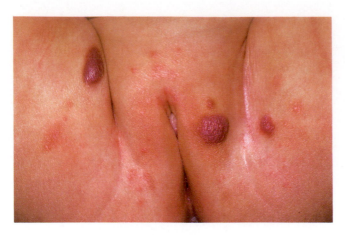

Plate 21-8-1 GRANULOMA GLUTEALE INFANTUM: Violaceous nodules in deeper area.

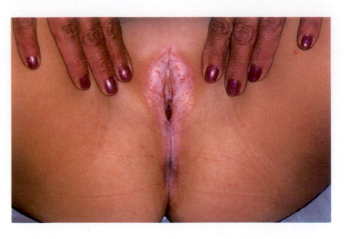

Plate 21-9-1 LICHEN SCLEROSIS ET ATROPHICUS: Atrophic hypopigmented figure-of-eight around child's vagina and rectum.

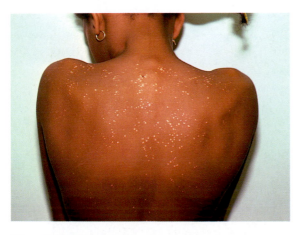

Plate 21-9-2 LICHEN SCLEROSIS ET ATROPHICUS: Depigmented atrophic lesions on trunk.

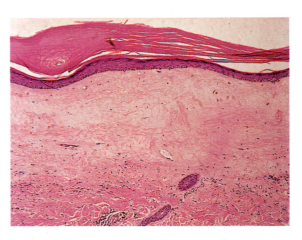

Plate 21-9-3 LICHEN SCLEROSIS ET ATROPHICUS: Beneath a hyperorthokeratotic stratum corneum is an atrophic, effaced epidermis. The papillary dermis is homogenized and there is an underlying lymphocytic infiltrate. (20×)

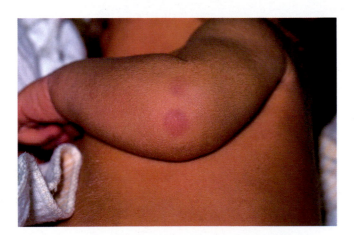

Plate 21-11-1 DERMAL HEMATOPOIESIS: Erythematous dermal nodules on the elbow of a neonate with dermal hematopoiesis.

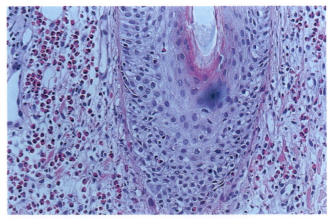

Plate 21-12-1 EOSINOPHILIC PUSTULAR FOLLICULITIS: The dermal infiltrate with marked eosinophilia. Eosinophils have invaded the follicular epithelium. (200×) (Courtesy of C. Darmstadt, M.D.)

usually in postpubertal individuals. Affected males and females have jet black hair, patchy alopecia, and sparse facial hair and lack body hair. Mental deficiency has been associated with this disorder.

A third form, known as Menkes' kinky or steely hair disease, is inherited as an X-linked recessive disorder and therefore occurs exclusively in males. Defective copper metabolism causes multisystem aberrations. Death usually occurs by the age of three years. This disorder is further discussed elsewhere in this chapter.

Finally, pili torti has been reported as an acquired change in areas of scarring alopecias, such as lupus erythematosus and pseudopelade. Perifollicular fibrosis may distort the hair follicle and cause this localized hair shaft abnormality.

Differential Diagnosis
Monilethrix
Bjornstad's syndrome
Menkes' kinky hair syndrome

HISTOLOGICAL DESCRIPTION

Microscopic examination shows flattened hair with clusters of three to ten twists along the length of the shaft in irregular intervals (Figure 15-3-1). Scanning electron microscopic studies indicate closer overlapping of the cuticle in comparison to normal hair. Pili torti is most often confused with monilethrix, in which there is narrowing rather than twisting of the hair shaft at variable intervals.

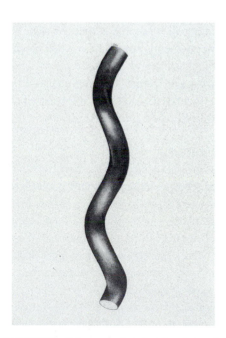

15-3-1 PILI TORTI: Schematic drawing showing twisting along the length of the hair shaft. (Courtesy of Michael Ioffreda, M.D.)

Differential Diagnosis
Monilethrix
Other hair shaft abnormalities

15-4 TRICHOTHIODYSTROPHY

CLINICAL DESCRIPTION

Translated from Greek, this term means sulfur malnourishment of hair.

Etiology and Incidence
This is a rare congenital disorder thought to be caused by one or more mutations of a regulatory gene that changes the synthetic pattern of high-sulfur proteins.

Clinical Features
Scalp and facial hair (eyebrow and eyelashes) are sparse, short, brittle, and of uneven length. Two types of hair fractures occur: trichorrhexislike breaks and complete breaks (trichoschisis). Identifying the hair defect is key in discerning patients who have associated clinical findings. Various eponyms for such associations exist in the literature: BIDS (brittle hair, intellectual impairment, decreased fertility, short stature); IBIDS (ichthyosis + BIDS); PIBIDS (photosensitivity + IBIDS); and PIBI(D)S, in which decreased fertility may be absent.

Correlation of clinical findings, microscopic examination of hair with polariscopy, and measurement of total sulfur content of affected hair are essential to establish the diagnosis of trichothiodystrophy.

Differential Diagnosis
Trichorrhexis nodosa
Other hair shaft defects

HISTOLOGICAL DESCRIPTION

The hair is flat and may appear ribbonlike. Hairs have an irregular outline and areas of complete fracture as well as trichorrhexis nodosalike fracture. The latter areas do not show prominent splaying of cortical cells, as seen in classic trichorrhexis nodosa.

Polariscopic examination of thiodystrophic hair shows characteristic patterns of birefringence: alternating areas of refringence and nonrefringence when polarizers are crossed, with the exact opposite pattern seen when the hairs are slightly rotated to either side of this position. These changes indicate the zigzag orientation of cortical microfibrils.

Scanning electron microscopy of affected hair shows both cuticular and cortical degeneration with a diminished or absent cuticle pattern, as well as abnormal ridging. These changes reflect the decreased cystine content of the cuticular layer.

Differential Diagnosis

Trichorrhexis nodosa

15-5 MONILETHRIX

CLINICAL DESCRIPTION

This disorder is characterized by hair that has a beaded appearance.

Etiology and Incidence

The cause of the disorder is unknown. It may be inherited as an autosomal dominant trait with a high degree of penetrance but variable expressivity.

Clinical Features

Although hair at birth may be normal, brittle and lusterless hair replaces the lanugo hair. Scalp hair as well as facial, axillary, pubic, and extremity hair may show similar alterations. When the entire scalp is affected, it appears bald because of the sparse covering provided by short, broken hair. Affected individuals show variable degrees of change and may also have trichorrhexis nodosa.

Associated cutaneous findings include keratosis pilaris. Various ectodermal defects, including cataracts and dental and neurological abnormalities, have been reported but appear to represent chance occurrences.

Differential Diagnosis

Trichotillomania

Pili torti

HISTOLOGICAL DESCRIPTION

The outline of affected hair is undulating because of the alternating pattern of swellings and constrictions along the length of the shaft (Figure 15-5-1). The swellings occur at intervals of 0.7 to 1 mm, have the diameter of normal hair, and contain a medulla. They are separated by constrictions that lack a medulla and are the points of weakness and fracture. (Figure 15-5-1). Lack of twisting of the shaft separates this entity from pili torti.

Disparate histological findings reported include no abnormalities in the follicular architecture to undulations of the inner surfaces of follicles, which parallel swellings and constrictions of the hair shafts. Ultrastructural and biochemical studies have not yet identified the etiology of this disorder.

Differential Diagnosis

Pili torti

Trichorrhexis nodosa

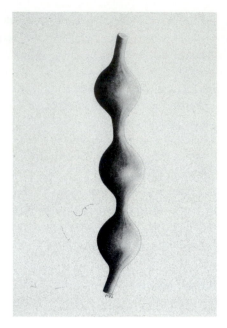

15-5-1 MONILETHRIX: Schematic drawing. The hair has an undulating outline because of swellings and constrictions along the length of the hair shaft. (Courtesy of Michael Ioffreda, M.D.)

15-6 MENKES' KINKY HAIR SYNDROME

CLINICAL DESCRIPTION

This disorder is characterized by multiple hair abnormalities previously described (pili torti, monilethrix, trichorrhexis nodosa), seizures, developmental and growth retardation, and radiologic findings simulating battering.

Etiology and Incidence

Menkes' kinky hair syndrome is thought to be caused by an abnormal copper metabolism. There is decreased serum copper and ceruloplasmin and decreased copper in the liver and brain, but increased copper in other organs. Copper metallothionein is increased in cultured fibroblasts. The disorder is inherited in an X-linked recessive manner.

Clinical Features

Affected children show signs of the syndrome in the neonatal period: they feed poorly, gain weight poorly, and are hypothermic. Characteristically they have coarse, scanty blond to whitish hair, pallor, pudgy cheeks, a blank expression, and twisted horizontal eyebrows (Plate 15-6-1; Figure 15-6-1). Progressive deterioration of all neurologic function occurs shortly after birth. Wormian bones occur in the posterior sagittal sutures and there is subperiosteal new bone formation. In the brain, limbs, and internal organs the arteries are tortuous because of changes in the internal elastic lamina and the intima. Affected children usually die between the ages of one and four years.

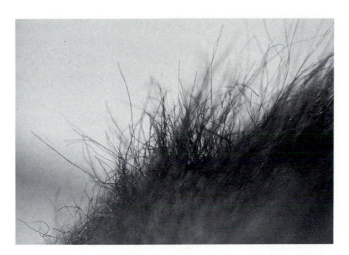

15-6-1 MENKES' KINKY HAIR SYNDROME: Close-up view of the kinky hair of the child in Plate 15-6-1.

Differential Diagnosis
Accidental trauma
Battering (based on radiographs)
Osteogenesis imperfecta
Scurvy
Infantile cortical hyperostosis
Syphilis
Leukemia

HISTOLOGICAL FEATURES

Hair shaft defects observed in Menkes' kinky hair syndrome include trichorrhexis nodosa (Figure 15-2-1), pili torti (Figures 15-3-1 and 15-6-2), and monilethrix (Figure 15-5-1). Of note, polariscopic examination of monilethrix shows irregular periodic constrictions that give the hair the appearance of multiple hourglasses connected in a chain (Plate 15-6-2).

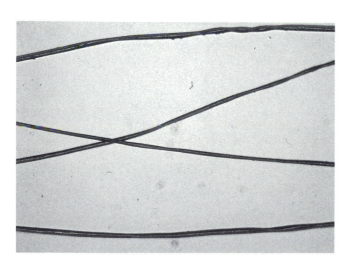

15-6-2 MENKES' KINKY HAIR SYNDROME: Hair mount, showing hair twisted in its axis from the child in Plate 15-6-1. (20×)

Differential Diagnosis
Various hair shaft defects

15-7 PILI ANNULATI

CLINICAL DESCRIPTION

Pili annulati, or ringed hair, is a hair shaft anomaly not associated with increased hair fragility.

Etiology and Incidence
This rare anomaly may occur in a sporadic or familial form with an autosomal dominant inheritance pattern. Its pathogenesis is unknown.

Clinical Features
This abnormality is clinically appreciated as random alternating light and dark banding of hair in reflected light. This finding is apparent only in light-colored hair. There is no increased fragility, thus the hair is able to attain normal length.

Coexistence of this abnormality with alopecia areata and woolly hair has been reported. There appear to be no other ectodermal disorders associated with pili annulati. Clinically, pseudo-pili annulati mimics this disorder but appears to be a variant of normal hair, where the banded reflection pattern is due to twisted and flattened surfaces of hair rather than an internal defect.

Differential Diagnosis
Pseudo-pili annulati

HISTOLOGICAL DESCRIPTION

Hair affected by pili annulati has clusters of air-filled cavities, which cause light to be scattered. This scattering of light is perceived as bright bands, in contrast to normal zones of hair shaft formation, which appear darker. Since pigmented hair absorbs most of the incident light, the variation in light absorption is appreciated only in light-colored hair. On microscopic examination the air spaces appear as dark areas (Figure 15-7-1).

Scanning electron microscopy shows slight variation in the width of shafts and less overlap in the cuticle as compared with normal hair. Transmission electron microscopy confirms the presence of variably sized spaces randomly arranged within the cortex. It is unknown how these air-filled cavities arise within the hair shaft.

Differential Diagnosis
Trichophyton schoenleineii infection

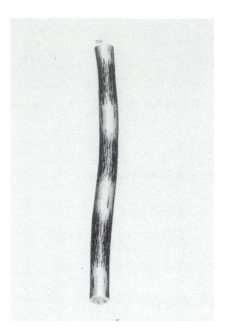

15-7-1 PILI ANNULATI: Schematic drawing. Alternating bands of normal and reduced pigmentation characterize these hair shafts. (Courtesy of Michael Ioffreda, M.D.)

15-8 WOOLLY HAIR

CLINICAL DESCRIPTION

This descriptive term refers to the tightly curled hair of sheep's wool.

Etiology and Incidence

The etiology of woolly hair is not known with certainty. Speculations include axial twisting of the hair shaft, variable rates of keratinization, variations in internal structure, and action of arrector pili muscles. Familial and sporadic occurrences have been reported. Localized patches of such hair within normal scalp hair can also be seen.

Clinical Features

Familial forms of woolly hair have been reported with both autosomal dominant and recessive inheritance patterns. Neither form is usually associated with skin, tooth, or nail abnormalities. In the autosomal dominant form the hair color of affected individuals is the same as that of unaffected family members, while in the recessive form it is significantly lighter. In general, affected individuals have shorter hair because of a shorter anagen growth phase or hair breakage. The hair is tightly curled together in groups, making combing difficult. This is a problem particularly in childhood but may improve in adulthood.

    In the localized form, known as woolly hair nevus (Figure 15-8-1), there is similar hair in a circumscribed zone of the scalp, surrounded by normal hair. The affected hair is shorter,

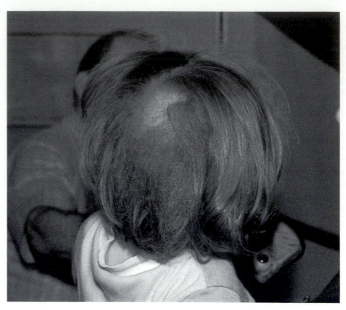

15-8-1 WOOLLY HAIR NEVUS: A localized zone of scalp hair with tightly curved hair. Note the contrast with normal surrounding scalp hair.

of smaller diameter, and often lighter than surrounding hair. Linear nevi are often found in affected patients, but other ectodermal and mesodermal anomalies may be found as well.

Differential Diagnosis

Menkes' kinky hair syndrome
Spun-glass hair

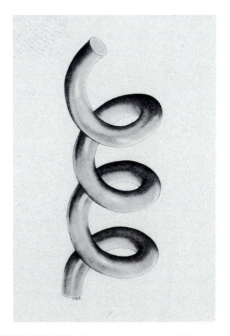

15-8-2 WOOLLY HAIR: Schematic drawing. The tight curvature of this hair is reminiscent of tightly curved hair of sheep's wool, hence its name. (Courtesy, Michael Ioffreda, M.D.)

HISTOLOGICAL DESCRIPTION

Microscopically, hairs appear elliptical in cross sections. They twist on their axes (Figure 15-8-2) and focally show changes of trichorrhexis nodosa. Often the anagen hair bulb appears dystrophic and lacks a root sheath.

Differential Diagnosis
Hair of African-American individuals
Trichorrhexis nodosa

15-9 UNCOMBABLE (SPUN-GLASS) HAIR

This unusual anomaly of hair has characteristic clinical and histological findings. It is also known as pili trianguli et canaliculi.

Etiology and Incidence
Uncombable hair appears to be caused by an abnormal configuration and faulty keratinization of the internal root sheath.

Clinical Features
The clinical presentation is striking. The hair has the appearnace of spun glass: it is frizzy and stands up off the scalp. It sharply contrasts with normal hair of other family members in reported cases. Despite its unusual appearance, the hair is not more fragile than normal.

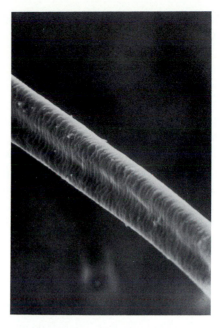

15-9-2 UNCOMBABLE HAIR: Electron micrograph. Note the central groove. (320×)

The problem may be evident in infancy but is usually present by the age of three years; spontaneous improvement may occur later in childhood. Familial cases are thought to be transmitted in an autosomal dominant pattern. There are occasional reports of concomitant ectodermal dysplasia.

Differential Diagnosis
Other hair shaft anomalies

HISTOLOGICAL DESCRIPTION

In cross section, hair shafts have triangular and kidney-shaped contours in contrast to the round or oval shapes of normal hair; they may show longitudinal grooving (Figures 15-9-1 and 15-9-2). This altered shape gives the hair a flattened surface, which changes orientation along the axis. This, in turn, variably reflects light and gives hair the appearance of spun glass.

Scalp biopsy shows internal root sheaths that conform to the abnormal shapes of the hair shaft. Study of cross sections of paraffin-embedded hair shafts, scalp biopsies, and/or scanning electron microscopy may be necessary to diagnose the disorder accurately.

Differential Diagnosis
Monilethrix

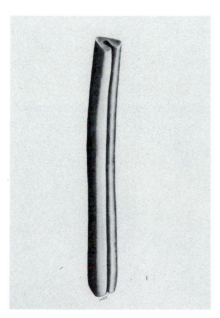

15-9-1 UNCOMBABLE HAIR: Schematic drawing. This hair has a kidney-shaped or triangular outline in cross section. (Courtesy of Michael Ioffreda, M.D.)

15-10 HAIR CASTS

CLINICAL DESCRIPTION

Hair casts are small concretions or nodules found at various intervals along the length of hair shafts. They are caused by various infectious organisms and on occasion by applied cosmetic agents, such as lacquers.

Etiology and Incidence

One variety of hair casts, white piedra, is caused by infection with the fungus *Trichosporon beigelii*. This disorder is rare. A similar but distinguishable process is black piedra, infection of hair with *Piedraia hortai*. These infections are rare and more often seen in tropical climates. *Corynebacterium tenuis* infection is the cause of trichomycosis axillaris. The nits of pediculosis capitis must be distinguished from the above-mentioned infectious processes. Of these, pediculosis capitis is the most common in the pediatric age group.

Clinical Features

White Piedra

Minute white dots irregularly stud otherwise normal-appearing hair shafts. They may be localized within the scalp or involve facial and/or pubic hair. There is no increase in hair fragility. Potassium hydroxide preparations (see below) guide the clinician to obtain fungal cultures that grow *T. beigelii* organisms in approximately one week.

Black Piedra

Jet-black or brown stony concretions surround hair shafts of the scalp at variable intervals. These findings are more noticeable along the distal half of the hair shaft and, as with white piedra, are not associated with increased hair fragility.

Trichomycosis Axillaris

Since this infection occurs on axillary and pubic hair, this disorder does not occur prior to puberty. Colonization of hair with *C. tenuis* causes the beaded appearance of axillary hair. The concretions may be yellow, red, or, rarely, black and may transmit this color into sweat of pubic or axillary hair. Under Wood's light the affected areas fluoresce, a finding not observed with either white or black piedra.

Pediculosis Capitis

Infestation of hair with lice is known as pediculosis capitis. The causative parasite, *Pediculus humanus* var. *capitis*, has a worldwide distribution, affects children as well as adults, and occurs more commonly with poor hygiene. Lice are transmitted by physical contact with infested persons or their hats, combs, or brushes.

Head lice infestation can cause widespread erythema and excoriation, as well as secondary pyoderma. The number of mites infesting the scalp is usually five to ten but can occasionally exceed several hundred. Nits are gray-white oval capsules that contain eggs of mites. Nits are firmly attached to the hair shaft. Their presence close to the scalp indicates recent deposition by mites.

Differential Diagnosis

Trichorrhexis nodosa
Trichonodosis

HISTOLOGICAL DESCRIPTION

White Piedra

Potassium hydroxide preparation of an affected hair shows large numbers of 10 to 12 μm spores and short hyphae embedded in an amorphous matrix.

Black Piedra

Potassium hydroxide preparation shows darkly pigmented amorphous material surrounding hair shafts admixed with 4 to 6 μm arthrospores and septate hyphae. The fungal elements are also Gram-positive and show white birefringence on polaroscopy. Scanning electron microscopy of the surface of these concretions reveals openings that resemble a sponge. The underlying cuticle may be damaged by growth of the organism, but the cortex is spared.

Trichomycosis Axillaris

Gram stains reveal the presence of *C. tenuis* Gram-positive bacilli within the concretions. The diagnosis should be confirmed with culture studies of affected hair. Electron microscopy shows tightly packed bacteria within the concretions, growing into the cuticle but not damaging the cortex.

Pediculosis Capitis

Mites can be identified with a hand lens as well as on microscopy. Head lice are distinguished from pubic lice by their distribution on the body (pubic lice may be found on the eyebrows and eyelashes (Figure 15-10-1) but are virtually never seen in the scalp) and their configuration (pubic lice are broader, flatter, and have claws on their second and third

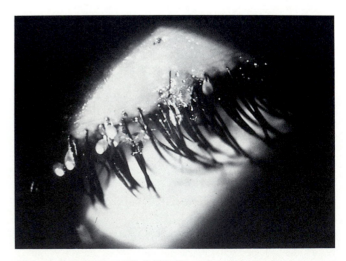

15-10-1 PEDICULOSIS CAPITIS: Lice on the eyelashes.

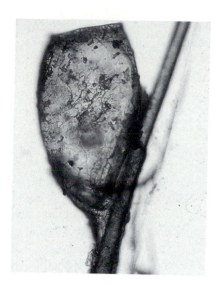

15-10-2 PEDICULOSIS CAPITIS: The appearance of an adherent nit without the egg inside it. (200×)

legs). Nits are grayish-white ovoid structures attached to hair shafts at an angle. Microscopic examination of their contents may reveal nymphs (Plate 15-10-1; Figure 15-10-2).

Differential Diagnosis

Trichorrhexis nodosa
Trichonodosis

15-11 FOLLICULITIS

CLINICAL DESCRIPTION

Folliculitis is a broad term that refers to inflammation of hair follicles.

Etiology and Incidence

Folliculitis may occur as a result of bacterial, viral, fungal, or parasitic infection or noninfectious causes. It is therefore a common problem. Of these causes, infection of hair follicles with parasites, in particular *Demodex* organisms, is virtually nonexistent in the pediatric age group, and thus is not further addressed here. Viral infections that arise in follicular epithelium include molluscum contagiosum and herpes virus infections (Chapter 17).

Clinical Features

Perifollicular erythema with crusting often indicates follicular inflammation with or without infection. An assortment of lesions may be seen, ranging from papules to pustules to indurated plaques. Inflammation may be so intense that it disrupts the follicular epithelium. In such cases the follicular

contents may escape into the dermis and cause a persistent granulomatous host response, which eventuates in scarring.

Bacterial Folliculitis

Superficial bacterial folliculitis is most often secondary to *Staphylococcus aureus* infection and is known as Bockhart's impetigo. Other organisms may cause folliculitis, but this usually occurs in patients with altered flora (concurrent antibiotic therapy) or immunosuppression (steroid therapy, AIDS). Clinically, the lesions are perifollicular pustules.

Deep folliculitis of the face (pyoderma faciale) or bearded area in adolescents (sycosis barbae) is also most often caused by *S. aureus*. Some authors consider folliculitis decalvans, a scarring alopecia, to be caused by chronic *S. aureus* infection, however the etiology of this disorder is still uncertain. Deep folliculitides are frequently accompanied by scarring, particularly when treatment is delayed.

Fungal Folliculitis

Fungal folliculitis is referred to as tinea capitis. It occurs most often in school-aged children, where infections have occasionally reached epidemic proportions. *Trichophyton* and *Microsporum* species are the causative agents of this disorder, with *Trichophyton tonsurans* being the most common causative organism currently in the United States.

Infections start as variably scaly erythematous patches, which may become alopecic. *Microsporum* infection is characterized by scaly annular patches in the scalp, while infection with *Trichophyton* causes slight scaling with ill-defined borders. Some *Microsporum* species (*M. audouinii, canis, ferrugineum, distortum*) produce pteridines. These substances fluoresce under Wood's light, a feature used to advantage to make the diagnosis of infection with these organisms. A rather distinct clinical picture occurs with *Trichophyton schoenleinii* infection: yellowish cup-shaped crusts (scutulae) form around the follicular ostia of infected hair follicles. These crusts contain abundant matted fungal organisms. This form of infection, however, is unusual in the United States.

Fungal spores may replicate within hair shafts and weaken them, causing breakage. In particular, the type of fungi that multiply within the hair medulla (endothrix) often cause breakage of hair as it exits onto the scalp surface, leaving behind "black dots."

Infected individuals mount variable host responses to the organisms. An intense inflammatory response known as kerion may accompany infection. Kerion appears as boggy induration of the scalp accompanied by variable erythema and the formation of perifollicular pustules (Figure 15-11-1). Although in such cases the host response may clear the infection without therapeutic intervention, secondary bacterial infection often supervenes and leads to significant scarring and permanent alopecia.

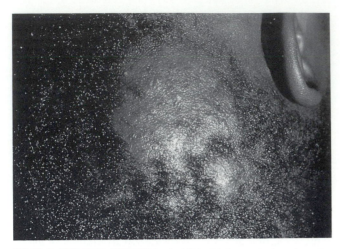

15-11-1 FUNGAL KERION: A child with boggy induration of the left posterior scalp with occasional pustules and a large zone of alopecia.

Noninfectious Folliculitides

Entities in which there is follicular inflammation of noninfectious etiology include: (1) pseudofolliculitis barbae and acne keloidalis nuchae; (2) folliculitis decalvans; and (3) dissecting cellulitis of the scalp (perifolliculitis capitis abscedens et suffodiens), which forms a triad with acne vulgaris and hidradentitis suppurativa. These disorders are not seen before puberty.

    Pseudofolliculitis barbae and acne keloidalis nuchae occur when a tightly curved hair reenters the skin as it grows, causing intense perifollicular inflammation and scarring. This commonly occurs in black adolescents in the bearded area (pseudofolliculitis barbae; Figure 15-11-2) and along the posterior hairline (acne keloidalis nuchae). Affected areas show

localized pustules around hairs; over time, small papular scars arise in these sites. Papules may coalesce to form large hypertrophic scars, which continue to discharge purulent material.

    Folliculitis decalvans is a deep-seated suppurative folliculitis thought by some to be related to persistent staphylococcal infection. It consists of perifollicular pustules within discrete areas of scarring (Plate 15-11-1).

    Dissecting cellulitis, acne, and hidradenitis suppurativa constitute the "follicular occlusion triad" and are characterized by occlusion and inflammation of the folliculosebaceous units. Dissecting cellulitis of the scalp presents as large zones of boggy induration and confluent dermal abscesses. Sinus tracts and scarring often develop. Acne, a common problem in young adolescents, occurs as erythematous papules, pustules, comedones, cysts, and nodules arising on the face, chest, and back. Hidradenitis suppurativa presents as deep-seated erythematous nodules and abscesses in apocrine gland-bearing sites: the axillary, inguinal, and perianal areas. It is thought to result from follicular occlusion and secondary bacterial infection of apocrine glands at affected sites. As all these processes persist, sinus tracts, fistulas, and scars form.

Differential Diagnosis

Miliaria rubra
Furuncles
Carbuncles

HISTOLOGICAL DESCRIPTION

Bacterial Folliculitis

Acute bacterial folliculitis shows spongiosis and infiltration of follicular epithelium by neutrophils. Neutrophils may coalesce to form follicular infundibular abscesses. Occasionally,

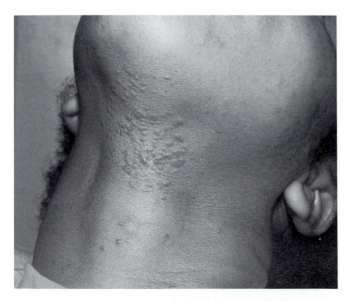

15-11-2 PSEUDOFOLLICULITIS BARBAE: Perifollicular papules in the beard area. Similar clinical lesions located along the occiput are characteristic of acne keloidalis nuchae.

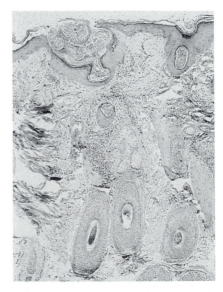

15-11-3 TINEA CAPITIS: Low power shows the large number of organisms in keratin-plugged follicular infundibulae. (100×)

Gram stains of such lesions may disclose the presence of Gram-positive cocci, however cultures are usually more informative in identifying the infecting organism.

When follicular epithelium is permeated by eosinophils rather than neutrophils, eosinophilic pustular folliculitis should be considered. This disorder does not have an infectious etiology and has been reported in individuals infected with the human immunodeficiency virus.

Fungal Folliculitis

Fungal folliculitis may be subdivided into ectothrix and endothrix infections, depending on where spores proliferate in the hair shaft. Ectothrix infections, caused most often by *Trichophyton mentagrophytes* or, less often, *Trichophyton rubrum*, shows spores invading the cuticle and surrounding the hair shaft. In contrast, endothrix infections, caused by *Trichophyton tonsurans* and *Trichophyton violaceum*, are present within the medulla of hair shafts. Although location of changes gives a clue to the type of the invading organism, cultures are optimal for positive identification of organisms (Figure 15-11-3; Plate 15-11-2).

Scutulae show an abundance of fungal organisms matted among keratinocytes. Special stains, such as periodic acid-Schiff or Gomori methenamine silver, will highlight the presence of fungal hyphae and spores in tissue sections.

Noninfectious Folliculitis

Histologically, acne keloidalis nuchae is a small nodule surrounded by variably hyperplastic squamous epithelium (Fig-

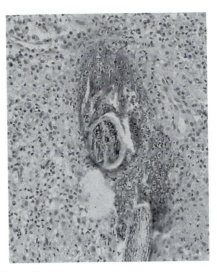

15-11-5 ACNE KELOIDALIS: A hair shaft without associated follicular epithelium is surrounded by a brisk neutrophilic infiltrate. (200×)

ure 15-11-4). In the dermis, hair shafts without intact follicular epithelium are surrounded by neutrophils (Figure 15-11-5). Peripheral to such areas there are areas of dermal fibrosis and inflammatory infiltrates composed of lymphocytes, histiocytes, plasma cells, and/or multinucleated giant cells.

Pseudofolliculitis barbae shows similar inflammatory infiltrates, which may be situated deeper within reticular dermal stroma.

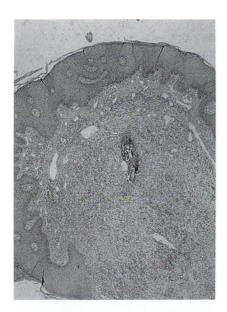

15-11-4 ACNE KELOIDALIS: A papule surrounded by a collarette of hyperplastic squamous epithelium. In the stroma there are entrapped hair shafts surrounded by neutrophilic inflammatory infiltrates. Away from the hair there is evidence of fibrosis and a chronic lymphoplasmacytic inflammatory infiltrate. (40×)

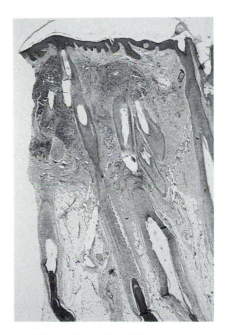

15-11-6 FOLLICULITIS DECALVANS: Low power shows perifollicular location of inflammatory infiltrates in the reticular dermis. (40×)

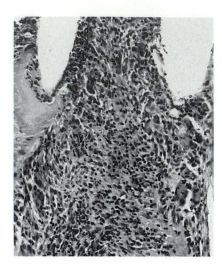

15-11-7 FOLLICULITIS DECALVANS: Neutrophils, lymphocytes, plasma cells, histiocytes, and multinucleated giant cells surround ruptured follicular epithelium. There is also evidence of early fibrosis of adjacent dermal stroma. (200 ×)

Folliculitis decalvans begins with perifollicular neutrophilic abscesses, which cause follicular epithelial disruption and perifollicular fibrosis. Depending on the intensity of the infiltrate and duration of the process there is scarring and hair loss (Figures 15-11-6 and 15-11-7).

Dissecting cellulitis (as well as acne and hidradenitis suppurativa) shows dermal abscesses separated by zones of granulation tissue and variable fibrosis. Epithelial-lined sinus tracts may form in long-standing lesions.

Differential Diagnosis
Eosinophilic pustular folliculitis
Follicular eczema
Alopecia mucinosa
Seborrheic dermatitis

15-12 ALOPECIA AREATA

CLINICAL DESCRIPTION
Alopecia areata is thought to be an immunologically mediated disorder. The hair and nails are target organs.

Etiology and Incidence
The etiology of this disorder is unknown. It has been estimated that between 1% and 4% of all outpatient dermatology visits are cases of alopecia areata. Alopecia areata is a common disorder, estimated to affect 1 in 1,000 individuals at any given point in time. The disorder has equal distribution between the sexes and races. There is a high familial incidence, which ranges from 5% to 25%.

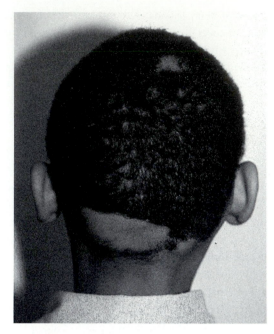

15-12-1 ALOPECIA AREATA: Note patchy hair loss without scaling, forming round patches on the scalp.

Clinical Features
Alopecia areata may affect any hair-bearing area and has a high degree of variability in extent and pattern of expression. Although most commonly alopecia areata presents as circular nonscaly patches of acute hair loss in the scalp (Figure 15-12-1), it may also present as diffuse scalp hair loss, a confluent band around the occiput extending to the temporal scalp (ophiasis pattern), complete loss of scalp hair (alopecia totalis; Figure 15-12-2), or complete loss of scalp and body hair (alopecia universalis). The hair loss may be accompanied by symptoms such as itching or burning. A highly characteristic

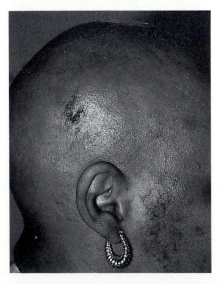

15-12-2 ALOPECIA AREATA (ALOPECIA TOTALIS): Complete loss of scalp hair with a small patch of regrowth.

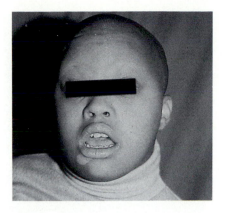

15-12-3 ALOPECIA AREATA: Association of alopecia areata (alopecia universalis) with vitiligo (note patch on chin) and Down's syndrome.

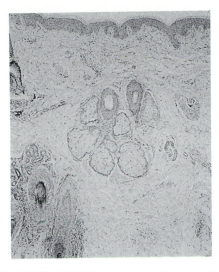

15-12-4 ALOPECIA AREATA: Low magnification of scalp with reduced numbers of hair follicles and peribulbar inflammation. (40×)

finding of alopecia areata is the presence of exclamation point hairs along the periphery of active lesions. Such hairs have normal distal shaft diameters and proximally thinned diameters indicative of disturbed hair formation. Reduced pigment formation may also cause hair to lose its pigment (poliosis).

Nail changes occur in at least 10% of affected patients. Close examination of the nails may disclose fine pitting, ridging, koilonychia, or thinning and increased friability. These changes may arise in a synchronous or asynchronous manner with hair loss. They may persist or resolve as the hair loss subsides.

Alopecia areata occurs more frequently in association with Down's syndrome (Figure 15-12-3), in families with atopy (asthma, eczema, hayfever), and in individuals with autoimmune disorders, such as Hashimoto's thyroiditis, vitiligo, and pernicious anemia. In general, localized disease resolves. The problem may or may not recur. Extensive hair loss at an early age often indicates a persistent relentless course. The course of disease in a given individual, however, is highly variable and difficult to predict.

Differential Diagnosis

Trichotillomania
Traction alopecia
Tinea capitis
Androgenetic alopecia (diffuse alopecia areata)

Histological Description

As may be expected, the histological findings of alopecia areata vary with the duration of the lesions. Early lesions are characterized by lymphocytic infiltrates surrounding hair papillae of anagen (actively growing) hairs. This finding has been called the swarm of bees pattern (Figure 15-12-4 and 15-12-5). The infiltrate in this stage is composed of T lymphocytes in a helper/inducer (CD4) to suppressor/cytotoxic

(CD8) ratio ranging from 2:1 to 8:1. These cells express the activation antigen HLA-DR on their surfaces. B lymphocytes and natural killer cells are not detected in these infiltrates.

The longer the duration of the process the greater the number of hair follicles affected and the greater the degree of matrix injury sustained. This results in cessation of active growth in affected follicles: hairs convert to catagen (transitional) and telogen (resting) follicles. Hair follicles may then become dystrophic and miniaturized.

Established lesions show less intense inflammatory infiltrates and fewer anagen hair follicles. The infiltrate in this stage is composed of T lymphocytes in a decreased CD4 to CD8 ratio of 2:1 to 3:1, as compared with the acute active phase. The typical findings of the early inflammatory phase

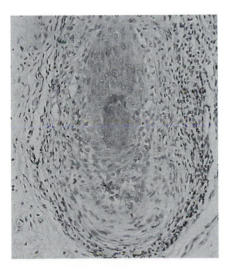

15-12-5 ALOPECIA AREATA: High magnification shows the "swarm of bees"—dense peribulbar lymphocytic infiltrate—characteristic of active lesions. (200×)

may be absent. There may be mild thickening of connective tissue sheaths. Reticular dermal fibrosis of the type seen in classic scarring alopecias is not seen.

Differential Diagnosis

Androgenetic alopecia (long-standing lesions with follicular miniaturization)

15-13 TELOGEN EFFLUVIUM

CLINICAL DESCRIPTION

A diffuse nonscarring alopecia of sudden onset should suggest the possibility of telogen effluvium.

Etiology and Incidence

The abrupt conversion of large numbers of anagen hairs (actively growing) to catagen and telogen (resting) results in telogen effluvium. A large variety of factors can trigger this changed growth pattern. Although this type of hair loss is most common postpartum, it is often seen after febrile illnesses, with ingestion of certain medications (e.g., isotretinoin, etretinate, lithium carbonate, valproic acid) and after crash/starvation diets.

Clinical Features

Patients with telogen effluvium or their parents notice shedding of large numbers of hairs with daily grooming or shampooing. Counts of shed hair consistently show a loss in excess of 100 hairs per day. Occasionally this may lead to thinning of scalp hair in a diffuse pattern. Examination of shed hairs under the microscope shows them to be club or telogen hairs. As telogen effluvium resolves, normal hair growth resumes and is apparent as short hair shafts of similar length between long hairs that were not shed. The key to making the diagnosis is correlating the clinical findings with a history of stress that occurred two to four months prior to shedding (Figure 15-13-1). The process usually spontaneously resolves over several months to a year if the underlying cause is removed.

Differential Diagnosis

Diffuse alopecia areata
Alopecia associated with hypothyroidism
Nutritional alopecia (e.g., malabsorption states, zinc deficiency)

HISTOLOGICAL DESCRIPTION

Since the diagnosis of telogen effluvium is frequently made on the basis of history and clinical findings, biopsy study for this condition is uncommon. If biopsies are performed early on they show an increased percentage of hair in catagen and telogen phases, usually in excess of 30% of all hairs. With

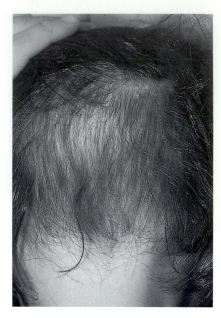

15-13-1 TELOGEN EFFLUVIUM: Diffuse thinning of the scalp three months after surgery under general anesthesia.

increased duration of the process, these hairs are shed, leaving empty follicular canals; as hair regenerates the growth pattern reverts to normal.

Differential Diagnosis

Early stages of androgenetic alopecia
Nutritional deficiencies

15-14 ANDROGENETIC ALOPECIA

CLINICAL DESCRIPTION

Androgenic or androgenetic alopecia refers to hair loss influenced by androgenic hormones in genetically predisposed individuals. In postpubertal individuals it commonly occurs in the absence of gross hormonal abnormalities. In prepubertal children it is an indicator of excess systemic androgens and should trigger a search for the source.

Etiology and Incidence

Androgenic alopecia is rare in prepubertal children; it is more common in the postpubertal adolescent male population, but can also occur in females. In addition to a hereditary predisposition and circulating androgens, end-organ metabolism of testosterone may be a factor in this type of hair loss.

Clinical Features

Recession of the frontal hairline as well as thinning of the temporal angles, vertex, and/or crown (Figure 15-14-1) is characteristic of early androgenic alopecia. Affected sites

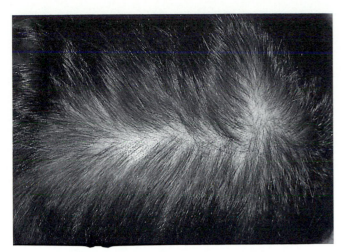

15-14-1 ANDROGENETIC ALOPECIA: Thinning of the crown of the scalp in an adolescent male.

show loss of terminal hairs and replacement by small, fine vellus hairs. Androgenic alopecia resulting from excess systemic androgens may be accompanied by increased hair growth in androgen-dependent sites (hirsutism) such as the beard area, areolae, and lower abdomen. The presence of androgenic alopecia, hirsutism, severe acne, and/or virilization in a prepubertal patient should trigger a search for the source (adrenal glands and/or gonads) and cause (hyperplasia, enzymatic defect, tumor) of increased androgen output.

Differential Diagnosis
Telogen effluvium
Alopecia associated with thyroid disease
Alopecia associated with nutritional disorders

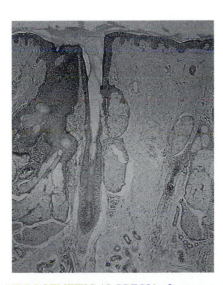

15-14-2 ANDROGENETIC ALOPECIA: Low power early disease shows normal, large-caliber anagen follicle to the left and miniaturized follicle to the right. (100 ×)

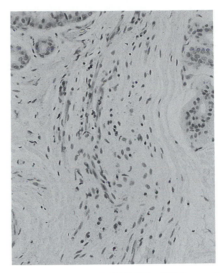

15-14-3 ANDROGENETIC ALOPECIA: High magnification of follicular tract, a residual follicular adventitial sheath of a previously cycling hair follicle. (400 ×)

HISTOLOGICAL DESCRIPTION

Early changes of androgenic alopecia are subtle: there is inflammation around folliculosebaceous junctions and diminished caliber of occasional anagen hair follicles. As the process evolves there is an overall reduction in number and miniaturization of anagen follicles (Figures 15-14-2 and 15-14-3). Where the process is well-established, there is extensive replacement of normal terminal hairs by miniaturized vellus-type hairs.

Differential Diagnosis
Telogen effluvium

15-15 ALOPECIA MUCINOSA

CLINICAL DESCRIPTION

This term refers to hair loss associated with intercellular deposition of mucopolysaccharides in hair follicles and sebaceous glands.

Etiology and Incidence
The etiology of alopecia mucinosa is unknown. It may be speculated that inflammation may induce mucin deposition in follicular sheaths and thus produce hair loss, but the primary cause for inflammation is unknown. Alopecia mucinosa most often is a benign, reactive inflammatory process but has occurred in association with lymphoma (mainly in adults). It rarely occurs in children; when it does, it usually has a self-limited benign course.

Clinical Features
Children with alopecia mucinosa present with erythematous perifollicular papules, scaly patches, or boggy indurated

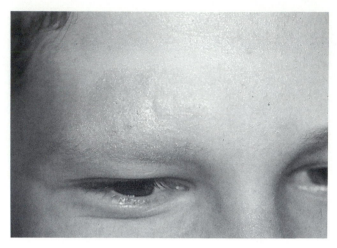

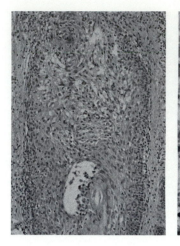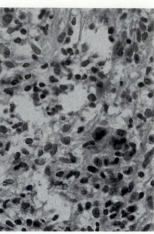

A   B

15-15-1 ALOPECIA MUCINOSA: Erythematous, scaling, plaque above child's left eye. Important to note is the hair loss in the involved eyebrow.

15-15-3 ALOPECIA MUCINOSA: (A) Higher magnification of 15-15-2 shows deposition of mucopolysaccharides between epithelial cells. (200×) (B) A lymphohistiocytic inflammatory infiltrate with eosinophils is present in the stroma and infiltrates the epithelium of hair follicles and sebaceous glands. (400×)

plaques. Affected sites characteristically show hair loss. Alopecia mucinosa most commonly affects the scalp, face, and upper trunk and upper extremities, and less often the lower trunk and lower extremities. In most instances, the process spontaneously resolves over several weeks to months. A small number of cases in children have occurred synchronously or asynchronously with lymphoreticular neoplasms (Hodgkin's disease and cutaneous T cell lymphoma).

Differential Diagnosis
Tinea infection
Pityriasis rubra pilaris
Granulomatous folliculitis

HISTOLOGICAL DESCRIPTION

Sections characteristically show deposition of basophilic mucopolysaccharides between epithelial cells of follicular outer

root sheaths and sebaceous glands. Multiple hair follicles are usually affected by this process (Figures 15-15-1 and 15-15-2). By contrast, follicular mucinosis describes those cases where similar changes are seen in random follicles without associated alopecia. Mucopolysaccharides are highlighted by stains such as Alcian blue or colloidal iron. A lymphocytic infiltrate with or without eosinophils surrounds and/or infiltrates affected epithelium (Figure 15-15-3). If cytologic atypia of lymphocytes is discernible in routine sections, immunophenotyping should be performed to exclude associated cutaneous T cell lymphoma. Similar inflammatory infiltrates may be seen in follicular eczema, however edema (not mucin) separates epithelial cells.

Differential Diagnosis
Follicular mucinosis
Follicular eczema

15-16 TRAUMATICALLY INDUCED ALOPECIA

CLINICAL DESCRIPTION

Traction alopecia and trichotillomania are two types of traumatically induced alopecia.

Etiology and Incidence
Traction alopecia and trichotillomania are similar in that they result in hair loss by continued mechanical pull on hair shafts. They differ in distribution on the scalp and cause. Traction alopecia results from repetitive tight braiding, rolling, or pulling hair with styling. It is thus common in individuals who use

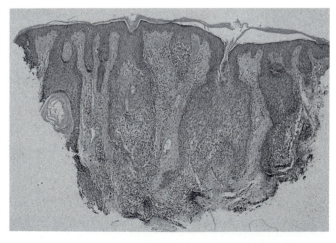

15-15-2 ALOPECIA MUCINOSA: Multiple hair follicles show expansion of follicular sheaths. (40×)

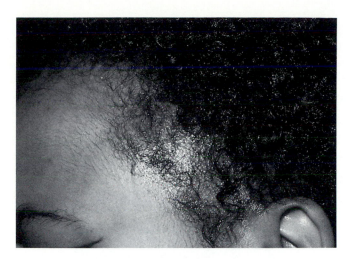

15-16-1 TRACTION ALOPECIA: Thinning along the lateral hairline from tight curling.

such styling techniques and is probably the most common cause of scarring alopecia in children. Trichotillomania is a compulsive disorder of pulling, twisting, or fracturing one's own hair commonly seen by pediatricians and other primary care physicians. It likely occurs in many individuals who do not seek help for this problem. It is considered to be a sign of underlying emotional distress.

Clinical Features

Traction Alopecia

Traction alopecia is detected commonly in females as hair thins along scalp margins (Figure 15-16-1) or as parts widen. In children who have long hair worn back in a braid, continued pull can result in a recession of the frontal hairline, giving the child an appearance of a large forehead. Sideways pull results in hair loss perceived as widened parts. Occasionally, diffuse

15-16-2 TRICHOTILLOMANIA: Irregular patches of incomplete hair loss with a roughly geometric shape.

thinning can be seen with constant pull with blow drying, vigorous combing, and rolling of hair.

Trichotillomania

Trichotillomania is more common in children than in adults and is frequently associated with other compulsive disorders, such as nail biting and thumbsucking. It can affect eyebrow, eyelash, axillary, and pubic hair, but most commonly it affects the scalp. The crown and occiput show asymmetric oval, linear, or irregular patches of incomplete hair loss (Figure 15-16-2). Hair shafts of variable lengths can be discerned within such patches. There is lack of associated inflammation. If the process has been present for several years, scarring may be present.

Differential Diagnosis

Alopecia areata
Noninflammatory tinea capitis

HISTOLOGICAL DESCRIPTION

Trichotillomania has been noted to coexist with alopecia areata, thus distinction between these two disorders may necessitate biopsy study. In such cases, sampling of the most recently noted areas of alopecia is most informative.

Significant hair loss may not be apparent in histological sections. More often, increased numbers of catagen follicles are seen. Subtle clues to trichotillomania include empty follicular tracts from which hairs were avulsed and corkscrewlike collections of keratin containing variable amounts of melanin (pigment casts) impacted within follicular canals (Figure 15-16-3). These findings, along with perifollicular hemorrhage or

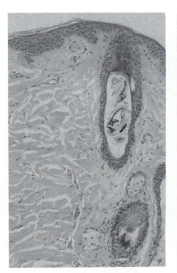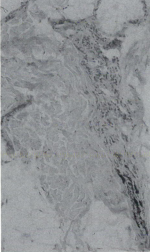

A   B

15-16-3 TRAUMATICALLY INDUCED ALOPECIA: (left) Low magnification shows a corkscrewlike hair in an ectatic follicular infundibulum. (40×) (right) Pigment incontinence in a follicular tract. (200×)

hemosiderin deposition from traumatization of the surrounding vasculature, are relatively rare and must be meticulously sought.

Traction alopecia may show similar features, thus histological findings may suggest a diagnosis of traumatically induced alopecia. The cause must be correlated with clinical findings.

Differential Diagnosis
Tinea capitis
Alopecia areata

15-17 LICHEN PLANOPILARIS

CLINICAL DESCRIPTION

This disorder has clinical and histological similarities to lichen planus, hence its name.

Etiology and Incidence
The etiology of lichen planopilaris is unknown. It is uncommon in children; it more commonly affects women more than men in the age ranges of 30 to 70 years.

Clinical Features
Lichen planopilaris may affect any hair-bearing area of the skin. Most commonly it is noticed in the scalp because of associated hair loss. Lesions begin as erythematous to violaceous papules surrounding hair follicles. The inflammatory phase causes destruction and loss of affected hairs. Lesions resolve with scarring patches where hair is absent. Such areas may be localized to an area of the scalp or affect the scalp in a

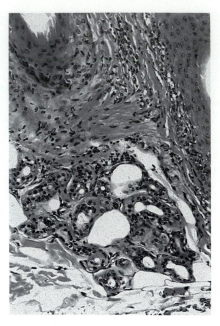

15-17-2 LICHEN PLANOPILARIS: There is individual keratinocyte necrosis in follicular epithelium. Note relative lack of inflammatory cells in eccrine apparatus, a finding that contrasts with lesions of lupus erythematosus. (200×)

more diffuse distribution. Lesions typical of lichen planus found elsewhere on the body suggest the diagnosis.

Differential Diagnosis
Lupus erythematosus
Other scarring alopecias
Brocq's pseudopelade (end-stage lesions)

HISTOLOGICAL DESCRIPTION

Early lesions of lichen planopilaris show a lymphocytic infiltrate closely apposed to follicular epithelium, a feature reminiscent of the interfollicular inflammation seen in lichen planus. Usually the upper half of the hair follicle shows involvement (Figure 15-17-1): lymphocytes infiltrate the epithelium, surround keratinocytes, and cause individual cell necrosis (Figure 15-17-2). Depending on the degree of involvement there may be destruction of the basement membrane and accumulation of degenerated keratinocytes (colloid or Civatte bodies) in the surrounding dermal stroma. As inflammatory infiltrates recede, follicular tracts (remnants of preexisting hair follicles) indicate the degree of follicular injury and death. Dermal fibrosis may also be apparent.

Since lupus erythematosus and lichen planus may appear similar or coexist clinically and histologically, it is important to assess inflammatory follicular processes accurately. Characteristically, basement membrane zone thickening occurs in lupus erythematosus and not in lichen planopilaris

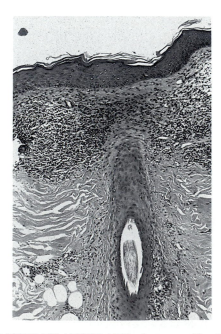

15-17-1 LICHEN PLANOPILARIS: Low magnification shows inflammation surrounding the upper half of a hair follicle and perifollicular fibrosis. (100×)

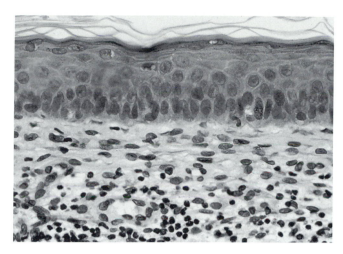

15-17-3 LICHEN PLANOPILARIS: Note lack of basement membrane thickening of interfollicular epithelium, a finding that assists in excluding lupus erythematosus. (200×)

(Figure 15-17-3), thus special stains (e.g., periodic acid-Schiff) are often helpful in ascertaining the thickness of basement membranes. In addition, increased ground substance deposition in the dermis and lymphoplasmacytic infiltrates surrounding eccrine coils are seen in lupus erythematosus and not in lichen planopilaris.

If histological findings do not permit a definitive diagnosis, immunofluorescence studies may be helpful. Colloid bodies nonspecifically fluoresce with IgM, IgG, IgA, and/or C3. This pattern is similar to the one seen in lichen planus. It has been shown that there are linear deposits of IgG and/or IgA around hair follicles in lichen planopilaris, a pattern not seen in lichen planus. Both types of deposits differ from the continuous granular immunoreactant deposits (interfollicular and perifollicular) seen in lupus erythematosus. Where lupus and lichen planus coexist, both fluorescence patterns can be seen.

Differential Diagnosis
Lupus erythematosus
Traumatically induced alopecia
Brocq's pseudopelade (late lesions)

15-18 LUPUS ERYTHEMATOSUS

CLINICAL DESCRIPTION

When lupus erythematosus affects the scalp it commonly produces hair loss associated with scarring.

Etiology and Incidence
Lupus erythematosus is an autoimmune disorder modified by hereditary factors. It can affect the scalp in discrete lesions or diffusely but rarely does so (less than 10% of patients) with-out evidence of disease elsewhere. Since lupus is uncommon in children, alopecia due to lupus is rare.

Clinical Features
Close examination of lesions shows localized or diffuse zones of hair loss associated with erythema and scaling. If the lesion is well established the skin often shows follicular plugging and scarring; there may be mottled pigmentation (hyper- and hypopigmentation) in areas of involvement (Figure 15-18-1). These findings should trigger a search for lesions elsewhere on the body as well as systemic workup for the presence of systemic lupus erythematosus.

Differential Diagnosis
Lichen planopilaris
Pseudopelade
Traumatically induced alopecias

HISTOLOGICAL DESCRIPTION

The histological features of discoid lupus erythematosus on the scalp are similar to those of discoid lesions elsewhere on the skin. Lymphocytic inflammatory infiltrates admixed with plasma cells are present at interfaces of epithelium and stroma: they approximate the dermal-epidermal junction, and follicular epithelium and are usually present around eccrine glands (Figures 15-18-2 to 15-18-4). Along the dermal-epidermal interface there is loss of the rete ridge pattern and variable tortuosity and thickening of the basement membrane zone. Follicular ostial plugging and ectasia and hyperkeratosis accompany well-established lesions. Stromal mucin deposition varies with the duration of lesions: it is scant initially and abundant in long-standing lesions.

Direct immunofluorescence studies of untreated established lesions (at least eight weeks' duration) usually show

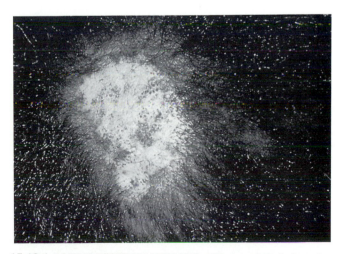

15-18-1 LUPUS ERYTHEMATOSUS: Characteristic lesion of discoid lupus erythematosus in the scalp: there is alopecia associated with follicular plugging, erythema and scarring.

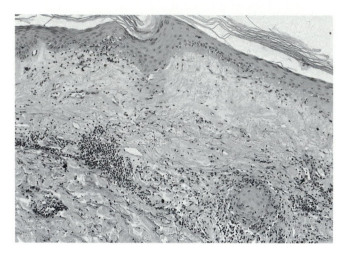

15-18-2 LUPUS ERYTHEMATOSUS: Low magnification shows thinning of epidermis and loss of rete ridge pattern. There is also follicular plugging. A mononuclear inflammatory infiltrate is present in the dermal stroma and focally surrounds appendages. Only a rare hair follicle is seen in this section. (40×)

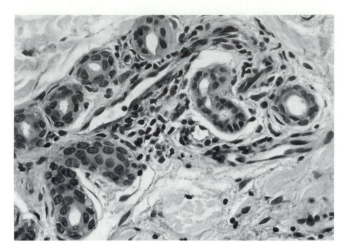

15-18-4 LUPUS ERYTHEMATOSUS: Dermal appendages, including eccrine coils, are surrounded by a lymphoplasmacytic inflammatory infiltrate. (400×)

finely or coarsely granular deposits of immunoreactants (C3, IgG, IgA, and/or IgM) in a continuous pattern along the dermal-epidermal junction. Such deposits can frequently be seen along the midreticular dermal basement membrane zones of hair follicles as well.

Differential Diagnosis
Lichen planopilaris
Syphilitic alopecia
Pseudopelade (late-stage, "burned-out" lesions)

15-19 MORPHEA (EN COUPE DE SABRE)

CLINICAL DESCRIPTION
The appearance of this form of morphea mimics that of a blow to the forehead with a saber.

Etiology and Incidence
As with morphea elsewhere on the body, the cause of this process is unknown. Although uncommon, it is seen in children. Girls are more often affected than boys; there is no recognized hereditary predisposition. This localized process is only rarely associated with systemic scleroderma. There has been association with Lyme disease described in Europe. However, the association of morphea and Lyme disease in the United States is controversial.

Clinical Features
Patients are, on average, five to six years old. They or their parents notice localized itching and hardening of skin of the frontoparietal scalp. Although early lesions appear as erythematous to violaceous patches or plaques, these areas quickly develop into linear, white, indurated plaques that extend from the scalp onto the face (Figure 15-19-1). A violaceous rim about these plaques indicates ongoing disease activity and probable peripheral extension of the process. Affected skin becomes taut, shiny, and hairless. These changes are thus most easily discerned on the scalp.

Morphea may cause skin to be bound down to underlying bone and impede its normal growth. Occasionally, en coup de sabre may extend from the forehead to the chin; when associated with hemiatrophy of the tongue and/or face it may

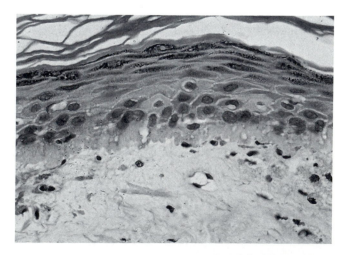

15-18-3 LUPUS ERYTHEMATOSUS: The basement membrane shows striking thickening, and the subjacent stroma contains abundant mucin and extravasated erythrocytes. (200×)

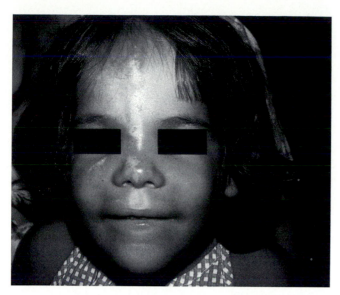

15-19-1 EN COUP DE SABRE: A white sclerotic plaque of the forehead extends onto the nose in this six-year-old girl.

represent a limited form of Parry-Romberg syndrome. Once the inflammatory phase subsides, white, hairless sclerotic plaques with mottled hypo- or hyperpigmentation remain.

Differential Diagnosis
Progressive systemic sclerosis
Eosinophilic fasciitis

HISTOLOGICAL DESCRIPTION

Early histological findings include a lymphoplasmacytic inflammatory infiltrate in the deep reticular dermis, usually near the dermal-subcutaneous interface and around eccrine coils. The reticular dermal collagen bundles become thick-

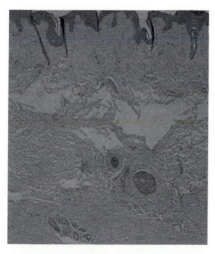

15-19-2 EN COUPE DE SABRE: Scalp biopsy of a lesion in the noninflammatory phase. There is a tremendous reduction in the number of hair follicles at this site, and dermal stroma completely surrounds eccrine glands. (20×)

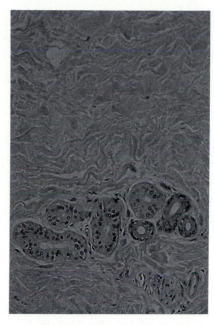

15-19-3 EN COUPE DE SABRE: Higher magnification of lesion in Figure 15-19-2 shows acellular eosinophilic collagen bundles surrounding eccrine glands. Remnant adipocytes, which usually are present around eccrine glands, are lost as well. (200×)

ened: they appear homogenous, eosinophilic, and less cellular than adjacent normal bundles. As the process evolves, sclerotic collagen bundles entrap eccrine glands and gradually replace reticular dermal stroma. Eventually, both eccrine glands and hair follicles are destroyed by this process.

As morphea extends down into subcutaneous adipose tissue, normal adipocytes are replaced by thickened collagen bundles as well. If eosinophils are present in the deep dermal infiltrate, underlying eosinophilic fasciitis should be excluded. The sclerotic plaques of "burned out" morphea lack an inflammatory infiltrate and show replacement of stroma by hyalinized bundles of collagen and loss of normal appendageal structures (Figures 15-19-2 and 15-19-3). These histological changes are indistinguishable from those of systemic sclerosis (scleroderma), which must be excluded on clinical grounds.

Differential Diagnosis
Scleroderma
Necrobiosis lipoidica

15-20 PSEUDOPELADE

CLINICAL DESCRIPTION

Many consider pseudopelade an end-stage scarring alopecia subsequent to lupus erythematosus, morphea, or follicular lichen planus. Others reserve this term for scarring alopecia without an antecedent inflammatory process (idiopathic). The latter form of alopecia is rare.

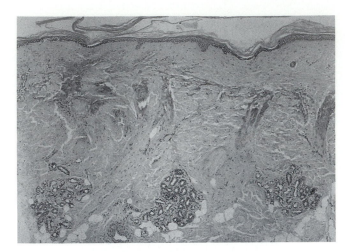

15-20-1 PSEUDOPELADE: There is a complete absence of folliculosebaceous apparatus. Only pilar muscle and eccrine glands remain intact. (20×)

Etiology and Incidence
This entity is rare in children and is likely to be of the type associated with a preexisting inflammatory process.

Clinical Features
Where associated with a preexisting inflammatory alopecia, primary lesions of lupus erythematosus, morphea, folliculitis decalvans, or lichen planopilaris either are identifiable or have been previously documented. The idiopathic form of pseudopelade starts as small patches of alopecia with irregular angulated borders that blend into adjacent normal scalp. Perifollicular inflammation is minimal and a primary inflammatory process is not identifiable. The alopecic areas coalesce into larger patches over time, producing diffuse patches of alopecia with scarring but without follicular plugging. This diagnosis is made by exclusion of other scarring alopecias.

Differential Diagnosis
Other scarring alopecias

HISTOLOGICAL DESCRIPTION
Lesions associated with inflammatory disorders such as lupus show histological features of the primary process. Idiopathic forms have been noted to have minimal lymphocytic infiltrates around folliculosebaceous units. Follicular atrophy and replacement of viable hair follicles by fibrous tracts are apparent. In long-standing lesions the dermis is devoid of viable hair follicles and shows dermal fibrosis (Figures 15-20-1, and 15-20-2). Immunofluorescence studies have found IgM deposits at the basement membrane zone or no deposits at all.

Differential Diagnosis
Scarring alopecias

15-21 PITTED NAILS

CLINICAL DESCRIPTION
Pitting of the nails occurs most commonly in psoriasis, lichen planus, and alopecia areata; although it may be seen with eczematous dermatitides, the latter type is rarely biopsied.

Etiology and Incidence
Focal inflammation in the nail matrix causes defective nail-plate formation in a corresponding discrete punctate pattern. Although random pitting is common in the general population, large numbers of pits on multiple digits are uncommon. Multiple pits are most often seen in association with psoriasis, alopecia areata, and eczema.

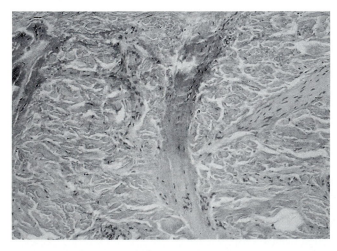

15-20-2 PSEUDOPELADE: Higher magnification shows a follicular adventitial tract, where a hair used to cycle in the past. (200×)

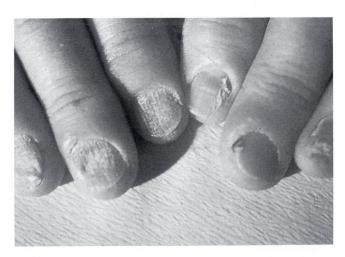

15-21-1 PSORIATIC NAILS: Multiple fine pits of the nail-plates.

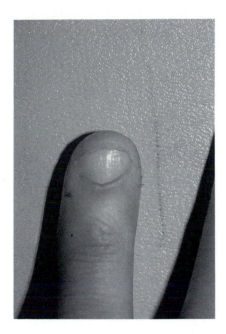

15-21-2 ALOPECIA AREATA: Pitting of a child's nail.

Clinical Features

Psoriasis

Pitting is the most common psoriatic nail change and has been reported in 7% to 79% of children with psoriasis. Pits may be numerous and form a gridlike pattern on the nailplate. There may also be discoloration of the nailbed, subungual hyperkeratosis, and onycholysis. Chronic inflammation of the proximal nailfold is commonly seen in nail psoriasis (Figure 15-21-1).

Alopecia Areata

Pitting may appear synchronously or asynchronously with hair loss in alopecia areata (15-21-2). The degree of nail change

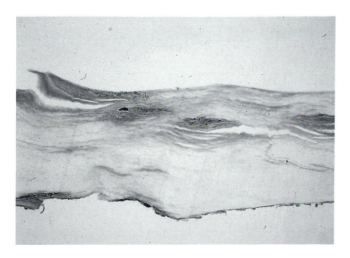

15-21-3 PSORIASIS: Nailplate. Note parakeratotic foci admixed with neutrophils, findings reminiscent of psoriatic scale on glabrous skin. (100×) (Courtesy of R. Rudolph, M.D., and L. Dzubow, M.D.)

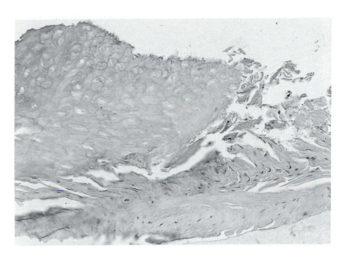

15-21-4 PSORIASIS: Focal hemorrhage and columns of parakeratin in psoriatic nailplate. (200×) (Courtesy of R. Rudolph, M.D., and L. Dzubow, M.D.)

does not correlate with the extent or prognosis of the loss of hair. Clinical differences between pits of alopecia areata and psoriasis have been subject to debate. Pitting is more common in children than in adults. Other nail changes seen in alopecia areata include dystrophy, with thickening of all twenty nails; vertical striations, which give the surface a "sandpaper" surface; and longitudinal ridging and stippling of all twenty nails.

Differential Diagnosis

Onychomycosis

HISTOLOGICAL DESCRIPTION

Psoriasis

Pitting results from inflammation of the proximal nail matrix. The result is defective keratinization of the nailplate surface: focal aggregates of parakeratotic cells on the surface are dyshesive and separate from the surrounding normal orthokeratotic plate, leaving behind pits. Histologically, such areas appear as parakeratotic foci in the plate (Figures 15-21-3 and 15-21-4). When they are accompanied by neutrophils, they mimic Munro's microabscesses of glabrous skin. Fungal infection must be ruled out in each case, since both may have the same histological features.

Alopecia Areata

Nail pits associated with alopecia areata do not show parakeratosis as they do in psoriasis. There appear to be alternating zones of hyperchromatic tissue surrounding pits, which can easily be shed with slight friction.

Differential Diagnosis

Onychomycosis

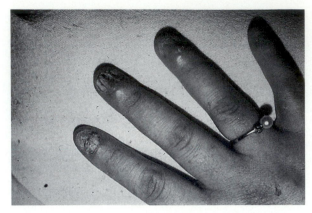

15-22-1 LICHEN PLANUS: Pterygium formation.

15-22 LICHEN PLANUS

CLINICAL DESCRIPTION

Lichen planus affects the nails less frequently in children than in adults.

Etiology and Incidence

The cause of this disorder is unknown. In children it rarely affects the nails without evidence of lesions elsewhere on the body (glabrous skin or mucosa).

Clinical Features

Nail changes vary from pitting, ridging, and grooving of the nailplate to pterygium formation and shedding of the nailplate. The degree of injury to the nail apparatus depends on the location (matrix versus nailbed) and intensity of local inflammation.

Inflammation of the matrix causes variable thinning and ridging of the nailplate. Severe inflammation of the nail matrix may prevent formation of a nailplate; the exposed nail bed then becomes attached to the proximal nailfold, forming a pterygium (Figure 15-22-1). Subungual hyperkeratosis and

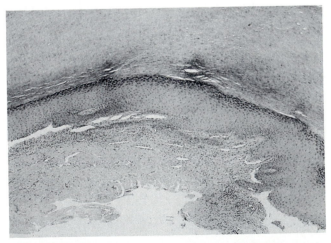

15-22-2 LICHEN PLANUS: An inflammatory infiltrate hugs the junction of nailbed with dermis and a broad zone of separation. (20×)

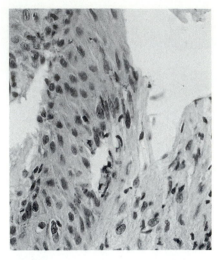

15-22-3 LICHEN PLANUS: Individually necrotic keratinocytes can be seen along the basilar layer of the nailbed. (200×)

separation of the nailplate from the underlying nailbed are associated with inflammation of the nailbed.

Differential Diagnosis

Trauma
Psoriasis
Dystrophic epidermolysis bullosa

HISTOLOGICAL DESCRIPTION

A bandlike dermal lymphocytic inflammatory infiltrate associated with basilar keratinocyte necrosis are the histological hallmarks of lichen planus (Figures 15-22-2 and 15-22-3). Sawtoothing of the dermal-epithelial junction and hypergranulosis may be seen as well.

Differential Diagnosis

Nail changes following Stevens-Johnson syndrome
Nail changes from cytotoxic agents

15-23 TWENTY NAIL DYSTROPHY

CLINICAL DESCRIPTION

Twenty nail dystrophy is a clinical entity in which all twenty nails show ridging and loss or lack of normal luster. It was first reported in 1977 as a self-limited nail dystrophy of unknown cause. Since then, however, it has been noted to include idiopathic and other causes of nail dystrophy affecting all the digits. It no longer represents a monomorphous condition.

Etiology and Incidence

The etiology varies from idiopathic to hereditary changes, lichen planus, and psoriasis. It is uncommon but is seen in pediatric patients.

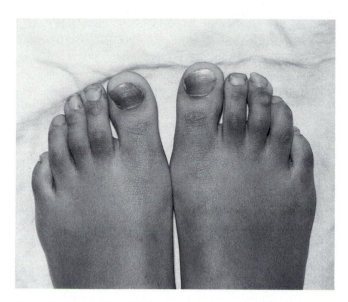

15-23-1 TWENTY NAIL DYSTROPHY: Nails of feet are abnormal.

Clinical Features

Longitudinal ridging and loss of luster are changes of idiopathic twenty nail dystrophy that begin insidiously in childhood and slowly improve or resolve with age (Plate 15-23-1; Figure 15-23-1). Other etiologies of this type of dystrophy should be considered, including lichen planus, alopecia areata, psoriasis, and ichthyosis.

Differential Diagnosis

Lichen planus
Psoriasis
Alopecia areata
Epidermolysis bullosa dystrophica

HISTOLOGICAL DESCRIPTION

The histological features vary with the cause of the dystrophy; for example, if it is due to psoriasis, the histological changes of psoriasis will be apparent.

Differential Diagnosis

Lichen planus
Psoriasis
Alopecia areata
Epidermolysis bullosa dystrophica

REFERENCES

Trichorrhexis Invaginata

Altman J, Stroud J: Netherton's syndrome and ichthyosis linearis circumflexa. Arch Dermatol 1969;100:550.

Stroud JD: Hair-shaft anomalies. Dermatol Clin North Am 1987;5:581.

Whiting DA: Structural abnormalities of the hair shaft. J Am Acad Dermatol 1987;16:1.

Trichorrhexis Nodosa

Chernosky ME, Owens DW: Trichorrhexis nodosa. Arch Dermatol 1966;94:577.

Pili Torti

Beare JM: Congenital pilar defect showing features of pili torti. J Dermatol 1952;65:366.

Kurwa AR, Abdel-Aziz A-HM: Pili torti: Congenital and acquired. Acta Derm Venereol (Stockh) 1973;53:385.

Menkes JH, Alter M, Steigleder GK, et al.: A sex-linked recessive disorder with retardation of growth, peculiar hair, and focal cerebral and cerebellar degeneration. Pediatrics 1962;29:764.

Ronchese F: Twisted hairs (pili torti). Arch Dermatol Syphilol 1932;26:98.

Trichothiodystrophy

Price VH, Odom RB, Ward WH, et al.: Trichothiodystrophy: Sulfur-deficient brittle hair as a marker for a neuroectodermal symptom complex. Arch Dermatol 1980;116:1375.

Monilethrix

Gummer CL, Dawber RPR, Swift JA: Monilethrix: An electron microscopic and electron histochemical study. Br J Dermatol 1981;105:529.

Summerly R, Donaldson EM: Monilethrix: A family study. Br J Dermatol 1962;74:387.

Menkes' Kinky Hair Syndrome

Danks DM, Campbell PE, Stevens BJ, et al.: Menkes' kinky hair syndrome. An inherited defect in copper absorption with widespread effects. Pediatrics 1972; 50:188.

Pili Annulati

Price VH, Thomas RS, Jones FT: Pili annulati: Optical and electron microscopic studies. Arch Dermatol 1968;98:640.

Woolly Hair

Hutchinson PE, Cairns RJ, Wells RS: Woolly hair: Clinical and general aspects. Trans St Johns Hosp Dermatol Soc 1974;60:160.

Jacobsen KU, Lowes M: Wooly hair naevus with ocular involvement. Dermatologica 1975;151:249.

Uncombable Hair

Larralde de Luna MM, Rubinson R, Gelman de Kohan ZB: Pili trianguli canaliculi: Uncombable hair syndrome in a family with apparent autosomal dominant inheritance. Pediatr Dermatol 1985;2:237.

Shelley WB, Shelley ED: Uncombable hair syndrome: Observation on response to biotin and occurrence in siblings with ectodermal dysplasia. Am Acad Dermatol 1985; 13:97.

Stroud JD, Mehregan AH: "Spun glass" hair. A clinicopathologic study of an unusual hair defect. In Proceedings of the first human hair symposium. New York: Medcom, 1973;103.

Hair Casts

Van Staey A, Suys E, Derumeaux L, et al.: Hair casts. Dermatologica 1991; 182:124.

White Piedra

Fishman HC: White piedra. Int J Dermatol 1987;26:538.

Steinman HK, Pappenfort RB: White piedra: A case report and review of the literature. Clin Exp Dermatol 1984;119:602.

Black Piedra

Adam BA, Soo Hoo TS, Chong KC: Black piedra in west Malaysia. Aust J Dermatol 1977;18:45.

Trichomycosis Axillaris

McBride ME, Freeman RG, Knox JM: The bacteriology of trichomycosis axillaris. Br J Dermatol 1968;80:509.

Shelly WB, Miller MA: Electron microscopy, histochemistry, and microbiology of bacterial adhesion in trichomycosis axillaris. J Am Acad Dermatol 1984;10:1005.

Pediculosis Capitis

Parish LC, Witkowski JA, Millikan LE: Pediculosis capitis and the stubborn nit. Int J Dermatol 1989;28:436.

Folliculitis

Caputo RV: Fungal infections in children. Dermatol Clin 1986;4:137.

Hebert AA: Tinea capitis: Current concepts. Arch Dermatol 1988;124:1554.

Swartz MN, Weinberg AN: Infections due to gram positive bacteria. In Fitzpatrick TB, Eisen AZ, Wolff K, et al., eds.: Dermatology in general medicine. New York: McGraw-Hill, 1994:2309.

Alopecia Areata

Drake LA, Ceilley RI, Cornelison RA, et al.: Guidelines of care for alopecia areata. J Am Acad Dermatol 1992;26:247.

Gollnick H, Orfanos CE: Alopecia areata: Pathogenesis and clinical picture. In Orfanos CE, Happle, eds.: Hair and hair diseases. Berlin: Springer-Verlag, 1990.

Perret C, Wiesner-Menzel L, Happle R: Immunohistochemical analysis of T-cell sunsets in peribulbar infiltrates of alopecia areata. Acta Derm Venereol (Stockh) 1984;64:26.

Ranki A, Kianto U Kanerva L, et al.: Immunohistochemical and electron microscopic characterization of the cellular infiltrate in alopecia areata, totalis, and universalis. J Invest Dermatol 1984;83:7.

Williams N, Riegert AL: Epidemic alopecia areata. J Occup Med 1971;13:535.

Telogen Effluvium

Bernstein B, Leyden JJ: Zinc deficiency and acrodermatitis after intravenous hyperalimentation. Arch Dermatol 1978;114:1070.

Goette DK, Odom RB: Alopecia in crash dieters. JAMA 1976;235:2622.

Kligman AM: Pathologic dynamics of human hair loss: I. Arch Dermatol 1961;83:175.

Androgenetic Alopecia

Lattanand A, Johnson WC: Male pattern alopecia: A histopathologic and histochemical study. J Cutan Pathol 1975;2:58.

Lucky AW: Disorders of androgen excess. In Schachner LA, Hansen RE, eds.: Pediatric dermatology. New York: Churchill Livingstone, 1988:1134.

Alopecia Mucinosa

Gibson LE, Muller SA, Leiferman KM, et al.: Follicular mucinosis: Clinical and histopathologic study. J Am Acad Dermatol 1989;20:441.

Hempstead RW, Ackerman AB: Follicular mucinosis. Am J Dermatopathol 1985;7:245.

Mehregan DA, Gibson LE, Muller SA: Follicular mucinosis: Histopathologic review of 33 cases. Mayo Clin Proc 1991;66:387.

Traumatically Induced Alopecia

Trichotillomania

Krishnan KRR, Davidson IRT, Guatardo C: Trichotillomania: A review. Compr Psychiatry 1985;26:123.

Muller SA, Winkelmann RK: Trichotillomania: A clinicopathologic study of 24 cases. Arch Dermatol 1972; 105:535.

Muller SA: Trichotillomania. Dermatol Clin North Am 1987;5:595.

Traction Alopecia

Halder RM: Hair and scalp disorders in blacks. Cutis 1983;32:378.

Newton RC, Hebert AA, Freese TW, et al.: Scarring alopecia. Dermatol Clin North Am 1987;5:603.

Slepyan AH: Traction alopecia. Arch Dermatol 1958;78:395.

Lichen Planopilaris

Ionnides D, Bystryn JC: Immunofluorescence abnormalities in lichen planopilaris. Arch Dermatol 1992;128:214.

Newton RC, Hebert AA, Freese TW, et al.: Scarring alopecia. Dermatol Clin North Am 1987; 5:603.

Lupus Erythematosus

Grossman J, Schwartz RH, Callerame ML, et al.: Systemic lupus erythematosus in a 1-year-old child. Am J Dis Child 1975;129:123.

Newton RC, Hebert AA, Freese TW, et al.: Scarring alopecia. Dermatol Clin North Am 1987;5:603.

Morphea

Hoesly J, Mertz LW, Winkelmann RK: Localized scleroderma (morphea) and antibody to borrelia burgdorferi. J Am Acad Dermatol 1987; 17:455.

Moynahan EJ: Morphoea (localized cutaneous scleroderma) treated with low-dosage penicillamine (4 cases, including coup de sabre). Proc R Soc Med 1973; 66:1083.

Rook A, Dawber D: Diseases of the hair and scalp. Oxford: Blackwell Scientific, 1982.

Serup J: Clinical appearance of skin lesions and disturbances of pigmentation in localized scleroderma. Acta Derm Venereol (Stockh) 1984;64:485.

Pseudopelade

Braun-Falco O, Lukas S, Goldschmidt H: Dermatologic radiotherapy. New York: Springer-Verlag, 1976.

Brocq L: Alopecia. J Cutan Venereol Dis 1885;3:49.

Prieto JG: Pseudopelade of Brocq: Its relationship to some forms of cicatricial alopecias and lichen planus. J Invest Dermatol 1955;24:323.

Pitted Nails

Baran R, Dawber RPR: The nail in dermatological diseases. In Baran R, Dawber RPR, eds: Diseases of the nails and their management. Oxford: Blackwell Scientific, 1984:157.

Farber EM, Jacobs AH: Infantile psoriasis. Am J Dis Child 1977;131:1266.

Horn RT, Odom RB: Twenty nail dystrophy of alopecia areata. Arch Dermatol 1980;116:573.

Puissant A: Psoriasis in children under the age of ten: A study of 100 observations. Gazz Sanita 1970;19:191.

Zaias N: Psoriasis of the nail. Arch Dermatol 1969;99:567.

Lichen Planus

Zaias N: The nail in lichen planus. Arch Dermatol 1970;101:264.

Twenty Nail Dystrophy

Hazzelrig DE, Duncan WC, Jarrat M: Twenty nail dystrophy of childhood. Arch Dermatol 1977;113:73.

Samman PD: The nails in disease. London: Heinemann, 1965;122.

16

Panniculitis

Contents

Panniculitis describes disorders in which there is inflammation of the subcutis (lipocytes, fibrous trabeculae, and blood vessels). These disorders usually appear as erythematous to violaceous deep-seated nodules, which may be painful and accompanied by systemic symptoms. Although clinical characteristics suggest the diagnosis, a skin biopsy is often required for more definitive answers.

The deep-seated inflammatory focus of panniculitis must be adequately represented for maximal diagnostic utility of the biopsy. Inflammatory infiltrates frequently disrupt the normal cohesiveness of tissue. Thus, if inflamed adipose tissue separates from intact overlying dermis, the diagnostic focus may escape histological evaluation. Careful sampling in panniculitis is therefore essential for adequate diagnostic assessment of the process.

Microscopically, the panniculitides may be categorized according to the dominant location of inflammatory infiltrate and the presence or absence of vascular injury (vasculitis). If infiltrates are concentrated among adipocytes, the process has a lobular pattern. If, on the other hand, they are concentrated in the fibrovascular septae separating adipose lobules, the process has a septal pattern. As lesions evolve over time, the original inflammatory patterns become obscured with extension of inflammation to adjacent structures. Therefore, biopsy of early lesions is optimal for histological study.

16-1 HISTIOCYTIC CYTOPHAGIC PANNICULITIS

CLINICAL DESCRIPTION

Etiology and Incidence
This inflammatory process of adipose tissue has been reported rarely in children and adolescents. The etiology of the benign variant is often unknown; in many instances this process is associated with viral infection or lymphoma.

Clinical Features
The process presents as large, inflamed subcutaneous nodules or plaques. They may be noted on the face, trunk, or proximal extremities; occasionally areas of involvement may be hemorrhagic (Plate 16-1-1). Fever, adenopathy, and hepatosplenomegaly may accompany histiocytic cytophagic panniculitis. Acute destruction of adipose tissue as well as involved viscera has been reported. The pattern of inflammation is not entirely specific: it may be seen within the reticuloendothelial system in reaction to viral, bacterial, fungal, and parasitic infections, with neoplasia (lymphoma, histiocytosis X), leukemia (Hodgkin's disease), familial syndromes, and drug intake. It is thus crucial to identify a cause for this process if

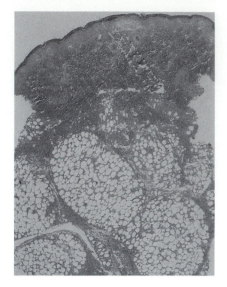

16-1-1 HISTIOCYTIC CYTOPHAGIC PANNICULITIS: Low-power view of inflamed deep reticular dermis and adipose tissue. (20×) (Courtesy of the Department of Pathology at the Children's Hospital of Philadelphia)

possible and to treat cases associated with neoplasia, since the latter often have a fatal outcome.

Differential Diagnosis
Lupus panniculitis
Erythema induratum
Factitial panniculitis

HISTOLOGICAL DESCRIPTION

The histological hallmark of this entity is phagocytosis of lymphocytes and/or erythrocytes by histiocytes, which then acquire the appearance of beanbags (Figures 16-1-1 and 16-1-2). These

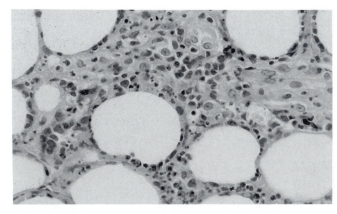

16-1-2 HISTIOCYTIC CYTOPHAGIC PANNICULITIS: Adipose lobules show the inflammatory infiltrate to contain highly pleomorphic mononuclear cells. Note the rims of adipocytes, where histiocytes contain intact and partially degraded leukocytes and erythrocytes. (200×)

changes are found in subcutaneous adipose tissue in a lobular pattern, with involvement of septae as well. Staining for intra-histiocytic lymphocytes may be positive (Plate 16-1-2).

Differential Diagnosis

Reactive histiocytic cytophagic panniculitis
Histiocytic cytophagic panniculitis associated with
  malignancy

16-2 IDIOPATHIC LOBULAR PANNICULITIS (WEBER-CHRISTIAN DISEASE)

CLINICAL DESCRIPTION

Etiology and Incidence

Although the disease occurs mainly in adult women, infants and children manifest this disorder also. The etiology is unknown, but many have hypothesized immunologically mediated reactions to varied immunologic stimuli.

Clinical Features

The disease is characterized by the appearance of crops of 1 to 2 cm subcutaneous nodules (Plate 16-2-1) on the thighs and lower extremities. The arms, trunk, and face may be involved as well. The overlying skin is red, warm, and sometimes tender. The lesions regress over the course of several weeks, leaving a hyperpigmented depression. New crops of lesions may occur at intervals of weeks to months, but generally they subside over time. Associated systemic symptoms, including fever, arthralgia, arthritis, abdominal pain, hepatosplenomegaly, and episcleritis, have been reported. Rarely, inflammatory infiltrates of the type seen in skin can also involve visceral organs.

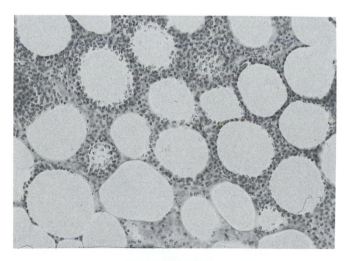

16-2-1 WEBER-CHRISTIAN PANNICULITIS: Individual lipocytes are outlined by large numbers of neutrophils, without associated necrosis. (200×) (Courtesy of Arlene Herzberg, M.D.)

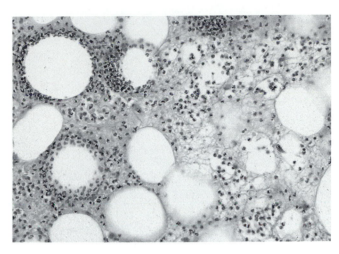

16-2-2 WEBER-CHRISTIAN PANNICULITIS: Injured lipocytes are evident as foam cells in the later stage. (200×) (Courtesy of Arlene Herzberg, M.D.)

Differential Diagnosis

Erythema induratum
Sarcoidosis
Postinjection fat necrosis
Other panniculitides

HISTOLOGICAL DESCRIPTION

The earliest lesions of idiopathic nodular panniculitis show neutrophils infiltrating adipose lobules (Figure 16-2-1), sparing the septal and vascular networks. Lipid escapes from injured adipocytes and is engulfed by macrophages. As a result, large numbers of variably sized foam cells appear to replace adipose lobules (Figure 16-2-2). As the acute and subacute phases resolve, fibrosis of injured tissue ensues. These findings may be seen in many forms of panniculitis to varying degrees, thus exclusion of possible underlying factors, including infection or infarction, is essential.

Differential Diagnosis

Erythema nodosum (early lesions where neutrophils
  predominate)
Panniculitis secondary to infectious organisms
alpha-1 antitrypsin deficiency panniculitis
Pancreatic fat necrosis
Factitial panniculitis

16-3 LUPUS PROFUNDUS

CLINICAL DESCRIPTION

Involvement of subcutaneous fat by lupus erythematosus describes lupus panniculitis.

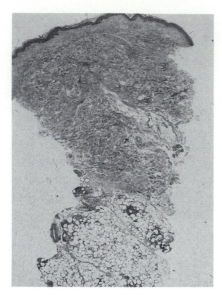

16-3-1 LUPUS PANNICULITIS: An early lesion shows ==patchy== mononuclear infiltrates within the deep reticular dermis and subjacent adipose lobules. (20×)

Etiology and Incidence

This disorder is an unusual variant of cutaneous lupus erythematosus. As with lupus, it occurs more frequently in females than males and is thought to be an autoimmune disorder modified by hereditary factors. It is rare in children; those affected often develop systemic disease. Occasionally it may be the presenting sign of cutaneous or systemic lupus erythematosus.

Clinical Features

Lupus profundus presents as firm, well-defined nodules on the face, breast, upper arms and legs, and buttocks. ==Overlying epidermal changes vary from none to characteristic discoid lesions to ulceration.== As lesions resolve, the loss of normal adipose tissue appears as disfiguring deep depressions (Plate 16-3-1). When such lesions have linear configurations they may closely mimic linear morphea.

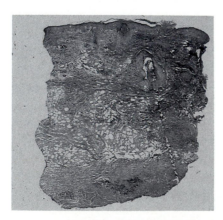

16-3-2 LUPUS PROFUNDUS: Well-established lesions may show altered dermal-epidermal junctions, perifollicular inflammation, and profound alterations of subcutaneous fat. (20×)

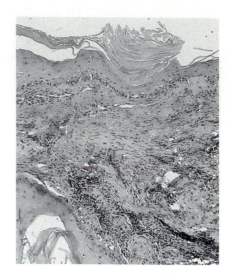

16-3-3 LUPUS PROFUNDUS: There is hyperkeratosis, follicular plugging, effacement of the rete ridge pattern, subepidermal vacuolization, and extension of the process to involve middermal follicular epithelium. These findings are characteristic of discoid-type lesions of cutaneous lupus erythematosus. (40×)

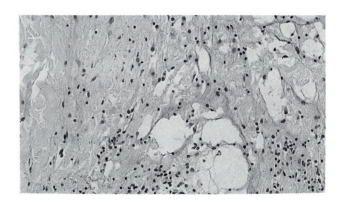

16-3-4 LUPUS PROFUNDUS: At the dermal-subcutaneous junction there are pools of mucin surrounded by mononuclear cells. (40×)

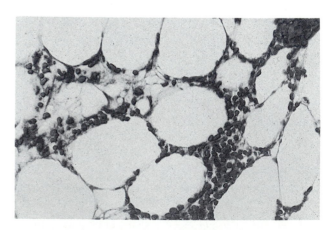

16-3-5 LUPUS PROFUNDUS: Individual adipocytes are outlined by aggregates of lymphocytes and plasma cells. (200×)

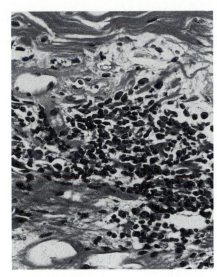

16-3-6 LUPUS PROFUNDUS: The inflammatory infiltrate contains plasma cells admixed with lymphocytes and is associated with mucin deposition. (200×)

Differential Diagnosis
Necrobiosis lipoidica involving the panniculus
Morphea profunda
Poststeroid panniculitis

HISTOLOGICAL DESCRIPTION

The epidermis may be entirely normal (Figure 16-3-1) or may show focal vacuolar alteration with thickening of the basement membrane (Figures 16-3-2 and 16-3-3). Subjacent dermal mucin deposition may be present as well (Figure 16-3-4). Within the deep dermis and subcutis there are localized dense collections of lymphocytes, histiocytes, and plasma cells among adipose lobules (Figures 16-3-5 and 16-3-6). Interstitial mucin deposition, hyalinization, and sclerosis of adipocytes may be observed (Figure 16-3-7). The histological picture in early lesions is dominated by inflammatory infiltrates. Advanced lesions are dominated by fat necrosis and sclerosis.

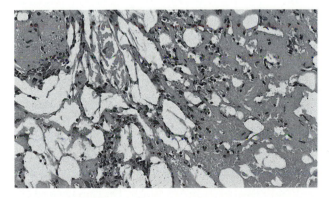

16-3-7 LUPUS PROFUNDUS: The adipose tissue shows a lobular inflammatory infiltrate of plasma cells and lymphocytes. There is necrosis and hyalinization of adipose lobules. (100×)

In cases where the dermal-epidermal junction shows alterations of lupus erythematosus, direct immunofluorescence studies show granular deposits of IgG, IgM, and/or C3 (positive lupus band test; Chapter 7). When the epidermis is unaltered, immunoreactant deposits are lacking at the dermal-epidermal interface but may be found in deep dermal vessel walls, indicating vasculitis.

Differential Diagnosis
Necrobiosis lipoidica involving the panniculus
Morphea profunda
Poststeroid panniculitis
Traumatic panniculitis

16-4 POSTSTEROID PANNICULITIS

CLINICAL DESCRIPTION

Patients with this disorder have received high doses of corticosteroids for prolonged periods of time.

Etiology and Incidence
This rare condition occurs in children within two weeks of discontinuation of steroid therapy. The reason for this phenomenon is unclear. Since the panniculitis occurs in areas of greatest fat deposition, it has been suggested that rapid removal of lipid following steroid withdrawal may lead to damage of lipocytes. The panniculitis disappears with reinstitution of steroid therapy.

Clinical Features
Subcutaneous nodules occur on the cheeks, arms, and trunk. The lesions are asymptomatic and range in size from 1 to 4 cm in diameter. Although other causes of panniculitis may be considered, the history of recent steroid withdrawal and resolution with reinstatement of this therapy are diagnostic.

Differential Diagnosis
Postinjection panniculitis
Erythema nodosum
Other panniculitides

HISTOLOGICAL DESCRIPTION

Needle-shaped clefts are observed within the adipocytes and histiocytes. These clefts are thought to result from crystallization of triglycerides in the adipose tissue of children, which has a higher ratio of unsaturated to saturated fatty acids as compared with adults. The crystals are removed by routine processing, leaving behind intracellular radial arrays of needlelike clefts. This histological feature is not unique to post-steroid panniculitis; it is also observed in subcutaneous fat necrosis of the newborn and sclerema neonatorum. In post-steroid panniculitis there is an associated patchy lymphohistiocytic infiltrate within the adipose lobules admixed with occasional multinucleated giant cells. Lipocytes may have spokelike, needleshaped clefts.

Differential Diagnosis

Subcutaneous fat necrosis of the newborn
Sclerema neonatorum
Cold panniculitis

16-5 COLD PANNICULITIS (POPSICLE STICK PANNICULITIS)

CLINICAL DESCRIPTION

This entity is a result of cold injury to fat.

Etiology and Incidence

The subcutaneous fat of infants and some children solidifies more readily at higher temperatures than that of adults, because of the higher relative concentration of saturated fats. Injury occurs mainly during the cold winter months, and at times during summer months when Popsicles, ice cubes, or cold fluids come in contact with an infant's cheek.

Clinical Features

The face and extremities are most frequently involved due to exposure to cold air (Plate 16-5-1). The cheeks are affected when cold substances are held in the buccal pouch. Following the insult the subcutaneous tissues become indurated while the overlying skin is red, violaceous, or blue. At times the area is tender. The lesions gradually soften and resolve over the course of one to several weeks.

Differential Diagnosis

Facial cellulitis
Traumatic hematoma
Direct trauma
Reaction to DPT injection (if thigh is involved)
Factitial panniculitis

HISTOLOGICAL DESCRIPTION

Within hours of cold exposure there is necrosis of lipocytes. This injury is more apparent near the junction of the dermis with the subcutis than in the deep panniculus. Foamy macrophages become surrounded by neutrophils, lymphocytes, and histiocytes. These changes occur predominantly in adipose lobules. Vasculitis is not a feature of this disorder.

Differential Diagnosis

Traumatic fat necrosis
Panniculitis secondary to infectious agents
Factitial panniculitis

16-6 SCLEREMA NEONATORUM

This condition is seen in seriously ill premature or full-term infants.

Etiology and Incidence

Sclerema neonatorum afflicts debilitated infants with serious underlying conditions (e.g., congenital heart disease, respiratory distress syndrome, necrotizing enterocolitis) during the first few weeks of life. One-fourth of women who deliver these infants are ill. Hypothermia, shock, and sepsis have been identified as predisposing factors. The high ratio of saturated to unsaturated fats in newborns is thought to make newborns susceptible to this process. The mortality rate is high.

Clinical Features

A diffuse, rapidly spreading hardening of the skin is noted within the first few weeks of life. The skin appears waxy and feels very cold. This process eventually involves all subcutaneous tissues. The infant becomes immobilized with a fixed masklike facies.

Differential Diagnosis

Subcutaneous fat necrosis of the newborn
Systemic sclerosis of the newborn
Scleredema neonatorum

HISTOLOGICAL DESCRIPTION

Within poorly developed lobules of adipose tissue there are large numbers of adipocytes that contain needle-shaped clefts arranged in radial patterns (Figure 16-6-1). Such clefts may also be noted in histiocytes. In frozen sections, rather than

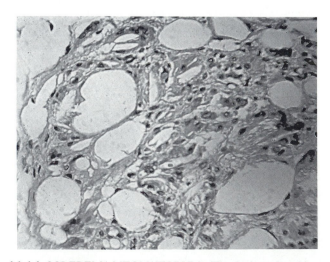

16-6-1 SCLEREMA NEONATORUM: The fat is replaced by variably sized cystic cavities. A rare adipocyte shows radially arranged shadows of washed-out crystals. There is a minimal host response. (200×)

routine histological study, they contain doubly refractile crystals. Inflammatory infiltrates, if present, are sparse and composed of neutrophils, eosinophils, lymphocytes, or histiocytes. The relative paucity of an inflammatory response to this process has been attributed to the short interval between disease onset and fatal outcome or inability to mount a host response to this process.

Differential Diagnosis
Subcutaneous fat necrosis of the newborn
Cold panniculitis

16-7 SUBCUTANEOUS FAT NECROSIS OF THE NEWBORN

CLINICAL DESCRIPTION

This condition occurs in healthy full-term infants.

Etiology and Incidence
As with sclerema neonatorum, the specific cause of subcutaneous fat necrosis is unknown. It has been associated with hypothermia, asphyxia, traumatic deliveries, and maternal diabetes mellitus. Infants are predisposed to this problem because of the increased ratio of unsaturated to saturated fat in the newborn.

Clinical Features
Subcutaneous indurated nodules occur in the first two weeks of life in single or multiple locations. A number of lesions may coalesce to form large plaques, which can feel lobulated (Plate 16-7-1). The overlying skin is frequently erythematous to violaceous. The areas most often affected are the cheeks, buttocks, arms, and thighs. As the lesions resolve, they may

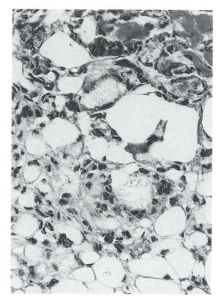

16-7-2 SUBCUTANEOUS FAT NECROSIS OF THE NEWBORN: Closer examination shows a lymphohistiocytic inflammatory infiltrate with eosinophils surrounding lipocytes, which contain radially arranged projections. These projections are remnants of crystalline material removed by routine processing. (200×)

become fluctuant. Significant hypercalcemia may occur as the lesions disappear. Infants with this condition should be screened for hypercalcemia for the first six weeks of life.

Differential Diagnosis
Sclerema neonatorum

HISTOLOGICAL DESCRIPTION

Adipocytes in subcutaneous fat necrosis of the newborn show radially arranged, needlelike crystals similar to those observed in cold panniculitis and sclerema neonatorum (Figures 16-7-1 and 16-7-2). In contrast to sclerema, mixed inflammatory infiltrates with multinucleated giant cells accompany fat necrosis.

Differential Diagnosis
Subcutaneous fat necrosis of the newborn
Cold panniculitis

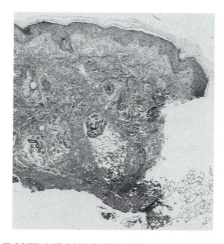

16-7-1 SUBCUTANEOUS FAT NECROSIS OF THE NEWBORN: At the very edge of the deep dermis there is inflammation of the attached fragment of adipose tissue. (20×)

16-8 NODULAR VASCULITIS (ERYTHEMA INDURATUM)

CLINICAL DESCRIPTION

Etiology and Incidence
This entity is rarely seen in childhood. The cause and treatment of this disorder are subjects of controversy. The etiology has been attributed to an immune complex-mediated vasculitis.

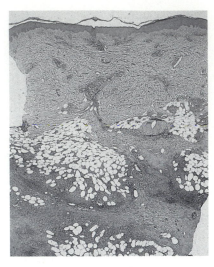

16-8-1 NODULAR VASCULITIS (ERYTHEMA INDURATUM): Scanning magnification shows intense inflammation of adipose lobules with extension into adjacent septae. (20×)

Clinical Features

These lesions appear as violaceous, indurated nodules, 1 to 2 cm in diameter, on the lower legs. They occasionally ulcerate and heal with scarring. Often they occur in crops and are painful. In some cases there is a history of recent or remote infection with *Mycobacterium tuberculosis.* In such instances this panniculitis is thought to be related to heightened delayed hypersensitivity to components of tubercle bacilli released from latent foci of infection. Since idiopathic cases have been reported as well, the term *nodular vasculitis* is preferred.

Differential Diagnosis

Erythema nodosum
Panniculitis secondary to infectious causes
Other panniculitides

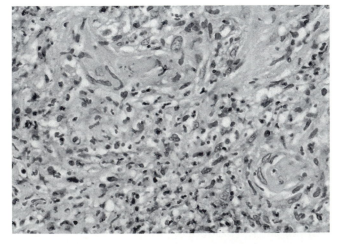

16-8-2 NODULAR VASCULITIS: In areas there are collections of neutrophils, nuclear dust, and extravasated erythrocytes surrounding injured vessels. These are characteristic findings. (200×)

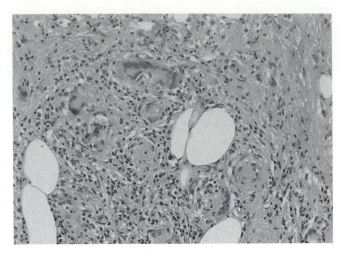

16-8-3 NODULAR VASCULITIS: In other areas there is fibrosis and granulomatous inflammation containing multinucleated giant cells. (200×)

HISTOLOGICAL DESCRIPTION

Early lesions of erythema induratum show lymphocytes and plasma cells infiltrating adipose lobules. Vascular changes are pronounced: there is invasion of small to medium-sized vessel walls by neutrophilic and mononuclear cells associated with swelling of endothelial cells (Figures 16-8-1 and 16-8-2). Thrombosis and occlusion of affected vessels may be noted.

Later lesions show formation of epithelioid granulomas in the subcutis with or without involvement of the deep dermis (Figure 16-8-3). In such areas, caseation necrosis may be seen. Immunohistochemical studies have shown these granulomas to have a predominance of Leu-1 and Leu 3a-bearing T cells, which express the activation marker HLA-DR. Where lesions contain brisk inflammatory infiltrates, special stains to exclude an infectious etiology should be performed. In late resolving phases, as with other panniculitides, fibrosis predominates.

Differential Diagnosis

Polyarteritis nodosa
Panniculitis secondary to infectious organisms (bacterial, mycobacterial, fungal)

16-9 ERYTHEMA NODOSUM

CLINICAL DESCRIPTION

The presence of erythema nodosum should trigger an investigation for one of the many associated disorders.

Etiology and Incidence

Erythema nodosum seems to be a hypersensitivity response to infection (Group A beta streptococci, tuberculosis, histoplasmosis, coccidioidomycosis, cat-scratch fever), inflammatory

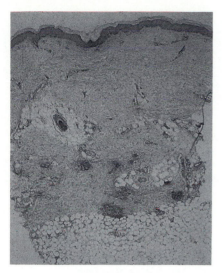

16-9-1 ERYTHEMA NODOSUM: An early lesion displays patchy inflammatory infiltrates in widened subcutaneous adipose septae. (20×)

bowel disease, sarcoidosis, or drugs. The exact immunologic mechanism has not been clarified. Although it occurs at any age, it is most commonly seen in adolescents during the spring and fall. Females are more often affected than males.

Clinical Features

The lesions of erythema nodosum appear as symmetric deep, tender, erythematous nodules (1 to 5 cm) or plaques on an extensor surface (Plate 16-9-1). The extensors of the extremities, face, and neck may be involved. With time, the overlying skin acquires a blue violaceous, resembling a bruise. The lesions last three to six weeks. Seventy percent of patients have associated arthralgias and other systemic symptoms. Recurrences can occur.

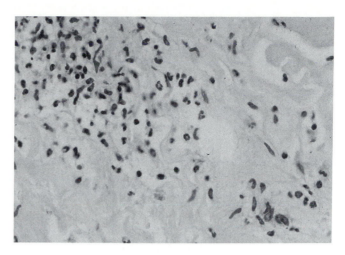

16-9-3 ERYTHEMA NODOSUM: The infiltrate contains neutrophils, eosinophils, and mononuclear cells. (400×)

Differential Diagnosis

Bruise
Cellulitis
Erysipelas
Insect bite
Vasculitis
Erythema induratum

HISTOLOGICAL DESCRIPTION

Erythema nodosum is the classic example of a septal panniculitis. In the late lesions, lobules are usually involved secondarily.

Early lesions show infiltrates dominated by polymorphonuclear leukocytes. Eosinophils may be seen as well. Septae often appear edematous (Figures 16-9-1 to 16-9-3). As lesions evolve, the composition of the infiltrate changes to

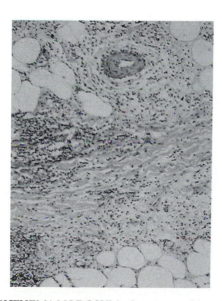

16-9-2 ERYTHEMA NODOSUM: Septae are widened by edema and inflammation. (100×)

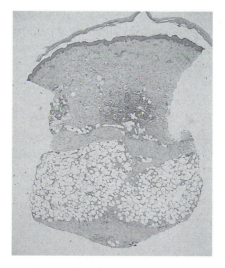

16-9-4 ERYTHEMA NODOSUM: A late lesion. Note the fibrotic septae outlining adipose lobules. (20×)

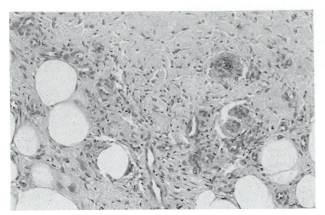

16-9-5 ERYTHEMA NODOSUM: The fibrotic septae contain multinucleated giant cells, mononuclear cells, and rare eosinophils. The fibrosis impinges on adjacent adipose lobules. (400×)

histiocytes admixed with multinucleated giant cells. Widened fibrous septae show less edema and the beginnings of fibrosis (Figures 16-9-4 and 16-9-5). Late lesions show less intense infiltrates of mononuclear cells, prominent septal fibrosis, and microcyst formation in previously inflamed adjacent adipose lobules.

Differential Diagnosis
Early stages:
    Panniculitis secondary to infectious organisms
Late (fibrotic) stage:
    Morphea profunda

16-10 EOSINOPHILIC FASCIITIS

CLINICAL DESCRIPTION

Etiology and Incidence
This sclerodermalike disorder is seen in children as well as adults, although it is rare in childhood. It has a sudden onset, frequently following strenuous exercise. Its cause and specific relationship to scleroderma have yet to be elucidated.

Clinical Features
The disorder affects primarily the skin of the arms and legs. Tenderness, edema, and induration of acute onset characterize this condition. The skin in affected areas is tightly bound to the underlying tissues, acquires a yellow-red hue, and has a cobblestonelike surface. An associated transient eosinophilia and elevated sedimentation rate are present in the early stages of this process. Eosinophilic fasciitis frequently resolves spontaneously.

Differential Diagnosis
Scleroderma

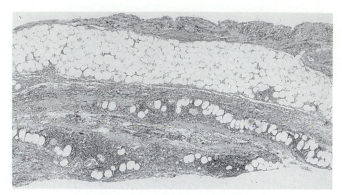

16-10-1 EOSINOPHILIC FASCIITIS: Low power view of a large excisional biopsy shows that inflammatory infiltrates expand the muscular fascia beneath the panniculus. (20×)

HISTOLOGICAL DESCRIPTION

As its name implies, the inflammatory focus of eosinophilic fasciitis is the muscular fascia. This necessitates a deep biopsy specimen to detect diagnostic changes.

Characteristically, lymphocytes, plasma cells, and eosinophils are observed permeating variably thickened collagen bundles of the fascia (Figures 16-10-1 and 16-10-2). Infiltrates of similar composition may be observed extending into adjacent adipose lobules (Plate 16-10-1). Late lesions, where inflammatory infiltrates are not as intense, may mimic scleroderma because of the presence of sclerotic collagen bundles (Figures 16-10-3 to 16-10-5). Although fibrosis dominates this stage, eosinophils among thickened collagen bundles are highly suggestive of eosinophilic fasciitis. If eosinophils are absent but the index of suspicion is high, stains for myelin basic protein may be useful in detecting the degranulation products of eosinophils.

Differential Diagnosis
Scleroderma

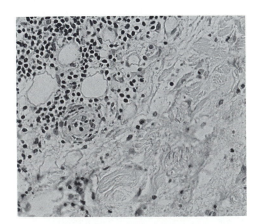

16-10-2 EOSINOPHILIC FASCIITIS: High magnification shows lymphocytes, plasma cells, and eosinophils embedded in a mucinous stroma. (100×)

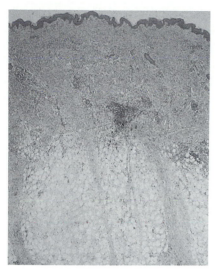

16-10-3 EOSINOPHILIC FASCIITIS: A well-established lesion, showing extensive subcutaneous fibrosis within adipose septae. (20×)

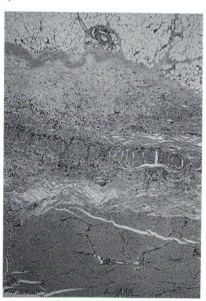

16-10-4 EOSINOPHILIC FASCIITIS: The fascia overlying muscle shows widening and fibrosis with only sparse inflammation. (40×)

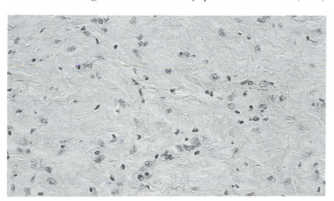

16-10-5 EOSINOPHILIC FASCIITIS: A residual inflammatory infiltrate of eosinophils and plasma cells is enmeshed in thickened, sclerotic collagen bundles. (200×)

16-11 POLYARTERITIS NODOSA

CLINICAL DESCRIPTION

Polyarteritis nodosa occurs in two forms in childhood: infantile (the first two years of life) and adult (after the second year of life).

Etiology and Incidence

An immune complex-mediated vasculitis is theorized as the cause of this process. The specific cause is unknown. The infantile form affects both sexes equally and is now thought to be Kawasaki's disease. Cutaneous changes may be found in 25% to 50% of children with the adult form.

Clinical Features

Dermatologic findings of the infantile form of polyarteritis nodosa are similar to those of Kawasaki's disease (Chapter 6). Arteritis of vessels in the heart leads to aneurysms, infarction, and congestive heart failure. The kidneys and central nervous system are also severely affected.

Cutaneous changes in the adult form include tender erythematous subcutaneous nodules in a linear array following the course of superficial arteries. The lesions are most frequently found on the lower legs and feet, however the upper extremities and trunk may be affected. Other skin findings include livedo reticularis, purpura, urticaria, vesicles, pustules, and ulcers. Ecchymoses and peripheral gangrene may ensue. Systemic symptoms similar to those in the infantile form are also a prominent feature. The triad of spiking fever, calf pain, and tender nodules on the legs with a linear distribution should raise suspicion of polyarteritis nodosa.

Differential Diagnosis

Vasculitis of other causes

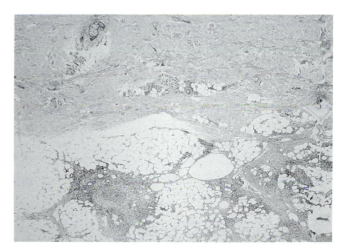

16-11-1 POLYARTERITIS NODOSA: A medium- to large-caliber vessel within a subcutaneous adipose septum is surrounded by an intense inflammatory infiltrate. (20×)

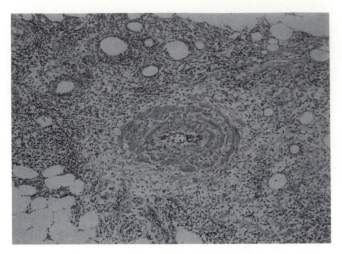

16-11-2 POLYARTERITIS NODOSA: The vessel wall is expanded and surrounded by large numbers of neutrophils admixed with cellular debris and extravasated erythrocytes. (200×)

HISTOLOGICAL DESCRIPTION

It is important to select a tender nodule for biopsy because involvement of vessels in this disorder is segmental. Affected vessels are arterioles of small and medium caliber. Their walls are infiltrated by neutrophils and eosinophils and display necrosis and thickening. Intraluminal thrombosis is apparent. There are extravasated erythrocytes and collections of nuclear dust around affected vessels (Figures 16-11-1 and 16-11-2). Late lesions show recanalization of lumina, perivascular fibrosis, and mononuclear inflammatory infiltrates.

Differential Diagnosis
Nodular vasculitis

REFERENCES

Histiocytic Cytophagic Panniculitis
Alegre VA, Winkelmann RK: Histiocytic cytophagic panniculitis. J Am Acad Dermatol 1989;20:177.

Smith JK, Skelton HG, Yeager J, et al.: Cutaneous histopathologic, immunohistochemical, and clinical manifestations in patients with hemophagocytic syndrome. Arch Dermatol 1992;128:193.

Winkelmann RK, Bowie EJ: Hemorrhagic diathesis associated with benign histiocytic cytophagic panniculitis and systemic histiocytosis. Arch Intern Med 1980;140:1460.

Idiopathic Lobular Panniculitis (Weber-Christian Disease)
Abid S, Memon K: Weber-Christian disease. J Pak Med Assoc 1988;38:330.

Aronson IK, Zeitz HJ, Variakojis D: Panniculitis in childhood. Pediatr Dermatol 1988;5:216.

Christian HA: Relapsing febrile nodular nonsuppurative panniculitis. Arch Intern Med 1928;42:338.

Sorensen RU, Abramsky CR, Stern RC: Ten year course of early onset Weber-Christian syndrome with recurrent pneumonia: A suggestion for pathogenesis. Pediatrics 1986;78:115.

Weber FP: A case of relapsing nonsuppurative panniculitis showing phagocytosis of subcutaneous fat cells by macrophages. Br J Syphilol 1925;37:301.

Lupus Profundus
Ackerman AB: Histologic diagnosis of inflammatory skin diseases. Philadelphia: Lea & Febiger, 1978:813.

Fox JN, Klapman MH, Rowe L: Lupus profundus in children: Treatment with hydroxychloroquine. J Am Acad Dermatol 1987;16:839.

Koransky JS, Esterly NB: Lupus panniculitis (profundus). J Pediatr 1981;98:241.

Sanchez NP: The histology of lupus erythematosus panniculitis. J Am Acad Dermatol 1981;5:673.

Tuffanelli DL: Lupus erythematosus panniculitis (profundus). Arch Dermatol 1971;103:231.

Poststeroid Panniculitis
Ackerman AB: Histologic diagnosis of inflammatory skin diseases. Philadelphia: Lea & Febiger, 1978:779.

Roenigk HM, Roeniga HH, Haserick JR, and Drundell FD: Post steroid panniculitis. Arch Dermatol 1964;90:387.

Saxena AK: Poststeroid panniculitis. Aust J Dermatol 1986;27:143.

Spagnvolo M, Taranta A: Post-steroid panniculitis. Ann Intern Med 1961;54:1181.

Cold Panniculitis (Popsicle Stick Panniculitis)
Epstein EH Jr, Oren MF: Popsicle panniculitis. N Engl J Med. 1970;282:966.

Hultercrantz E: Haxthausen's disease: Cold panniculitis in children. J Laryngol Otol 1986;100:1329.

Page EH, Shear NH: Temperature-dependent skin disorders. J Am Acad Dermatol 1988;18:1003.

Silverman AK, Michels EH, Rasmussen JE: Subcutaneous fat necrosis in an infant, occurring after hypothermic cardiac surgery: Case report and analysis of etiological factors. J Am Acad Dermatol 1986;15:331.

Sclerema Neonatorum
Fretzin DF, Arias A: Sclerema neonatorum and subcutaneous fat necrosis of the newborn. Pediatr Dermatol 1987;4:112.

Subcutaneous Fat Necrosis of the Newborn

Balasz M: Subcutaneous fat necrosis of the newborn with emphasis on ultrastructural studies. Int J Dermatol 1987;26:227.

Cook JS, Stone MS, Hansen JR: Hypercalcemia in association with subcutaneous fat necrosis of the newborn: Studies of calcium. Reg Norm Pediatr 1992;90:93.

Fretzin DF, Arias A: Sclerema neonatorum and subcutaneous fat necrosis of the newborn. Pediatr Dermatol 1987; 4:112.

Friedman SJ, Winkelmann RK: Subcutaneous fat necrosis of the newborn: Light, ultrastructural and histochemical microscopic studies. J Cutan Pathol 1989;16:99.

Nodular Vasculitis (Erythema Induratum)

Kuramoto Y, Aiba S, Tagami H: Erythema induratum of Bazin as a type of tuberculid. J Am Acad Dermatol 1990; 22: 612.

Lebel M, Lassonde M: Erythema induratum of Bazin. J Am Acad Dermatol 1986;14:738.

Rademaker M, Lowe DG, Munro DD: Erythema induratum (Bazin's disease). J Am Acad Dermatol 1989;21:710.

Erythema Nodosum

Hannuksela M: Erythema nodosum. Clin Dermatol 1985;4:88.

Paller AS: Cutaneous changes associated with inflammatory bowel disease. Pediatr Dermatol 1986;3:139.

Reed RJ, Clark WH, Mihm MC: Disorders of the panniculus adiposus. Hum Pathol 1973;4:219.

Eosinophilic Fasciitis

Grisanti WM, Moore TL, Osborne TG, Haber PL: Eosinophilic fasciitis in children. Semin Arthritis Rheum 1989;19:151.

Krauser RE, Tuthill RJ: Eosinophilic fasciitis. Arch Dermatol 1977;113:1092.

Lakhanpal S, Ginsburg WW, Michet CJ, et al.: Eosinophilic fasciitis: clinical spectrum and therapeutic response in 52 cases. Semin Arthritis Rheum 1988;7:221.

Polyarteritis Nodosa

Dillon MJ: Classification and pathogenesis of arteritis in children. Toxicol Pathol 1989;17:214.

Golitz LE: The vasculitides and their significance in the pediatric age group. Dermatol Clin North Am 1986;4: 117.

Goodless DR, Dhawan SS, Alexis J, Wiszniak J: Cutaneous polyarteritis nodosa. Int J Dermatol 1990;29:611.

Moreland LW, Ball GV: Cutaneous polyarteritis nodosa. Am J Med 1990;88:426.

17

Infectious Diseases

Contents

17-1 MYCOBACTERIAL INFECTIONS

CLINICAL DESCRIPTION

Mycobacterial skin infections, though uncommon, must be included in the discussion of pediatric dermatology. Many daily activities (e.g., swimming in pools, hobbies that include tropical fish) predispose children to some of these acid-fast infections. In addition, the immigration of significant numbers of Southeast Asians has increased the number of cases of leprosy in the United States. Table 17-1-1 describes mycobacterial skin infections.

Differential Diagnosis

Granuloma or ulcer of any origin
Systemic lupus erythematosus
See Sporotrichosis

HISTOLOGICAL DESCRIPTION

Tuberculosis (Lupus Vulgaris)

The histological features of infections with acid-fast organisms in children are the same as those in adults. The prototypical findings are granulomatous inflammation and tuberculoid granulomas with caseation. The epithelioid granulomas (tuberculoid granulomas) are composed of epithelioid histiocytes surrounding a varying amount of caseation. Surrounding the granulomas is an infiltrate composed of plasma cells with

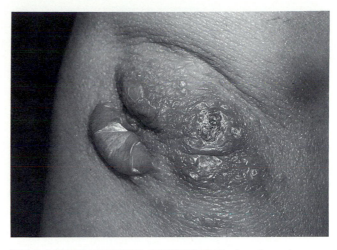

17-1-1 MYCOBACTERIAL INFECTIONS: A patient who scraped his knee on the swimming pool wall and developed *M. marinum* granulomas.

lymphocytes at the periphery. The epithelioid granulomas are almost always located in the superficial dermis (Figure 17-1-2). Giant cells can also be found in the infiltrate. They are most often the Langerhans' type, although foreign body types can be seen. The epidermis usually shows atrophy and/or ulceration and, at the periphery of an ulcer, there is pseudoepitheliomatous hyperplasia. Special stains for acid-fast organisms are usually unrewarding because of the small numbers of organisms present in lupus vulgaris.

17-1-1 Mycobacterial Skin Infections

Mycobacterium	Incidence	Clinical Features	Comments
M. tuberculosis	Although a rare infection, there has been an increase with HIV-infected patients	Primary inoculation with lupus vulgaris; direct extension from infected node; all associated with brownish red plaques, ulcers with bluish red margins, and apple jelly color on diascopy	Most common form is lupus vulgaris; 90% occur on head and neck
Atypical			
Group I (photochromogen):		Inoculation into abrasion produces	Colonies in culture
M. kansasii		reddish papules and pustules;	produce pigment in
M. balnei (*marinum*; most common form in U.S.)		after 3 wk size of pea; solitary or multiple lesions may ulcerate;	light
M. ulcerans		look granulomatous (Fig. 17-1-1);	
Group II (scotochromogens)		may ascend proximally and resemble sporotrichoid infection	Pigment produced in dark
Group III (nonphotochromogens)			No pigment produced
Group IV (rapid growers)			Culture positive in < 1 wk
Leprosy			
M. leprae	Common in endemic areas: Africa, India, SE Asia; most cases brought into U.S.	Lepromatous (nodular); tuberculoid (Plate 17-1-1) (circular, hypopigmented, concave); borderline (circular convex)	Frequently skin is anesthetic

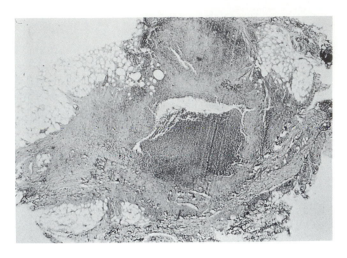

17-1-2 LUPUS VULGARIS: A deep-seated granuloma within the reticular dermis abuts the panniculus. (20×)

Atypical Mycobacterial Infections

The histological features of atypical mycobacterial infection vary depending on the time of the biopsy in the evolution of the lesion. Lesions older than seven to eight months show the typical histological picture described for lupus vulgaris (Figure 17-1-3). Early lesions (less than three months) have a mixed inflammatory infiltrate that includes acute inflammatory cells as well as histiocytes, lymphocytes, and plasma cells. No granulomas are seen in this stage. Organisms can be identified on acid-fast stains. Midduration lesions (four months or greater) show the transition from the nonspecific mixed infiltrate to the development of small granulomas with caseation. Demonstration of organisms becomes more difficult as the lesion ages. The epidermal reaction is greatest in this stage. When there is epidermal hyperplasia with hyperkeratosis, ulceration can occur.

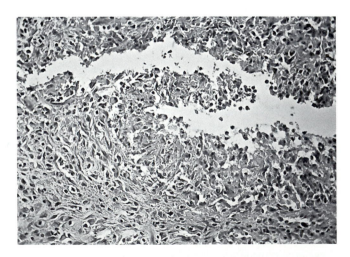

17-1-3 ATYPICAL MYCOBACTERIAL INFECTIONS: Higher magnification of *M. marinum* granuloma: large numbers of histiocytes admixed with giant cells are arranged in epithelioid granulomas. (400×)

Leprosy

Indeterminate

On histological study, indeterminate leprosy is, as the name implies, one that does not have features of either polar group (tuberculoid or lepromatous). There are a few collections of chronic inflammatory cells about blood vessels, as well as appendages, and small cutaneous nerves. Granulomas have not yet developed. Demonstration of organisms at this stage is difficult.

Tuberculoid

Granulomas are well developed in tuberculoid leprosy. There are epithelioid granulomas that follow the neurovascular bundles, giving them an oblong sausage shape that helps distinguish them from the more rounded granulomas of sarcoid. The granulomas may show slight central necrosis, especially those about cutaneous nerves. Organisms, although difficult to demonstrate, can be found in the granulomas in the superficial dermis or in those granulomas that show some necrosis.

Lepromatous

There is a diffuse infiltrate of foamy epithelioid histiocytes separated from the epidermis by a zone of uninvolved collagen (Figure 17-1-4). Organisms can be demonstrated readily in these histiocytes using acid-fast stains (Plate 17-1-2). In lepromatous leprosy, histiocytes filled with acid-fast-positive bacilli are called globi.

Differential Diagnosis

Sarcoidosis
Deep mycosis
Foreign body granuloma

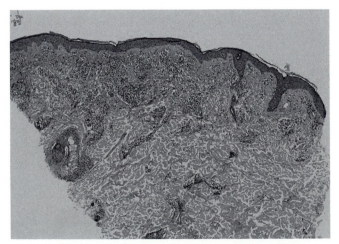

17-1-4 LEPROMATOUS LEPROSY: Lymphohistiocytic inflammatory infiltrate in a serpentine array in the dermis. (40×)

17-2 CAT-SCRATCH DISEASE

CLINICAL DESCRIPTION

Cat-scratch disease consists of subacute adenitis following inoculation of bacillus into the skin by a cat scratch or bite.

Etiology and Incidence

The gram negative bacillus that causes cat-scratch disease has recently been described to be Rochalimaea henselae. The bacillus can be observed in lymph nodes with the use of Warthin-Starry silver stain. The disorder is more common in children (five to fourteen years) than adults and occurs mostly between September and March. Skin findings have been reported in up to 90% of cases.

Clinical Features

After an incubation period of three to thirty days, one or more erythematous papules (Figure 17-2-1) appear at the site of inoculation. They persist for one to four weeks and disappear with the appearance of regional lymphadenopathy (Plate 17-2-1). Nodes last, on average, four to six weeks but may remain for one year. Most patients have little in the way of constitutional symptoms. Conjunctivitis followed by preauricular adenitis is called Parinaud's syndrome. On occasion encephalopathy or encephalitis appears six weeks after adenopathy is found. Cerebrospinal fluid pleocytosis may occur. Recovery is usually complete.

Differential Diagnosis

Any disorder associated with lymphadenopathy

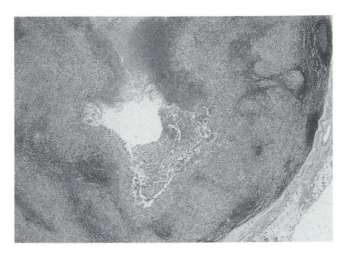

17-2-2 CAT-SCRATCH DISEASE: Lymph node with stellate zones of necrosis. (20×)

HISTOLOGICAL DESCRIPTION

The dermis shows multiple areas of necrosis of varying configurations (Figures 17-2-2 and 17-2-3), frequently triangular, surrounded by epithelioid histiocytes, plasma cells, and lymphocytes. The epidermis may be thinned or show acanthosis with focal parakeratosis. Regional nodes also show areas of necrosis that can be stellate in configuration. These necrotic centers are surrounded by epithelioid histiocytes. These, in turn, are surrounded by plasma cells, which are surrounded by lymphocytes (Figure 17-2-4). Warthin-Starry stains may identify Rochalimaea henselae in tissue.

Differential Diagnosis

Lymphogranuloma venereum

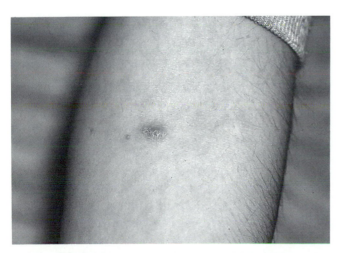

17-2-1 CAT-SCRATCH DISEASE: Erythematous papule on the volar aspect of the forearm in a child with cat-scratch disease at the site of inoculation.

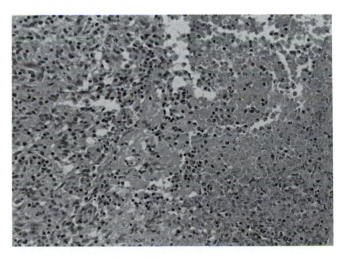

17-2-3 CAT-SCRATCH DISEASE: Central zones of necrosis admixed with neutrophils. (200×)

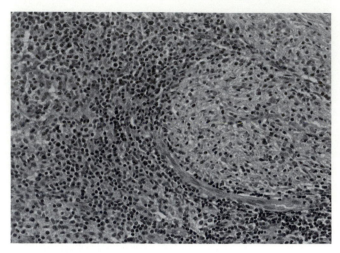

17-2-4 CAT-SCRATCH DISEASE: Peripheral to the necrosis there are epithelioid granulomas surrounded by lymphocytes and plasma cells. (200 ×)

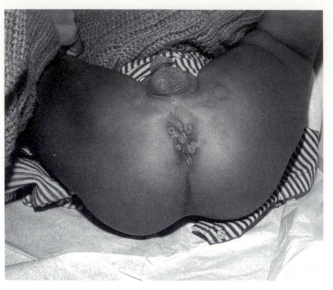

17-3-1 CONGENITAL SYPHILIS: Condylomata lata.

17-3 CONGENITAL SYPHILIS

CLINICAL DESCRIPTION

The incidence of syphilis declined in the 1950s with the widespread use of penicillin, and there was hope that it could be eliminated. Unfortunately, this has not been the case. Therefore, physicians must be familiar with the varying manifestations of the disease. One aspect is transplacental infection.

Etiology and Incidence

The causative organism is *Treponema pallidum.* The organism infects the fetus transplacentally. Transmission to the fetus occurs in almost all pregnant women with primary disease, 90% with secondary disease, and 30% with early latent disease. Intrauterine death occurs in 25% of untreated pregnancies. Another 25% to 30% of untreated infected babies die after birth.

Clinical Features

Congenital syphilis is divided into early manifestations (first two years of life) and late manifestations (after the second year of life and the result of scarring from early systemic disease).

Early manifestations appear between birth and three months (most in the first five weeks of life). A bloody rhinitis appears in the first week of life (up to three months) and is usually the first sign of the presence of congenital syphilis. The rash appears one to two weeks later and evolves over one to three weeks. Ham-colored maculopapular lesions appear, concentrated on the hands and feet (Plate 17-3-1). If a rash is present at birth it may be bullous (the only time bullae are seen in this disorder). Postinflammatory hyperpigmentation occurs as the rash fades, as does desquamation. Other skin

findings include shiny red palms and soles; fissures about the lips, anus (Plate 17-3-2) and nares (when scarred called rhagades); mucous patches in the mouth and genitalia; and condylomata lata (Figure 17-3-1) (moist, raised perianal lesions). Hair and nails may be lost. Associated findings include fever, hepatosplenomegaly, and periostitis.

Late congenital syphilis results in notched, tapered, central incisors (Hutchinson's teeth); maldevelopment of cusps of first molars (mulberry or Moon's molars); interstitial keratitis (four to thirty years later); saddle nose, saber shin, frontal bossing, perforation of hard palate, painless arthritis of knees (Clutton's joints), and rhagades.

Differential Diagnosis

Congenital infection

HISTOLOGICAL DESCRIPTION

The cutaneous manifestations of congenital syphilis are the same as those of secondary syphilis in adults. A singular difference is the involvement of the nasal mucosa in children, not a usual finding in adults. Also, syphilis in children can be bullous, an unusual finding in adults except in the elderly, in whom secondary syphilis may be bullous. The features of congenital syphilis in neonatal skin are an inflammatory dermatosis that shows an infiltrate at the dermal-epidermal junction around the dermal vessels and surrounding adnexae (Figure 17-3-2). The primary cell in the infiltrate is a lymphocyte, and this cell is always present. The characteristic cell in syphilis, the plasma cell, is variable in its presence within the inflammatory infiltrate and when present is helpful in the diagnosis, but its absence does not preclude the diagnosis of syphilis. Plasma cells can be found in the perivascular location

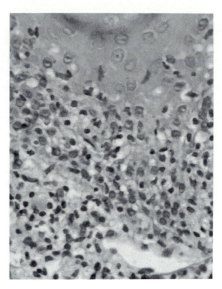

17-3-2 SYPHILIS: Lymphocytic inflammatory infiltrate in a bandlike configuration in the superficial dermis and infiltrating the epidermis. (200×)

as well as in the interstitial dermis. The inflammatory infiltrate also invades arrector pili muscles, and plasma cells may be seen in this location. When syphilis is bullous, the bulla is subepidermal and is produced because of the severe interface reaction that destroys the tenuous connection of dermis and epidermis in newborns. Mucosal involvement also shows a marked inflammatory response. Here plasma cells are usually plentiful. Inflammatory reactions can be severe enough to produce surface ulceration. Gummatous reactions are rare in children but when present show nodular granulomatous infiltration surrounding necrotic foci in the dermis (caseation necrosis). The nodules with central caseation in the surrounding infiltrate of lymphocytes, plasma cells, and histiocytes as well as giant cells are called gumma. Special stains in secondary syphilis can be helpful in determining the nature of the condition. The Steinert modification of the Dieterle stain is a variation of a silver precipitate stain and identifies spirochetes in the tissue (Plate 17-3-3). Spirochetes can be more readily visualized in the epidermis, the follicular epithelium, or the blood vessel wall. They are extremely difficult to identify in the dermis because of the fibrillar nature of the dermis and the confusion that can occur between small fibers and spirochetes. Mucosal lesions have abundant organisms within the epithelium, and in immunocompromised patients organisms are abundant.

Differential Diagnosis

Mycosis fungoides
Drug eruptions
Tuberculosis (late stage syphilis)
Lupus erythematosus

17-4 BACTERIAL INFECTIONS

CLINICAL DESCRIPTION

Bacterial infections of the skin include some of the most common infections of the skin in pediatric dermatology (Table 17-4-1).

HISTOLOGICAL DESCRIPTION

Erysipelas and Cellulitis

The histological features of erysipelas and cellulitis (all types) are the same. The epidermis may be thinned or show spongiosis without significant exocytosis. There is prominent dermal edema with vascular dilatation and discrete escape of red blood cells. The primary inflammatory cell is a neutrophil, which is found diffusely throughout the edematous dermis and may be found in the subcutis. The involvement of the lower dermis and subcutis is greater in cellulitis than in erysipelas. Streptococci can be found in vessel walls on gram-stained sections.

Differential Diagnosis

Fasciitis

Perianal Streptococcal Cellulitis

The histological features are marked dermal edema with associated mucosal edema and exocytosis. The exocytotic cells are the lymphocyte and neutrophil. The dermal features are similar to those seen in erysipelas and cellulitis. Streptococci can be found within the vessel walls. The inflammatory infiltrate, which is composed primarily of neutrophils, can extend into the subcutis.

Differential Diagnosis

Erysipelas
Contact dermatitis

Dermatitis/Arthritis (Chronic Gonococcemia)

The histological features are vasculitis with leukocytoclasis. The superficial and middermal vessels are usually surrounded by an infiltrate of lymphocytes, fragmented neutrophils, fibrin, hemorrhage, and histiocytoid cells.

The vessel walls are thickened and there is endothelial swelling. When the vascular injury is severe enough, a wedge-shaped area of necrosis occurs and the lesion ulcerates. In some cases bullae develop before ulceration and the bullous space may be filled with neutrophils. Organisms can rarely be identified in sections using special stains; when found they are seen within the walls of the blood vessels. Fluorescent antibody technique is more successful for organism identification, and confirmation with culture is best.

17-4-1   Bacterial Infections of the Skin

Condition	Most Common Infecting Bacteria	Incidence	Clinical Features	Differential Diagnosis
Cellulitis	S. aureus or S. pneumoniae	Common	Ill-defined area of erythema, swelling, and tenderness; tender regional nodes	Erysipelas
Facial	H. influenzae	3 mo–3 y	Central purplish hue	Cold panniculitis
Periorbital	H. influenzae, S. aureus, Group A beta hemolytic Streptococcus		Swelling and erythema of soft tissue around eye; EOM intact	Orbital cellulitis; insect bite
Orbital	Same organisms as periorbital	Uncommon	In addition to above, proptosis and ophthalmoplegia	Insect bite, periorbital cellulitis, cavernous sinus thrombosis
Perianal Streptococcal	Group A beta hemolytic Streptococcus (GABHS)	Uncommon	Intense to mild perianal erythema, pruritus, and painful defecation (blood at times) (Plate 17-4-1)	Moniliasis, psoriasis, inflammatory bowel disease and fissure
Dermatitis-arthritis	N. gonorrhoeae	1.9% of infections with this organism	Arthritis with acrally located erythematous papule or vesicopustules on a hemorrhagic base; few in number (2–9) (Plate 17-4-2)	Vasculitis
Ecthyma	GABHS	Common	Initial vesicle ruptures and forms thick adherent crust with surrounding indurated erythema; shallow ulcer that scars	Impetigo
Ecthyma gangrenosum	Pseudomonas, other bacteria and fungi	Uncommon	Erythematous macules that become vesicular, pustular, dark eschar, surrounding erythema	
Erysipelas	GABHS	Uncommon	Bright red plaque that spreads rapidly, distinct elevated borders, induration with shiny, warm surface; may develop bullae at surface	Non-GABHS cellulitis
Erythrasma	Corynebacterium minutissimum	Uncommon 15% between 5–14 y	Well-demarcated reddish brown, scaly intertriginous eruption; Coral-red fluorescence under Wood's light (Plate 17-4-3)	T. cruris, candidiasis
Impetigo (bullous)	S. aureus	Common	Bullous lesion; breaks, leaving collar of scale surrounding denuded moist erythematous base; formation of thick, soft honey-colored crusts	Flea bites, contact dermatitis
Meningococcemia	N. meningitidis	$\frac{2}{3}$ develop skin lesions	Early maculopapular eruption, petechiae, hemorrhagic lesions, necrosis acrally	Rubeola, scarlet fever, HSP gonococcemia, typhoid fever, rickettsial disease, EM, DIC

Differential Diagnosis
Vasculitis of other causes
Meningococcemia

Ecthyma

Ecthyma appears histologically as an ulcer that has an infiltrate of polymorphonuclear leukocytes, many of which may be fragmented. The epidermis at the margins of the ulcer is acanthotic with the presence of exocytotic neutrophils and lymphocytes. The ulcer base may show necrosis and in late lesions early fibrosis.

Differential Diagnosis
Ulcers of other causes

Ecthyma Gangrenosum (*Pseudomonas*)

The histological features are those of an ulcer secondary to a severe necrotizing vasculitis (Figure 17-4-1). These ulcers, unlike those of ecthyma, are less cellular and contain fewer inflammatory cells and areas of leukocytoclasis. The involved vessels contain many *Pseudomonas* organisms, which are visible on routine stains. In the dermis adjacent to the ulcer is seen, in addition to vascular necrosis, marked hemorrhage in association with the vascular invasion by the *Pseudomonas* organism.

Differential Diagnosis
Ecthyma
Traumatic ulceration
Ulceration of other causes

Erythrasma

The histological features of erythrasma can be initially disappointing, in that there does not appear to be significant

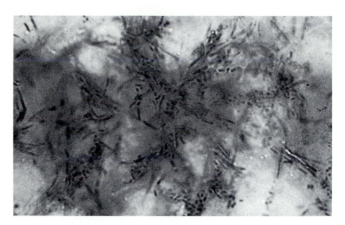

17-4-2 ERYTHRASMA: Gram stain shows Gram-positive rods arranged in chains. (20×)

change in the sections studied. The epidermis and dermis show slight alteration, and the salient histological features in the stratum corneum can be easily overlooked. The stratum corneum is thickened and there are filamentous forms and/or rods between the corneocytes. These Gram-positive organisms can best be demonstrated using tissue Gram stains (Figure 17-4-2).

Differential Diagnosis
Tinea versicolor

Impetigo

There is a subcorneal bulla (Figure 17-4-3) filled with neutrophils, fragmented keratin, serum, and debris. The epidermis is spongiotic and there is exocytosis of neutrophils and lymphocytes. The dermis has a perivascular infiltrate of lymphocytes and neutrophils. There are essentially no histological differences between nonbullous and bullous impetigo.

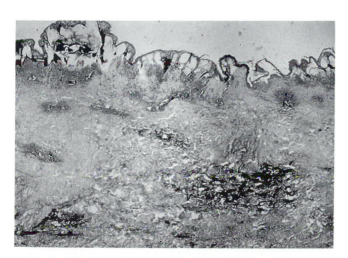

17-4-1 ECTHYMA GANGRENOSUM: Epidermal necrosis secondary to vascular necrosis. (20×)

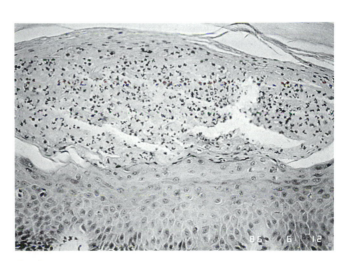

17-4-3 IMPETIGO: Sections show a large subcorneal collection of neutrophils, which on culture contained group A beta-hemolytic streptococci. (100×)

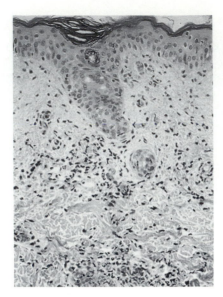

17-4-4 MENINGOCOCCEMIA: Neutrophils in the dermal stroma and surrounding damaged blood vessels, some of which contain small thrombi. There is prominent dermal edema and focal hemorrhage. (200×)

Differential Diagnosis

Subcorneal pustular dermatosis
Pustular psoriasis
Dyshidrosis

Meningococcemia

Meningococcemia, like gonococcemia, has vasculitis as the basic cause for the histological features (Figure 17-4-4). Here there is vessel damage with hemorrhage, endothelial swelling to the point of occlusion, fibrinoid necrosis, and leukocytoclasia. Subsequent to the vasculitis there is epidermal death and ulceration. Not all lesions progress to ulceration: some show only vasculitis with leukocytoclasia. Organisms can be demonstrated within the endothelial cells and are best demonstrated with the immunofluorescent technique. IgG, IgM, and IgA can also be found in vessel walls.

Differential Diagnosis

Gonococcemia
Vasculitis of other causes

17-5 LEISHMANIASIS

CLINICAL DESCRIPTION

The parasite *Leishmania* produces three different cutaneous disorders: cutaneous leishmaniasis, mucocutaneous leishmaniasis, and visceral leishmaniasis.

Etiology and Incidence

Cutaneous leishmaniasis is produced by the parasite *Leishmania tropica*. In this and all forms of leishmaniasis, humans are an accidental host: the parasite, which normally lives in animals, is transmitted to humans by the bite of the phlebotomus sandfly. Seen mainly in South and Central America, the disorder is manifested in the United States in immigrants and returning visitors from those continents. Mucocutaneous leishmaniasis is due to *Leishmania braziliensis* and also is seen principally in South and Central America. Visceral leishmaniasis is caused by exposure to *Leishmania donovani* in the Mediterranean, South America, and Asia.

Clinical Features

Cutaneous Leishmaniasis

There are four forms of cutaneous leishmaniasis, seen mainly on exposed areas, especially the face. The moist or rural type begins as a maculopapule, enlarges in months to a nodule, ulcerates, crusts, and resolves in six months to a year, leaving a pigmented depressed scar (Plate 17-5-1).

The dry or urban type begins as a small, brownish nodule, extends into a large plaque (1 to 2 cm in diameter) over six months, and then ulcerates centrally. Regression and scarring concludes a process that lasts longer than one year.

Lupoid leishmaniasis represents reactivation of the condition close to an old scar of previous disease. Lesions appear as red to yellowish-brown papules that coalesce into a ring or plaque which spreads outward. This is a very chronic form of leishmaniasis.

The lepromatoid form is nonulcerating and generalized. Papillomatous nodules involve the entire body (especially the face and ears).

Mucocutaneous Leishmaniasis

Nodules and ulcers that resemble the cutaneous form progress into fungating oral and nasopharyngeal lesions, which may produce considerable destruction. Secondary infection is common.

Visceral Leishmaniasis

Lesions are not limited to the skin. Lymph nodes, bone marrow, spleen, and spinal fluid can be involved with the organism.

Differential Diagnosis

Cat-scratch disease
Deep fungal disease
Foreign bodies
Mycobacterial disease
Sarcoidosis
Syphilis
Leprosy
South American blastomycosis
Chromomycosis
Yaws

HISTOLOGICAL DESCRIPTION

The hallmark of cutaneous leishmaniasis is the finding of parasitized histiocytes containing the *Leishmania* organisms within the dermis. *Leishmania* (*tropica, braziliensis,* or *donovani*) are the causative organisms. The epidermal response is variable, from hyper- and parakeratosis with acanthosis to epidermal atrophy. In the dermis in the acute form is a diffuse infiltrate of histiocytes associated with a sprinkling of lymphocytes and plasma cells (Figure 17-5-1). Organisms are found within histiocytes and can also be seen extracellularly. Within the macrophages are many organisms. The extracellular forms resemble fragmented neutrophils, although neutrophil fragments are usually larger than the *Leishmania* organisms. The organisms in tissue are 2 to 4 μm in diameter, are round to oval, and can be seen on routinely stained sections (Plate 17-5-2). The organisms have a basophilic staining nucleus with an associated rodlike paranucleus or kinetoplast that measures from 0.5 to 1 μm in diameter. The organisms are best visualized in Giemsa stain, where the nucleus and paranucleus usually stain red.

As leishmaniasis progresses from acute to chronic, the number of organisms decreases and they are often not found. Granulomas develop, consisting of epithelioid cells and giant cells surrounded by plasma cells and lymphocytes.

In lupoid leishmaniasis, the epidermal response is acanthosis with hyper- and parakeratosis. The dermal response is granulomatous with features similar to these in the chronic form. Typical tuberculoid granulomas can be seen. The number of organisms in this phase is variable and when present are best visualized with Giemsa stain.

Differential Diagnosis

Histoplasmosis
Rhinoscleroma
Granuloma

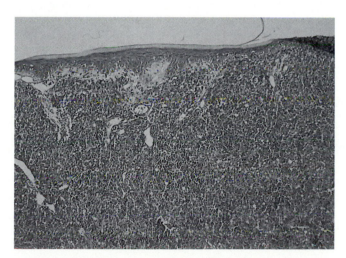

17-5-1 LEISHMANIASIS: Low-power view shows a dense lymphohistiocytic infiltrate throughout the dermis. (20×)

Tuberculosis
Late syphilis

17-6 NECROTIZING FASCIITIS

CLINICAL DESCRIPTION

Necrotizing fasciitis is a dangerous and infrequently reviewed soft tissue infection.

Incidence and Etiology

Necrotizing fasciitis is a rare infection of infants and children. Conditions that produce tissue anoxia allow a synergistic infection with endogenous anaerobes and facultative bacteria (nongroup A streptococci or enterobacteria) or *Streptococcus pyogenes* to overgrow and produce their effects. Therefore, gangrenous cellulitis in areas of trauma, surgery, ischemia, burns, malignancy, or foreign body introduction is seen. Tissue necrosis following infection occurs because inflammatory swelling produces necrosis in relatively closed spaces (e.g., fascia or skin), vessel thrombosis, or release of enzymes or toxins (e.g., lecithinase by *Clostridium perfringens*). Delay in diagnosis results in a 30% mortality rate.

Clinical Features

The clue to the presence of this condition is a rapidly spreading cellulitis in a very toxic individual, despite antibiotic therapy. Initially manifested are erythema and edema, which progress to brawny induration and cyanosis. Blister formation and gangrene eventually appear (Plate 17-6-1). Anesthesia of the skin is present as the gangrene progresses. Surgery reveals extensive undermining due to necrosis of fascia and subcutaneous tissue (lack of resistance to passage of a blunt instrument along the facial plane). When this condition involves the scrotum and penis it constitutes Fournier's disease.

Differential Diagnosis

Acute cellulitis
Erysipelas
Infected vascular gangrene
Phlegmasia cerulea dolens
Other gangrenous and crepitant cellulitis
Purpura fulminans

HISTOLOGICAL DESCRIPTION

The epidermis is usually not involved in this reaction, although in acute lesions subepidermal bullae may form. The significant finding is necrotizing vasculitis without an inflammatory response. The vasculitis is found throughout in the vessels of the dermis, subcutaneous fat, and fascia. In addition to noninflammatory intravascular coagulation, there is perivascular infiltration of lymphocytes, histiocytes, and plasma cells. The dermis can contain a diffuse infiltrate of neutrophils. Microorganisms can be seen in hematoxylin and eosin-Gram-stained and periodic acid-Schiff-stained sections. The fascia is edematous and necrotic. The necrosis can also involve all of the surrounding tissue, including fat, sweat glands, nerves, and dermis. The severely devitalized tissue is easily overgrown by opportunistic fungi, and often *Mucor* or other similar organisms can be seen. The bacteriology of necrotizing fasciitis is variable. Gram-positive or Gram-negative organisms, or both, may be found, although streptococci have been most commonly implicated in this condition. Early diagnosis and treatment are essential for patient survival.

Differential Diagnosis
Cellulitis
Leukocytoclastic vasculitis
Fungal infections and trauma

17-7 RICKETTSIAL DISEASES

CLINICAL DESCRIPTION

Humans are an accidental host in rickettsial infections. Rocky mountain spotted fever and rickettsialpox account for most of the clinical conditions produced by these organisms in the United States; the other entities are summarized in Table 17-7-1.

Etiology and Incidence
The rickettsial diseases are caused by pleomorphic Gram-negative coccobacillus organisms, which are obligate intracellular bacteria. They are spread to humans by blood-sucking insects. Rocky mountain spotted fever accounts for 95% of rickettsial infections and is potentially fatal. Mortality is 5% with treatment and 20% without treatment.

Clinical Features
Rocky mountain spotted fever begins with a prodrome of headache, malaise, and prominent myalgia following a five to seven day incubation period (range, three to twelve days). Significant conjunctival injection is a common early clinical finding. The rash appears two to four days after the onset of illness. It is first seen on the thenar eminences and flexural surfaces of the wrists and ankles. The maculopapular eruption then moves centrally and becomes hemorrhagic in one to three days (Plate 17-7-1). It may become confluent. Gangrene may develop on the fingers, toes, nose, and genitalia. The eruption eventually becomes pigmented and desquamates.

Rickettsialpox lesions develop after a ten to twenty-four day incubation period. Following introduction of the *Rickettsia*, an erythematous papule develops at the site of the mite bite. Two days later a vesicle appears, which progresses to an eschar that heals in three to four weeks. After three to seven days the patient experiences fevers, chills, headache, and myalgias. The rash appears three days after the onset of this syndrome. At first the eruption is maculopapular and discrete, without a characteristic distribution. Vesicles then form at the apex of the papules (Plate 17-7-2). These vesicles go on to crust and fall off without leaving a scar. Only on rare occasions are the palms and soles involved. The course of the illness is two weeks.

17-7-1 Rickettsial Disease

Disease	Vector	Infecting Agent	Animal Host	Proteus Agglutination	Distribution	Comments
RMSF	Ticks: West Wood tick (*D. andersoni*); East-dog tick (*D. variabolis*)	*R. rickettsii*	Rodents, mammals	OX₂ or OX₁₉	Western hemisphere; Rocky Mountains; Atlantic Coast	1–5% of ticks harbor organism in endemic regions
Rickettsialpox	Mite	*R. akari*	House mouse	Negative	New York City, Boston, Philadelphia, Delaware, Arkansas	Most commonly confused with varicella; only one with vesicles
Epidemic typhus	Body louse	*R. prowazekii*	None	OX₁₉	Worldwide, rarely U.S.	
Murine typhus	Louse, rat flea	*R. mooseri*	Rat	OX₁₉	Concentrated along Gulf of Mexico and Atlantic seaboard	50% of cases reported in Texas
Scrub typhus (tsutsugamushi fever)	Mite	*R. orientalis*	Rodents	OXK	Far East	Not seen in U.S.

Epidemic typhus has an incubation period of seven to fourteen days, followed by the onset of fever, chills, headache, and myalgias. The eruption appears four to six days into the illness. A maculopapular eruption appears initially on the trunk near the axillae and then spreads to the extremities. The face, palms, and soles are not involved. Petechiae and purpura appear in the second week of illness. Finally, a brownish pigmentation heralds the disappearance of the rash.

Murine typhus has an incubation period of one to two weeks. The syndrome is similar to epidemic typhus. The rash appears three to five days into the illness. The rash is sparse and rarely hemorrhagic.

The incubation period of scrub typhus is one to three weeks. An indurated papule appears after the usual prodrome of fever, chills, headache, and myalgia. The papule ulcerates and soon forms an eschar, with regional lymphadenopathy. One week after onset of fever, a macular or maculopapular rash is found on the trunk.

Differential Diagnosis

Rocky mountain spotted fever
Rickettsialpox
Typhus group
Meningococcemia
Varicella
Atypical measles
Herpes simplex
Epidemic typhus
Measles

HISTOLOGICAL DESCRIPTION

In Rocky mountain spotted fever, the epidermis does not show significant change. The dermal vessels and vessels in the subcutis show endothelial swelling, vessel wall necrosis, hemorrhage, and a surrounding infiltrate of lymphocytes and histiocytes. The involved vessels may have microthrombi that occlude some vessels (Figure 17-7-1). In spite of the marked vascular reaction, neutrophils are infrequently seen in the perivascular infiltrate. The organism (*Rickettsia rickettsii*) can sometimes be visualized in the endothelium with tissue Gram stains or Giemsa stain. Immunofluorescent techniques are the best method for identification of organisms in tissue. The histological findings in all rickettsial disease are due to the vascular damage caused by the action of the organism on the vessel wall. All conditions, including rickettsialpox and typhus, will show a varying degree of vascular injury with subsequent tissue reactions.

Differential Diagnosis

Vasculitis of other causes
Collagen vascular disease

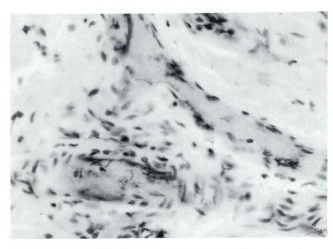

17-7-1 ROCKY MOUNTAIN SPOTTED FEVER: Dermal vessels show intravascular thrombosis and a sparse neutrophilic infiltrate. (400×)

17-8 SCARLET FEVER

CLINICAL DESCRIPTION

Although the incidence of scarlet fever and its severity have decreased, it still occurs with some frequency. Recent information suggests a return of the more severe form (i.e. streptococcal toxic shock syndrome) due to the fact that the A toxin, which was not being produced by Group A beta hemolytic streptococci, is now being produced more frequently by this organism.

Etiology and Incidence

Group A beta-hemolytic streptococcal infections produce this disorder. Following pharyngitis with this organism there is a two to four day incubation period. The rash appears within twelve to forty-eight hours after the onset of fever, vomiting, headache, chills, and malaise. Abdominal pain may be a prominent feature. Streptococcal pharyngitis occurs most frequently in late winter and early spring in temperate climates. Children between six and twelve years of age are most commonly infected.

Clinical Features

The rash first appears on the extensor surface as a blanchable, erythematous, punctate eruption with sandpaperlike texture (sunburn with goosebumps). It generalizes within twenty-four hours. The face is flushed. Circumoral pallor (Figure 17-8-1) is present but punctate lesions are absent on the face. The intensity of the rash is greatest in the skinfolds (e.g., axillae, groin). Transverse lines created by hyperpigmentation and petechiae occur in the creases of the antecubital spaces (Pastia's sign). These lines persist for several days following the disappearance of the rash. If the generalized

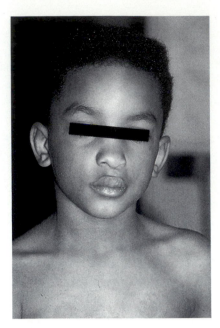

17-8-1 SCARLET FEVER: Circumoral pallor.

eruption is severe, minute vesicular lesions appear (miliaria, sudamina). Desquamation begins on the face (fine scales) after one week and then goes on to involve the trunk and extremities. The hands and feet peel by the second to third week.

    The enanthem includes reddened, edematous tonsils with patches of exudate, and petechiae on the soft palate. The tongue looks furry white on the first two days, with red edges and tip. On the third day, the papillae become edematous, producing white strawberry tongue. When the white coat peels off, on the fourth to fifth day, the red strawberry tongue remains.

Differential Diagnosis
Rubella
Rubeola
Drug eruption
Exanthem subitum
Erythema infectiosum
Infectious mononucleosis
Staphylococcal scalded skin syndrome
Kawasaki's disease
Toxic shock syndrome
Sunburn and nonspecific pharyngitis

HISTOLOGICAL DESCRIPTION

The histological features are not specific but involve the vasculature of the dermis more than other dermal elements. The epidermis is focally spongiotic with rare lymphocytic exocytosis. Parakeratosis is seen during the desquamative stage.

The superficial vessels in the papillary and upper reticular dermis are dilated and often congested with blood cells. The vessels around the adnexae show similar features.

Differential Diagnosis
Eczematous
Non-inflammatory purpuras

17-9 VIRAL DISEASES

Viruses infect the skin directly, causing localized or regional findings, or produce syndromes with more generalized skin changes. The morphologic changes vary greatly. Past history of infection or immunization, the prodrome, features of the rash, and other physical findings (Table 17-9-1) are used to distinguish these disorders from one another.

Rubeola

HISTOLOGICAL DESCRIPTION

The histological features of viral exanthema are nonspecific and may only show a perivascular infiltrate (Figure 17-9-1). Rubeola can show epithelial viral changes less severe than those of the herpes group in that vesicle formation is rare. The epidermis is acanthotic with focal parakeratosis. Intranuclear inclusion can sometimes be found within the parakeratotic nuclei. Viral multinucleated epithelial giant cells can be seen, as can necrotic keratinocytes. Ballooning and reticular degeneration do occur but are less intense than the herpetic group of viral infections. There is a perivascular reaction in the dermis of lymphocytes and histiocytes, the dermal vessels showing some endothelial swelling. The subcutaneous fat is not usually involved.

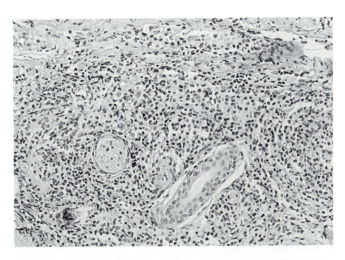

17-9-1 RUBEOLA: Perivascular lymphohistiocytic infiltrate of a viral exanthem. (20×)

Koplik's spots most commonly show mucosal ulceration secondary to epithelial necrosis. The infiltrate is mixed with lymphocytes, neutrophils, histiocytes, and plasma cells.

Differential Diagnosis
Herpes simplex
Herpes zoster

Rubella

HISTOLOGICAL DESCRIPTION

The histological findings in rubella are not specific. There is perivascular inflammation of lymphocytes and histiocytes without vessel wall damage. The epidermis may show focal spongiosis. The viral changes seen in rubeola are not seen in this condition.

Differential Diagnosis
Chronic dermatitis
Eczema

Coxsackie Virus, Echovirus, and Hand-Foot-Mouth Disease

HISTOLOGICAL DESCRIPTION

These conditions can be caused by Coxsackie virus A16 or other Coxsackie viruses, including A9 and echo-9. The histological features are similar, but in hand-foot-mouth disease there is more severe epidermal involvement than in Coxsackie virus infections. In hand-foot-mouth disease epidermal necrosis often occurs.

The vesicular change in these conditions is intraepidermal vesicle formation produced by spongiosis and individual cell necrosis. There is exocytosis of neutrophils as well as lymphocytes. Eosinophilic bodies can be seen in the epidermis; they may result from keratinocyte necrosis with the secondary deposition of immunoglobulin. As the infection proceeds, a subepidermal blister can develop subsequent to basal cell degeneration and dermal-epidermal separation. The epidermis adjacent to the blister shows spongiosis of the type frequently seen in dyshidrotic eczema, except that there may be more intracellular edema. Subsequent to vesicle formation the infiltrate in the dermis is mixed, containing lymphocytes, histiocytes, and polymorphonuclear leukocytes. Viral epithelial giant cells are not seen in these conditions.

Differential Diagnosis
Rubella
Herpes zoster
Herpes simplex
PLEVA (pityriasis lichenoides et varioliformis acuta)

Erythema Infectiosum

HISTOLOGICAL DESCRIPTION

The histological findings in this condition are similar to those of chronic inflammatory dermatoses and are not specific. The epidermis may show slight spongiosis with rare exocytosis of mononuclear cells. In the dermis there is a perivascular infiltrate of lymphocytes and histiocytes. Dermal edema is not striking and can be similar to that seen in urticaria. There are no viral changes seen within the epidermis.

Differential Diagnosis
Chronic dermatitis and eczema
Urticaria

Infectious Mononucleosis

HISTOLOGICAL DESCRIPTION

The epidermis may show focal discrete parakeratosis associated with either very discrete spongiosis or liquefaction degeneration of basal cells. Scattered in the epidermis there can be an occasional dyskeratotic keratinocyte. The dermis has the usual perivascular infiltrate of lymphocytes and histiocytes.

Differential Diagnosis
Graft versus host disease
Lupus erythematosus
Drug eruptions

Herpes Infections

CLINICAL DESCRIPTION

Herpes simplex virus infections range in severity from benign to life-threatening. Although herpes zoster occurs less frequently in children than in adults, it is not a rare disorder.

Etiology and Incidence
Herpes Simplex
Two significant DNA types are discussed: type I, traditionally associated with oral and other nongenital lesions; and type II, which occurs in conjunction with genital infections and, frequently, infections of the newborn. Primary infections may be localized or generalized. Unfortunately, recurrences occur, because antibody production does not totally eliminate the virus. Reactivation occurs following febrile illness, exposure to the sun, menstruation, and psychological disturbances.

Herpes Zoster
Herpes zoster is caused by the same virus that produces chickenpox, Varicella Zoster virus. This cutaneous disorder is the result of reactivation of Varicella Zoster virus that is latent in sensory ganglia. It can occur in normal children or those

17-9-1   Viral Infections

Infection	Etiology	Incidence	Incubation Period	Clinical Features
Rubeola	RNA paromyxovirus	Uncommon due to measles immunization	10–14 days	Maculopapular eruption on 4th day; head to feet in 3 days; becomes confluent; desquamates (Plate 17-9-1)
Atypical Measles	Exposure to above virus following inactivated measles vaccine received 2–4 years previously	Rare	Same	Resembles RMSF, urticarial maculopapular, petechial, purpura, or vesicular eruption concentrated on extremities; edema of hands and feet, myalgia, fever, pneumonitis, pleural effusion
Rubella	RNA virus or para-myxovirus	Uncommon since introduction of immunization	14–21 days	Maculopapular skin eruption; skin lesions remain discrete
Coxsackie and echo virus	Any coxsackie or echo virus; over 30 different types	Common	Variable	Generally rubellalike; may be associated with urticaria, vesicles, or petechiae (especially echo 9 and Coxsackie 9)
Hand-foot-mouth disease	Coxsackie A16	Common, isolated or epidemic form	3–6 days	Maculopapular and vesicular eruption concentrated on hands (palms), feet (soles), in the mouth; may be on erythematous bases (Plate 17-9-2)
Erythema infectiosum (fifth disease)	Parvovirus	Common, may occur in mini epidemics	6–14 days	Erythematous malar blush, erythematous maculopapular eruption on extremities going onto a reticulated or lacy eruption on proximal extremities (Plates 17-9-3 and 17-9-4)
Exanthem subitum (roseola)	Human herpes virus	Most common exanthem under 3 y	5–15 days	Discrete maculopapular eruption begins on trunk, spreads to neck and then extremities; frequently associated with a bulging fontanelle
Infectious mononucleosis	Epstein-Barr virus	Common, especially in adolescents; rash in 10–15% of cases	35–49 days	Rash is maculopapular (morbilliform); involves trunk and upper arms, occasionally face and extremities; 50% with lid edema; 25% have petechiae at junction of hard and soft palate; adenopathy, enlarged spleen, some enlarged liver; may have exudative tonsillitis
Varicella	Varicella zoster	50% of cases before 5 y; 80–90% by 15 y	14–16 days	Evolution of papules to vesicles to crusts within 24 h; vesicles may appear as "teardrop on a rose petal"; lesions appear in crops initially on trunk; may be in all stages in one location; go on to involve other areas, scalp, and mucous membranes

with an immunodeficiency. The majority of cases occur after the age of five years. The mean age at onset of varicella in these patients is younger than in the general population (68% younger than five years). Herpes zoster during the first year of life indicates intrauterine exposure of the fetus to varicella. Birth defects following herpes zoster during pregnancy have been described, but in most cases the fetus is unaffected.

Herpes zoster is a relatively benign condition during childhood and does not signal any underlying malignancy.

Clinical Features
Herpes Simplex
The typical change is a group of vesicles on an erythematous base. Clinical variants are described in Table 17-9-2.

17-9-1 continued

Course	*Comments*
Begins with cough, coryza and conjunctivitis; fever peaks 4–5 days; Koplik spots 1–2 days before rash	Koplik spots appear on buccal mucosa as blue-white specks on red background; hemorrhagic measles is rare; probably associated with DIC because often fatal
Prodrome of fever, cough, headache, myalgia, chest pain 2–4 days preceding rash	Not seen since inactivated measles vaccine no longer given; patients have very high hemagglutination inhibition titers (1:2,500 to 1:200,000), six times higher than seen following typical measles
Malaise, postauricular nodes initial finding; low-grade fever with rash on day 4; rash from head to feet, clears in 8 days	Exanthem (Forchheimer spots) seen during prodrome of first day of rash as pinpoint red spots on soft palate; suboccipital, postauricular, and cervical nodes
Variable; may have prodrome; fever and constitutional symptoms precede or coincide with appearance of rash	Mimics many viral entities
Begins with low-grade fever, anorexia, sore mouth, abdominal pain, followed in 2 days by rash; base clears in 2–7 days	Infections more common in late summer and fall
No prodrome; first sign of illness is skin eruption; initial sign is slapped-cheek appearance with circumoral pallor, followed by maculopapular eruption and then lacelike appearance; rash becomes evanescent and is precipitated by various stimuli (e.g., friction, sun, temperature changes); rash may last for 30 days	Produces hemolytic anemia of fetus and hydrops fetalis; affects 12-year-olds
3–4 days high fever; rash when fever resolves	Patient unusually well-appearing considering height of temperature (6% associated with seizures)
Eruption begins on day 4–6 of illness; lasts for only a few days	Infection frequently no more than a cold in young children or asymptomatic
Exanthems may be localized and concentrated on inflamed skin; noninfectious once all lesions are crusted; congenital varicella syndrome includes limb hypoplasia, cutaneous scars, microcephaly, cortical choreoretinitis, cataracts; secondary infections of primary lesions with toxin-producing *S. aureus* may produce rapid enlargement of vesicles and areas similar to the staphylococcal scalded skin syndrome (SSSS)	

Herpes Zoster

A cluster of papulovesicular lesions on an erythematous base, arranged in a bandlike distribution along dermatomes innervated by one or two spinal sensory nerves (thoracic in 77% of cases, the extremities in 18%, the head in 5%), indicates the presence of herpes zoster. Dysesthesia occurs in the affected dermatomes one to ten days prior to eruption of the rash. The first lesions appear nearest the central nervous system and erupt in crops along the course of the nerve over a seven-day period. Ninety percent of children clear within one to two weeks. Systemic reactions, such as fever, headache, and regional adenopathy, are common; pain and postherpetic neuralgia are not.

17-9-2   Herpes Simplex Variants

	Findings	Course	Comments
Gingivostomatitis	Oral ulcers and erosions, white plaques, gingiva red, swollen, and friable (bleeds easily); high fever, severe pain, increased salivation due to difficulty swallowing; cervical lymphadenopathy	Fever 3–7 days. Oral changes remain 10–14 days.	Most common presentation of HSV type I in childhood; peak incidence 1–3 y
Kaposi's varicelliform eruption	Umbilicated vesicles appear at site of atopic eczema; at times high fever and regional adenopathy	Lasts 7–14 days	May be life-threatening
Keratoconjunctivitis	Purulent conjunctivitis, marked inflammation of conjunctiva, corneal erosions; lid edema; severe pain, photophobia, tearing	Lasts 14 days	Primary infection of eye; corneal opacity a potential complication
Neonatorum	Single or grouped vesicles on erythematous base on presenting part at delivery; may appear septic; zosteriform distribution at times; pustules, large bullae, or skin denudation; infection during first trimester associated with hydranencephaly and choreoretinitis (Plate 17-9-5)		Incidence 1/2,500–10,000 deliveries, 50% have skin lesions; low risk if mother has recurrent HSV vaginal infection; mortality 15–50% with brain involvement or dissemination
Progenitalis	Involvement of any part of genitalia with characteristic lesions; no urethral discharge; shallow ulcers may appear	Primary infection 14–21 days; recurrences, 8 days	Type II HSV
Simplex (primary cutaneous)	Vesicles or bullae on fingertip (herpetic Whitlow)	21 days to resolve	Seen mainly in healthcare workers
Vulvovaginitis	Vesicles, superficial ulcerations, erythema, edema, pain; mucocutaneous involvement; fever and lymphadenopathy	Same as progenitalis	HSV type I or II; mean monthly recurrences of genital HSV I = 0.020, HSV II = 0.33

Two special situations should be kept in mind. First, when the distribution of the ophthalmic branch of the trigeminal nerve is involved with zoster, the eye is at risk. The risk for eye involvement is high (50%) when lesions appear on the tip of the nose (the distribution of the nasociliary branch). Second, blisters in the ear canal associated with facial palsy and hearing loss indicate the presence of Ramsay Hunt's syndrome.

Differential Diagnosis

Herpes Simplex
Gingivostomatitis
Trench mouth
Aphthous stomatitis
Gingivitis
Varicella
Hand-foot-mouth disease
Herpangina
Kaposi's varicelliform eruption
Coxsackie virus infection
Chlamydia
Herpes simplex virus keratoconjunctivitis

Gonorrheal conjunctivitis
Adenoviral infection
Vesicopustular lesions in the newborn:
   Erythema toxicum
   Staphylococcus pustulosis
   Varicella
   Cytomegolovirus
   Listeria or Pseudomonas sepsis
   Transient neonatal pustular melanosis
   Congenital cutaneous candidiasis
   Herpes zoster
Genital lesions:
   Aphthae
   Primary syphilis
   Warts
   Varicella
Herpetic whitlow
Distal blistering dactylitis

Herpes Zoster
Contact dermatitis
Herpes simplex infection of the neonate

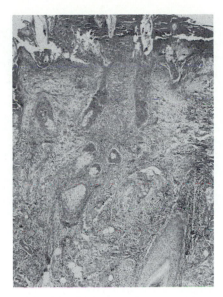

17-9-2 HERPES ZOSTER: Low-power view shows prominent epidermal necrosis and a mild to deep dermal inflammatory infiltrate. (20×)

HISTOLOGICAL DESCRIPTION

The histological features of herpes virus infections of the skin or mucosa vary somewhat depending on the site of infection. In all cases the epidermis or epithelium is most severely affected. The epidermis shows ballooning and reticular degeneration, with subsequent formation of intraepidermal vesicles; there may be epidermal ulceration (Figure 17-9-2). Acantholysis occurs within the epidermis, producing ballooned epidermal cells. Reticular degeneration results in multilocular intraepidermal vesicles. The balloon cells are large and pale, with condensed eosinophilic cytoplasm and a single

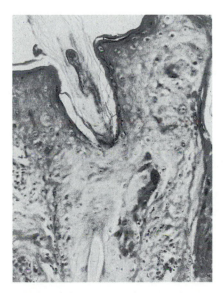

17-9-3 HERPES SIMPLEX/ZOSTER: Characteristic multinucleation of keratinocytes and nuclear moulding in keratinocytes of follicular epithelium. (200×)

large or multiple molded nuclei (Figure 17-9-3). The hallmark of herpes virus infections is the multinucleated epithelial giant cell. Intranuclear inclusions can be found in affected epidermal cells. In those lesions where there is no viable epidermis or epithelium, the crusted debris may show the characteristic balloon cells or multinucleated epithelial viral giant cells. The dermal response is usually marked perivascular inflammation with lymphocytes. The vessels may show some endothelial swelling, usually not to the point of occlusion. In herpes zoster the dermal reaction can be quite marked before there are epidermal changes (Figure 17-9-4). Ulceration secondary to severe destruction of the epidermis can occur (Figure 17-9-2). After ulceration the inflammatory infiltrate is mixed and contains many neutrophils.

Differential Diagnosis
Smallpox
Verruca

Varicella

HISTOLOGICAL DESCRIPTION

The histological features of varicella are the same as those seen in herpes simplex and herpes zoster. The severity of change in varicella may be even greater than in herpes simplex but the cytoplasmic changes within the epidermis are similar. The Tzanck smear in all of these infections is an important aid in diagnosis. The smear is made by opening and reflecting vesicles and scraping gently from the inner surface of the vesicle roof as well as the base of the vesicle and/or bulla. At least ten to fifteen vesicles should be sampled to ensure optimal results. The material is spread on a slide, dried, and stained with Wright's or Giemsa stain. The finding of multinucleated epithelial giant cells or balloon cell with one large or multiple nuclei is diagnostic.

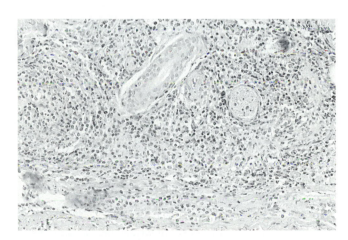

17-9-4 HERPES ZOSTER: The inflammatory infiltrate extends deeply and often surrounds nerves. (200×)

Differential Diagnosis
Herpes simplex
Herpes zoster

Molluscum Contagiosum

CLINICAL DESCRIPTION

This contagious disorder ranks with warts as being one of the most common skin disorders of childhood.

Etiology and Incidence

Molluscum contagiosum is produced by a DNA poxvirus. It is seen most frequently in childhood but can appear at any age. The epidemiology of this disorder is unknown, however swimmers and wrestlers are predisposed. Immunosuppressed patients are especially susceptible. Extensive lesions are seen in patients with atopic eczema and those taking prednisone or other immunosuppressants. Lesions last from several weeks to several years.

Clinical Features

The lesions are flesh-colored, dome-shaped or umbilicated papules with white centers. They can be found on any body surface. At times they coalesce into large sessile or pedunculated masses. Lesions may become inflamed or eczematous, indicating onset of immune rejection of the poxvirus.

Differential Diagnosis
Nonspecific papules
Acne

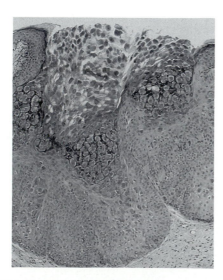

17-9-5 MOLLUSCUM CONTAGIOSUM: Lobular acanthosis of epithelium. Prominent eosinophilic inclusions of molluscum are present within keratinocytes and the stratum corneum. (40×)

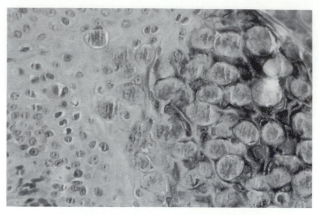

17-9-6 MOLLUSCUM CONTAGIOSUM: Higher magnification of molluscum bodies within keratinocytes. (100×)

HISTOLOGICAL DESCRIPTION

Molluscum contagiosum has distinctive histological features. There is lobular acanthosis of the epidermis with intervening papillomatosis of the dermis, the papillomatosis occurring between plump dependent lobules of epidermis. Within the epidermal cells at the sites of lobular acanthosis, there are large eosinophilic intracytoplasmic inclusion bodies (Figure 17-9-5) measuring up to 35 μm in diameter. Inclusion bodies are found beginning in the stratum Malpighi and upper layers of the epidermis, but are not found in the basal layer. The nuclei of the affected cells are pushed aside and become small hyperchromatic crescents (Figure 17-9-6). The center of the lesion disintegrates at the stratum corneum, releasing the infected cells (molluscum body), forming a crateriform lesion. Inflammation is variable and may be mixed, especially in lesions that become secondarily infected.

Differential Diagnosis
Verrucae (palmar or plantar)

Verrucae

CLINICAL DESCRIPTION

In the past, verrucae were not considered to be associated with serious health problems. As we learn more about this viral disorder, significant associations have been described. For example, wart virus in a woman's genital tract is associated with cervical cancer and has been found to produce laryngeal papillomas in the newborn.

Etiology and Incidence

Warts are caused by papillomavirus, a DNA virus. More than fifty different DNA types have been identified (Table 17-9-3). This is one of the most common skin disorders of childhood, with the highest incidence occurring in individuals between ten and nineteen years of age. Twenty-five percent of

17-9-3 Verrucae: DNA Types

HPV Type	Clinical Presentation
1, 4	Plantar verrucae
1, 2, 4, 7*, 26–29	Common verrucae
2, 3, 10, 26–29, 41	Flat warts
5, 8, 9, 12, 14, 15, 17, 19–25, 36–38, 46, 47, 49, 50	Epidermodysplasia
6, 11, 16, 18, 30, 31, 32, 42–44, 51–55	Genital warts
6, 11, 43, 44, 55	Laryngeal papillomas
13	Focal epithelial hyperplasia
16, 18, 31, 32, 33, 39, 42, 48, 51–54	Bowenoid papulosis
16, 18, 31, 32, 35, 42, 51–54	Cervical dysplasia
16, 18, 31, 32, 33, 35, 39, 42, 51–54	Cervical carcinoma
30	Laryngeal carcinoma

*In meat handlers

warts disappear three to six months after appearing, and 65% within two years.

Clinical Features

The clinical appearance of a wart is frequently determined by its location. Verrucae vulgaris are round, flesh-colored lesions with a rough papillomatous surface. Thrombosed superficial capillaries lead to the back pinpoint specks scattered at the surface. The lesions may have a broad base, as seen on fingers, lips, and on a narrow base with a filiform projection, as seen on the face and neck. Plantar warts are generally below the skin surface with small, raised openings at the surface (somewhat like an iceberg). The weight-bearing surfaces can be peppered with these lesions. The thick keratotic plaques of many warts are called mosaic warts. Flat warts are the most difficult to diagnose. Seen primarily on the face and extremities, these lesions are flesh-colored, yellow, or tan, dome-shaped to flat-topped, minimally elevated papules. They may be numerous in a single location and may appear in a linear distribution in scratch marks (Koebner phenomenon). Condyloma acuminata are warts that involve the mucocutaneous surfaces of the genitals. These lesions may be single fleshy lesions or large cauliflowerlike masses of numerous coalesced lesions.

Differential Diagnosis

Callus
Foreign body granuloma
Acne
Xanthoma
Molluscum contagiosum
Condyloma lata
Black heel

HISTOLOGICAL DESCRIPTION

Verrucae represent epithelium parasitized or infected by a variety of types of the human papilloma virus. All of the tissues respond in a similar manner, with hyper- and parakeratosis, acanthosis, papillomatosis, and vascular neogenesis.

Condyloma Acuminata

Condyloma do not exhibit significant hyperkeratosis because of their usual location in moist areas. They usually have scant parakeratosis and acanthosis (Figure 17-9-7) with vacuolated epidermal cells (koilocytes) (Figure 17-9-8) that extend to the midspinus level. These tumors may show significant cytological atypia and sometimes can be confused with epithelial malignancies. These verrucae can be caused by human papilloma virus types 1, 2, 4, 6, 11, 16, and 18.

Epidermodysplasia Verruciformis

These viral tumors resemble verruca plana. There is basket-weave hyperkeratosis without parakeratosis. The upper layers of the epidermis show vacuolated keratinocytes (koilocytes) with an increase in the thickness of the granular cell layer. The affected cells in this condition, in contrast to verruca plana, are larger and more irregularly shaped. Atypia can occur but is not common. Human papilloma virus 5 is most commonly associated with this condition.

Palmoplantar Verruca (Myrmecia)

These verrucae are most often confused with molluscum contagiosum because of the extensive presence of large eosinophilic keratohyaline granules, which may be confused with the cytoplasmic inclusions in molluscum contagiosum. The overall configuration is that of arborization of the rete at the margins, to give a cup-shaped appearance to this lesion that

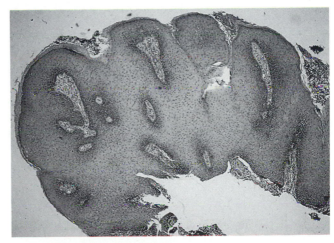

17-9-7 CONDYLOMA ACCUMINATA: Prominent acanthosis and rounding of papillae tips. (40×)

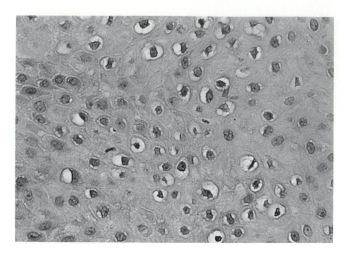

17-9-8 CONDYLOMA ACCUMINATA: Pernuclear halo formation in koilocytes indicates viral cytopathic effect. (100×)

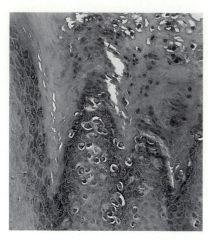

17-9-10 VERRUCA VULGARIS: In active verrucae there is prominent clumping of keratohyaline granules, especially at papillary tips. Note the parakeratotic columns above these tips. (100×)

has central hyper- and parakeratosis. Within the area of hyper- and parakeratosis there are large clumped eosinophilic granules. Keratohyaline granules normally stain basophilic but in this tumor are distinctly eosinophilic. The epidermis is acanthotic and there is distinct papillomatosis of the dermis with tall, thin papillary dermal blood vessels. The inflammatory response in the dermis is variable, usually mononuclear (lymphocytic). Intranuclear and intracytoplasmic inclusions can be seen in these tumors. Palmar-plantar verrucae are most associated with human papilloma virus 1 infections.

Verruca Plana

Verrucae plana have basket-weave orthokeratosis, hypergranulosis, and vacuolated cells with a centrally placed nucleus in the upper stratum Malpighi. Vacuolated cells are more uniform in appearance than in epidermal dysplasia. The vacuolar change is confined to the upper epidermis and does not ex-

tend to the midspinus layer, as in condyloma. Cellular atypia is rare. The tumor is frequently associated with human papilloma virus 3.

Verruca Vulgaris

Hyperkeratosis, parakeratosis, acanthosis, papillomatosis, vascular dilatation in the dermal papillae, arborization of acanthotic rete, and a chronic inflammatory infiltrate of dermal vessels characterize verruca vulgaris (Figure 17-9-9). Most characteristic are vacuolated cells in the epidermis under stacks of parakeratosis, in which the parakeratotic nuclei have been described as "fat cell" parakeratosis. The intervening crypts within the epidermis show hypergranulosis with clumping of keratohyalin granules. The keratohyalin granules in this tumor stain basophilic, in contrast to those of keratohyalin palmar-plantar verrucae (Figure 17-9-10). The vacuolated cells (koilocytes) are seen mainly in the upper stratum malpigi and are similar in appearance to those in verruca plana.

Differential Diagnosis

Molluscum contagiosum

17-10 FUNGAL DISEASES AND CANDIDIASIS

The deep fungal and systemic mycoses involve the skin secondarily. When skin lesions occur, especially in systemic mycosis, the prognosis is poor (Table 17-10-1).

Actinomycosis

HISTOLOGICAL DESCRIPTION

This is a rare condition in children, but when seen the histological features are the same as those in adults. There are

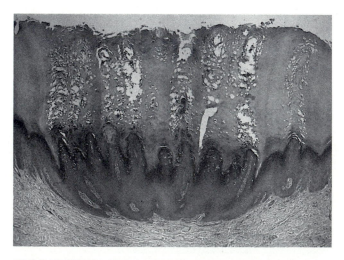

17-9-9 VERRUCA VULGARIS: Prominent papillomatosis and fusion of rete ridges that point inward (arborization). (20×)

colonies of organisms (sulfur granules) within abscesses in granulation tissue. The central abscesses are surrounded by histiocytes, plasma cells, and lymphocytes. The sulfur granules are composed of filaments (bacteria) that are, on average, 300 μm. The granules can attain macroscopic size and are seen in draining purulent sinuses. The organisms in tissue can be visualized with silver, Giemsa, or Gram stains. The organism is composed of multiple thin filaments with a clublike end or terminus (Plate 17-10-1). These organisms are not acid-fast. The cause of the organism in actinomycosis most commonly is *Actinomyces israelii*.

Differential Diagnosis

Nocardia

Mycetoma

Blastomycosis

HISTOLOGICAL DESCRIPTION

North American Blastomycosis

Primary skin infection is rare. The skin is usually involved secondary to pulmonary and subsequent systemic involvement. The causative organism is *Blastomyces dermatitidis*, a single budding large spore that measures 15 to 18 μm and has a thick refractile wall.

Infections in the skin show verrucous acanthosis to the point of pseudoepitheliomatous hyperplasia. The infiltrate is granulomatous with multinucleated giant cells, lymphocytes, histiocytes, plasma cells, and neutrophils in small dermal abscesses (Figure 17-10-1). Biopsy specimens from the active border best demonstrate the organisms found in giant cells as well as free in the tissue (Figure 17-10-2). In primary inoculation blastomycosis, organisms are plentiful and their inflam-

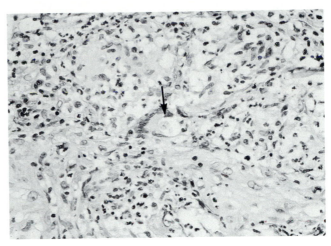

17-10-2 NORTH AMERICAN BLASTOMYCOSIS: Higher magnification discloses a brisk lymphohistiocytic infiltrate. A multinucleated giant cell contains a yeast form within its cytoplasm. (200×)

matory response is more lymphohistiocytic without such a pronounced granulomatous epithelioid or giant cell response. The organisms are best visualized with periodic acid-Schiff and/or silver stain. The spores are periodic acid-Schiff-positive diastase-resistant (Plate 17-10-2).

South American Blastomycosis (Paracoccidioidomycosis)

Infection of the skin is most commonly secondary to pulmonary infection. The causative organism is *Paracoccidioides braziliensis*, a spore that measures from 6 to 60 μm and in tissue diagnostically has multiple buds around the parent sporelike spokes of a wheel (Figure 17-10-3). Multiple budding organisms are difficult to find in tissue, and when the organism only has single buds or no buds it is very similar to the organism of North American blastomycosis. The tissue reaction is granulomatous inflammation with epithelioid histiocytes and giant cells. The organisms are found free in the tissue or within giant cells. The organisms are best visualized with periodic acid-Schiff or silver stains.

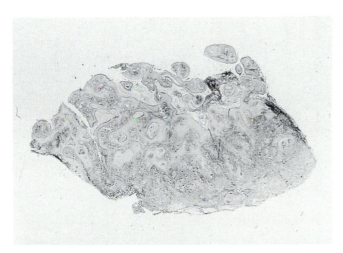

17-10-1 NORTH AMERICAN BLASTOMYCOSIS: Low magnification shows verrucous acanthosis simulating pseudocarcinomatous hyperplasia. (20×)

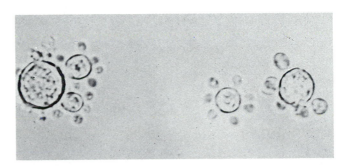

17-10-3 SOUTH AMERICAN BLASTOMYCOSIS: Spinal fluid preparation shows characteristic radiating buds from a large central yeast form. (200×)

17-10-1 Fungal Diseases

	Organism	Clinical Forms	Clinical Features	Incidence	Geographic Distribution	Source
Actinomycosis	Fungallike Gram-positive bacteria; *Actinomyces israelii* or *Actinomyces bovis*	Cervicofacial, pulmonary, intestinal	Painful suppurative draining sinuses, especially mandibular; sulfur yellow granular discharge	Rare in childhood	Worldwide	Saprophyte of tonsillar crypts or carious teeth
		NA, primary cutaneous pulmonary	Accidental inoculation produces ulcerated chancriform lesion with lymphangitis and adenopathy	Rare	Canada to Central America	
		Disseminated	Papules or nodules (hands, feet, face, wrist) ulcerate, or verrucous crusted lesion with active arciform or serpiginous border with violaceous margins, or nodule covered with pustules	Childhood	Central, Eastern, Midwestern U.S.	
Blastomycosis	*Blastomyces dermatitidis* (N. Am.) or *brasiliensis* (S. Am.)	South American cutaneous, disseminated	Progressive ulceration of face that destroys lips, nose, face; disseminated abscesses with nodes that drain	Uncommon	South & Central America (esp. Brazil)	Soil or vegetation
Chromoblasto-mycosis	*Phialophora, Cladosporium*	Chronic cutaneous, chronic subcutaneous	Verrucous nodules, plaques, or tumor masses of distal extremity (especially foot); reddish gray color, painless	Uncommon but seen in children	Tropical and subtropical countries	Soil or decaying vegetation
Coccidioidomy-cosis	*Coccidioides immitis*	Pulmonary	10% erythema macular exanthem during flulike illness; 20% Erythema multiforme or *E. nodosum*	Uncommon but seen in children	San Joaquin Valley, Mexico, parts of South America	Soil
		Systemic	Nondescript papules and pustules, nodules, abscesses, ulcers, vegetative surfaces			
		Primary cutaneous	Painless indurated ulcerated lesion with lymphangitis and adenopathy			

Disease	Organism	Clinical forms	Clinical description	Frequency in childhood	Distribution	Source
Cryptococcosis	*Cryptococcus neoformans*	Cutaneous, pulmonary, CNS	10–15% of cases with skin involvement; red to violaceous papules, pustules, arciform lesions on head and neck with surrounding inflammation; may develop into firm tumors, abscesses, or ulcers with papillomatous borders	Uncommon but does occur in childhood	Worldwide	Fruits, soil, pigeon feces, cow's milk
Histoplasmosis	*H. capsulatum*	Acute pulmonary, chronic pulmonary, disseminated	Cutaneous lesions uncommon and variable (e.g., *E. multiforme, E. nodosum*, purpura, papules)	Seen in childhood	Worldwide; Mississippi and Ohio Valleys	Soil contaminated with feathers and feces
Sporotrichosis	*Sporothrix schenkii*	Lymphocutaneous, fixed cutaneous, disseminated	75% of all cases: small papule that enlarges and ulcerates with subsequent nodules developing along lymphatic channels, producing a linear distribution; nodules violaceous; localized and disseminated lesions also may occur	Infrequent in childhood	Worldwide	Soil or vegetation
Mucormycosis	*Rhizopus and Mucor*	Subcutaneous, cutaneous, cerebral	Papular lesions, chronic ulcers, painless subcutaneous nodules	Rare	Worldwide	

Differential Diagnosis

North American blastomycosis

Candidiasis

CLINICAL DESCRIPTION

Candida albicans produces a variety of skin and mucous membrane changes.

Etiology and Incidence

Although many species of *Candida* exist, the most common is *C. albicans*. A regular inhabitant of the mouth, gastrointestinal tract, and vagina, the organism becomes pathogenic when conditions favoring its proliferation are present. Endocrinologic disorders (diabetes, hypothyroidism, Addison's disease), genetic disorders (Down's syndrome, acrodermatitis enteropathica), chronic illnesses, abnormal T cell function, and corticosteroid or systemic antibiotic therapy all predispose the patient to this infection, as do heat and moisture.

Superficial skin and mucosal infections are common, but systemic infections are not. About 50% of infants with positive oral cultures for *C. albicans* manifest thrush. These infants pick up the organism during delivery through an infected birth canal. Congenital cutaneous candidiasis is an uncommon condition thought to be caused by infected amniotic fluid from an ascending candidal vulvovaginitis. Most patients with chronic mucocutaneous candidiasis exhibit impaired, cell-mediated immunity, although 25% to 30% have no demonstrable immunologic defect.

Perlèche is produced by accumulation of moisture at the angles of the mouth. Predisposing factors include malocclusion, braces, and lip licking.

Clinical Features

Diaper candidiasis, candidal paronychia, and intertriginous candidiasis account for most cutaneous infections. Classically, candidal diaper dermatitis consists of erythematous papules and pustules that coalesce to form a sharply marginated, intensely erythematous eruption. Satellite papulopustules are frequently present. The eruption usually involves the inguinal folds.

Intertriginous infection with *C. albicans* is clinically similar to diaper involvement. Any skinfold can be involved.

Congenital cutaneous candidiasis manifests within the first twelve hours of birth. Initially there are erythematous macules, which evolve through papulovesicular and pustular stages. Although diffuse, the lesions usually spare the mouth and diaper areas. The lesions subsequently dry, causing widespread desquamation of the skin (Plate 17-10-3).

Disseminated systemic candidiasis occurs mainly in debilitated, immunosuppressed patients with chronically in-dwelling intravenous catheters. When skin lesions appear, there are scattered subcutaneous violaceous nodules. Patients are usually very toxic.

Chronic mucocutaneous candidiasis manifests with chronic recurrent thrush, recalcitrant candidal diaper dermatitis, and candidal intertrigo or paronychia. The infection involves large areas of skin with an erythematous, scaling eruption, which at times has polycyclic margins. Chronic changes include nail dystrophy and hair loss. Systemic spread is unusual.

Perlèche appears at the corners of the mouth and is characterized by painful fissures and inflammation.

Thrush is characterized by white, cheesy plaques on erythematous oral mucous membranes.

Differential Diagnosis

See Table 17-10-2.

HISTOLOGICAL DESCRIPTION

Candidiasis occurs in a variety of clinical syndromes, all of which share similar histological features. The causative organism, *C. albicans*, a normal inhabitant of the skin and gastrointestinal tract, becomes a pathogen under opportunistic circumstances. The organism is a single budding yeastlike form that measures approximately 2 to 5 μm, is round to oval in shape, and can produce filamentous forms (hyphae) in tissue.

In the mucosal syndromes, which are more common in children than in adults, there is edematous acanthotic mucosal epithelium with candidal spores and hyphae on the surface associated with cellular debris and other amorphous material. Usually the flora and fauna of the affected mucosa are also seen.

Cutaneous candidiasis in intertriginous areas will show the organism in the thinned stratum corneum as spores and budding spores with short hyphae.

In congenital cutaneous candidiasis there is hyperkeratosis and parakeratosis with the presence of subcorneal pustules. The epidermis is acanthotic and there is spongiosis and exocytosis. The exocytotic cells are mononuclear and neutrophils. Candidal organisms can be found in the stratum corneum and in the pustules. In systemic disseminated candidiasis the organism is found in the dermis. It can be found within dermal vessels that have been occluded by emboli of organisms. These occluded vessels contain spores as well as hyphae. Some vessels show leukocytoclastic vasculitis with occlusion and necrosis. Organisms can also be found within these areas.

The dermal response in cutaneous candidiasis is edema, perivascular inflammation of lymphocytes, and histiocytes. Organisms are not found below the stratum corneum in cutaneous candidiasis.

17-10-2   Candidiasis

Chronic Mucocutaneous Candidiasis	*Congenital Cutaneous Candidiasis*	*Diaper Rash*
Atopic dermatitis	Erythema toxicum	Primary irritant dermatitis
Seborrheic dermatitis	Staphylococcal pustulosis	Atopic dermatitis
Acrodermatitis enteropathica	Staphylococcal scalded skin syndrome	Seborrheic dermatitis
Biotin deficiency	HSV	Acrodermatitis enteropathica
Biotin-dependent carboxylase abnormalities		Histiocytosis X
		Kawasaki's disease
		Contact dermatitis

Disseminated Candidiasis	*Intertrigo*	*Perlèche*	*Thrush*
Lymphomatous disorder	Primary Irritant	Bacterial infection	Precipitated milk on mucous membrane
Granulomatous disorder	Contact dermatitis	Trauma	Chronic trauma (biting)
Infectious disorder	Seborrheic dermatitis	Viral infection	Lichen planus
			Pachyonychia congenita
			Dyskeratosis congenita
			White sponge nevus of Cannon

Differential Diagnosis

Tinea versicolor
Tinea nigra
Dermatophyte infection

Chromomycosis

HISTOLOGICAL DESCRIPTION

Chromomycosis is caused by direct inoculation of the organism into the skin. A variety of organisms cause the condition, the more common being Fonsecae species (Wangiella species) and the Phialophora species. The causative organism is a thick-walled, budding spore, brown on hematoxylin and eosin-stained sections, that aggregates after cell division. They range in size from 2 to 12 μm. The tissue reaction is acanthosis to the point of pseudoepitheliomatous hyperplasia. The dermis shows a granulomatous response with focal areas of abscess formation. The organisms are found in giant cells as well as free in the tissue. They usually occur in groups or chains and are likened to copper pennies (Plate 17-10-4). They can be seen readiliy without special stains but are also visualized with silver and periodic acid-Schiff stains.

Differential Diagnosis

North American blastomycosis
Coccidioidomycosis
South American blastomycosis
Squamous cell carcinoma

Coccidioidomycosis

HISTOLOGICAL DESCRIPTION

Infections with this organism is, as with most pathogenic fungi or systemic disease, with secondary skin involvement.

The organism is a large spore, 10 to 80 μm in diameter (Figure 17-10-4). It reproduces by endosporulation with endospores that are approximately 2 to 7 μm in diameter. The tissue reaction is similar to that in other deep mycotic infections, with pseudoepitheliomatous hyperplasia, exocytosis of mononuclear cells, and polymorphonuclear leukocytes and spongiosis. There is a granulomatous reaction in the dermis with giant cells, lymphocytes, histiocytes, and plasma cells. Neutrophil abscesses are also seen. The organisms are found free in the tissue and in giant cells. Due to their size, the organisms can be seen on routine stains but are better visualized with special stains such as a silver stain or periodic acid-Schiff.

Differential Diagnosis

See Chromomycosis

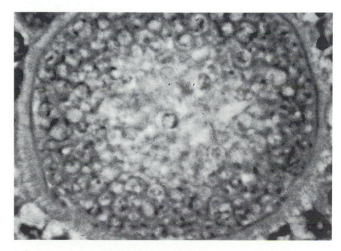

17-10-4 COCCIDIOIDOMYCOSIS: Large spherule contains many endospores of *Coccidioides immitis.* (600 ×)

Cryptococcosis

HISTOLOGICAL DESCRIPTION

Infection with this organism is usually by inhalation and is now more prevalent in the immunocompromised population. The causative organism is *Cryptococcus neoformans.*

The causative organism is a spore whose average size is 4 to 12 μm. It has a capsule and a centrally placed small nucleus (Figure 17-10-5). The tissue reaction is either a dense diffuse infiltration of the tissue by the organism without a significant host response, or a granulomatous reaction with histiocytes, lymphocytes, plasma cells, and giant cells, abscess formation, and necrosis. In the diffuse stage, the numerous organisms (gelatinous) cause the tissue to appear foamy, and the organisms are readily visualized. In the granulomatous response there are fewer organisms. The capsule does not stain on hematoxylin and eosin sections but can be visualized on periodic acid-Schiff stains with diastase digestion. With Alcian blue, the capsule stains blue-green. With mucicarmine stain, the organism has a red-pink capsule.

Differential Diagnosis
See Chromomycosis

Histoplasmosis

HISTOLOGICAL DESCRIPTION

Infection with *Histoplasma capsulatum* is via inhalation of spores, with the skin secondarily infected.

The causative organism is small, 2 to 4 μm in diameter, and reproduces by single buds that have a narrow neck at the point of attachment to the mother spore. In tissue the response is granulomatous, with histiocytes, plasma cells, lym-

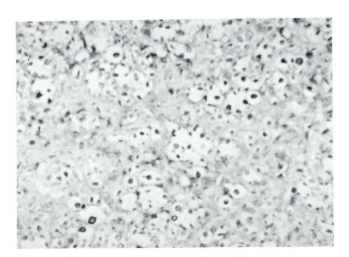

17-10-5 CRYPTOCOCCOSIS: Multiple spores surrounded by clear spaces characteristic of cutaneous infection with *Cryptococcus neoformans.* (200×)

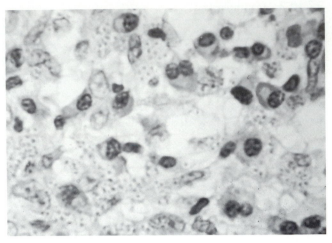

17-10-6 HISTOPLASMOSIS: Basophilic bodies surrounded by halos in parasitized histiocytes. (400×)

phocytes, and small neutrophilic abscesses. Epithelial giant cells can also be found. The organisms are found in the tissue and in the giant cells. The less immunity the patient has, the larger number of organisms that are found. The organism can be seen on hematoxylin and eosin-stained sections, staining as a basophilic body surrounded by a clear zone (Figure 17-10-6). Gram, Giemsa, or silver stains will show the organism in much more detail. On silver stain the clear zone is shown to be a part of the cell wall of the organism.

Differential Diagnosis
Leishmaniasis
Granuloma inguinale

Sporotrichosis

HISTOLOGICAL DESCRIPTION

Sporotrichosis, like chromomycosis, is caused by direct inoculation to the skin, producing a cutaneous eruption that is progressive from the site of the inoculation (Figure 17-10-7). In tissue there is an inflammatory response consisting of diffuse as well as perivascular lymphocytes, histiocytes, plasma cells, and giant cells (Figure 17-10-8). Small neutrophilic abscesses are frequently found. Organisms are not numerous in tissue but can be found within the neutrophilic abscesses as small spores, 3 to 5 μm in diameter, most commonly with single buds. Specialized forms of the organism can also be infrequently seen as a central spore with radiating elongate structures (asteroidlike bodies) (Plate 17-10-5). The causative organism, *Sporothrix schenckii,* is best visualized with silver stains. In the lymph nodes there is a characteristic neutrophilic abscess surrounded by a zone of lymphocytes and giant cells, which is, in turn, surrounded by a zone of plasma cells and lymphocytes.

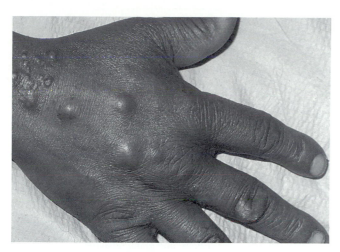

17-10-7 SPOROTRICHOSIS: Multiple subcutaneous nodules on the dorsum of the right hand and along the path of lymphatic drainage.

Differential Diagnosis

Tuberculosis
Atypical mycobacterial infection

Mucormycosis

HISTOLOGICAL DESCRIPTION

The striking features are large, segmented hyphae in areas of necrosis and lack of significant inflammatory response. The hyphae are large, some over 40 μm in diameter, and can be seen within vessels as well as emerging through the vessel walls. They are periodic acid-Schiff-positive and stain with silver stains. In areas within the tissue, granulomas can be seen about the large hyphae. The epidermis may be effaced, acanthotic, or ulcerated.

Differential Diagnosis

Foreign body granuloma

Dermatophytosis

CLINICAL DESCRIPTION

Dermatophytosis is an overgrowth of filamentous fungi in keratinized tissue. The severity and pattern of disease depend on the species of the dermatophyte and the host response. These infections are classified by the skin surface affected (Table 17-10-3).

Differential Diagnosis

Tinea Capitis
Atopic or seborrheic dermatitis
Psoriasis
Alopecia areata

Tinea Corporis
Granuloma annulare (no epidermal changes)
Nummular eczema
Herald patch of pityriasis rosea
Psoriasis
Allergic contact dermatitis
Tinea versicolor

Tinea Cruris
Intertrigo
Candidiasis
Erythrasma

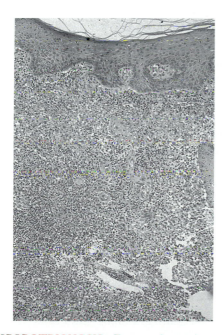

17-10-8 SPOROTRICHOSIS: Dense polymorphous dermal infiltrate. (40×)

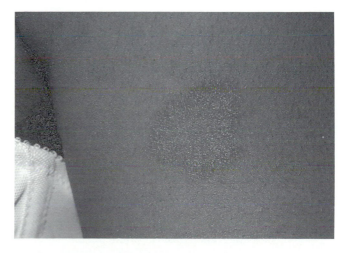

17-10-9 TINEA CORPORIS: A sharply demarcated scaly patch on the arm.

17-10-3   Etiology, Incidence, and Clinical Features of Dermatophytosis

Name	Body Part Involved	Infecting Organism	Prevalence	Clinical Features
Tinea capitis	Scalp, eyebrows, eyelashes	*Trichophyton tonsurans*	Common	Inflammatory: noninflammatory, 3:2; diffuse scaling with minimal hair loss or irregular, scaly patches of alopecia with black dots; pustular and crusted plaques of alopecia; kerions; nonfluorescent
		Microsporum audouinii	Uncommon	Annular, scaly patch of alopecia
		Microsporum canis	Uncommon	Kerions; fluorescent
Tinea corporis	Face, trunk, limbs	*T. tonsurans* *M. audouini* *Trichophyton mentagrophytes* (Figure 17-10-9)	Common Less common Less common	Circular lesions with scaling elevated borders and central clearing; border may be studded with vesicles; variants include eczematized plaques, crusted lesions, kerions, and granulomas; any scaling lesion on face may be tinea
Tinea cruris	Groin	*Epidermophyton floccosum* *Trichophyton rubrum* *T. mentagrophytes*	Seen mainly in adolescent males	Sharply delineated symmetrical, scaly plaques involve the intertriginous folds and proximal thighs; scrotum is usually spared
Tinea pedis	Feet	In preadolescents, same as tinea corporis; in adolescents, same as tinea cruris	Seen mainly in adolescents	Same as tinea corporis; maceration and scaling of 3rd and 4th interdigital spaces; itching and foul odor (due to bacterial infection) common
Tinea unguium	Nails	*T. rubrum, T. mentagrophytes*	Unusual in childhood; associated with immunosuppression	Yellow or white changes at distal edge of nail; gradually involves entire nailplate with subungual debris

Tinea Pedis
Contact shoe dermatitis
Atopic eczema
Dyshidrotic eczema
Simple maceration and peeling

Tinea Unguium
Twenty nail dystrophy
Pachyonychia congenita
Psoriasis
Lichen planus
Alopecia areata
Ectodermal dysplasia
Infection with *Candida albicans*
Infection with *Pseudomonas*

HISTOLOGICAL DESCRIPTION

Dermatophyte infection in the skin is caused by a host of organisms (most commonly *Trichophyton* species). The tissue response is variable. There may be severe inflammation that resembles contact dermatitis (Figure 17-10-10). Infection of the glabrous skin shows hyper- and parakeratosis with neu-trophils in the stratum corneum (a frequent finding). The sections may appear normal or have minimal reaction of a perivascular lymphohistiocytic inflammatory infiltrate in the dermis and only slight epidermal spongiosis and exocytosis. Organisms can rarely be seen on hematoxylin and eosin-stained sections but are readily visualized with silver or periodic acid-Schiff stains (Figure 17-10-10). Hyphae are found within the stratum corneum. When there is infection of the hair, hyphae are always found within the hair shaft and can be readily visualized on routine hematoxylin and eosin sections. Endothrix infections (*Trichophyton violaceum, tonsurans, schoenleinii*) develop spores in the follicular canal as the hyphae grow through the hairshaft. Hyphae should be seen within the hair and spores within the follicular canal surrounding the hairshaft. Ectothrix fungi (*Microsporum* species) have spores on the outside of the hairshaft. Hyphae can also be found in the scales on the scalp. The histological features of scalp infections are similar to those of glabrous skin (Figure 17-10-11).

Nail infections show similar features of hyphae found in the nailplate and are best visualized with periodic acid-Schiff technique.

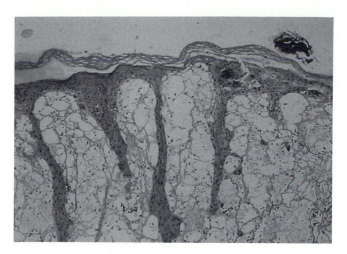

17-10-10 DERMATOPHYTOSIS: Using periodic acid-Schiff, the dermis shows striking edema and a sparse inflammatory infiltrate. The stratum corneum contains occasional characteristic septate hyphae. (100×)

Differential Diagnosis
Tinea versicolor
Candidiasis
Tinea nigra

Tinea Versicolor

CLINICAL DESCRIPTION
The varied presentations of this superficial yeast infection can be confusing.

Etiology and Incidence
Tinea versicolor is an extremely common superficial yeast infection produced by *Pityrosporum orbiculare* (*Malassezia furfur*). Although mainly seen during adolescence, it can be seen in younger children. Warm, humid climates and perspiration encourage growth of the filamentous form. Immunosuppression predisposes one to this eruption of the condition. Failure of the lesions to tan leads to increased recognition during the summer months.

Clinical Features
The disorder derives its name from the fact that the 5 to 10 mm oval scaling macules vary in color (hypopigmented, hyperpigmented, or erythematous) (Figure 17-10-12). The lesions may be isolated, numerous, or may coalesce into large plaques. They are found on the neck, shoulders, chest, back, and upper arms. The forehead and cheeks near the ears are most commonly involved in preadolescent children. Mild pruritus may be present.

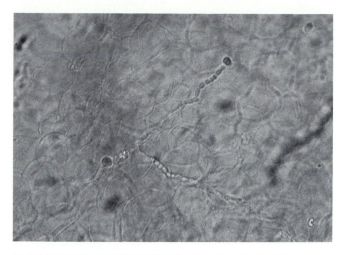

17-10-11 DERMATOPHYTOSIS: Potassium hydroxide preparation of dermatophyte-infected scale shows septate branching hyphae that cross cell borders. (100×)

Differential Diagnosis
Tinea corporis
Seborrheic dermatitis
Parapsoriasis
Atopic eczema
Pityriasis rosea
Secondary syphilis
Pityriasis alba
Vitiligo

HISTOLOGICAL DESCRIPTION
Tinea versicolor has subtle histological features. On initial viewing it is difficult to find a specific change that identifies the pathological process. On careful observation spores and hyphae are seen in the stratum corneum (Figure 17-10-13).

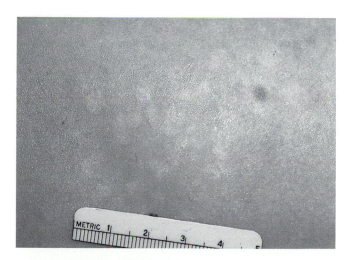

17-10-12 TINEA VERSICOLOR: Characteristic hypopigmented scaly macules on the trunk.

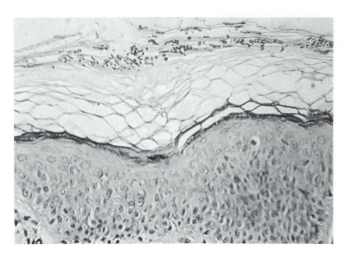

17-10-13 TINEA VERSICOLOR: Periodic acid-Schiff shows hyphae and spores within the stratum corneum. (100×)

The hyphae are short and broad and stain basophilic in hematoxylin and eosin. There is almost always an admixture of spores associated with hyphae, a feature that helps differentiate this condition from candidiasis. The epidermis and dermis do not show significant change.

Differential Diagnosis

Candidiasis

Tinea nigra

REFERENCES

Mycobacterial Infections

Ridley DS: Histological classification in the immunological spectrum of leprosy. Bull WHO 1974;51:451.

Saxe N: Mycobacterial infections. J Cutan Pathol 1985; 12:300.

Santa Cruz DJ, Strayer DS: The histologic spectrum of the cutaneous mycobacterioses. Hum Pathol 1982;13:485.

Cat-Scratch Disease

English CK, Wear DJ, Margileth AM, et al.: Cat-scratch disease. Isolation and culture of the bacterial agent. JAMA 1988;259:1347.

Johnson WT, Helwig EB: Cat-scratch disease: Histological changes in the skin. Arch Dermatol 1969;100:148.

Margileth AM: Antibiotic therapy for cat-scratch disease. Pediatr Inf Dis J 1992;11:474.

Congenital Syphilis

Abel LE, Marx R, Wilson Jones E: Secondary syphilis: A clinical pathologic review. Br J Dermatol 1975;93:53.

Matsuda-John SS, McElgunn PST, Ellis CN: Nodular late syphilis. J Am Acad Dermatol 1983;9:269.

Bacterial Diseases

Ackerman AB, Miller RC, Shapiro RL: Gonococcemia and its cutaneous manifestations. Arch Dermatol 1965;91:272.

Finch R: Soft tissue infections. Lancet 1988;1:164.

Goldberg GN, Hansen RC, Lynch PJ: Necrotizing fasciitis in infancy. Report of three cases and review of the literature. Pediatr Dermatol 1984;2:55.

Green SL, Su WP, Miller SA: Ecthyma gangrenosum: Report of clinical, histologic, and bacterial aspects of eight cases. J Am Acad Dermatol 1984;11:781.

Ignacio JU, Winkelman RK, Oliver GF, Peters MS: Necrotizing fasciitis: A clinical, microscopic, and histopathologic study of 14 patients. J Am Acad Dermatol 1989; 20:774.

Mandell JN, Feiner HP, Price NM, et al.: *Pseudomonas capacia* endocarditis and ecthyma gangrenosum. Arch Dermatol 1977;99:82.

Sarkany I, Taplin D, Blank H: Incidence and bacteriology of erythrasma. Arch Dermatol 1962;85:578.

Sotto MN, Langer B, Hoshino-Shimizu S, de brito T: Pathogenesis of cutaneous lesions in acute meningococcemia in humans: Light, immunofluorescent and electron microscopic studies of skin biopsy specimen. J Infect Dis 1976;133:506.

Stevens DL, Tanner MH, Winship J, et al.: Severe group A streptococcal infections associated with a toxic shock-like syndrome and scarlet fever toxin. N Engl J Med 1989;321:1.

Umbert IJ, Winkelmann RK, Oliver GF, et al.: Necrotizing fasciitis: A clinical, microbiological and histopathologic study of 14 patients. J Am Acad Dermatol 1989; 220:774.

Leishmaniasis

Farah FS, Malak JA: Cutaneous leishmaniasis. Arch Dermatol 1971;103:467.

Rickettsial Diseases

Walker DH, Cain BG, Olmstead M: Laboratory diagnosis of Rocky mountain spotted fever by immunofluorescent demonstration of rickettsia rickettsia in cutaneous lesions. Am J Clin Pathol 1978;69:619.

Viral Diseases

Bialeck C, Feder HM Jr, Grant-Kels JM: The sixth classic childhood exanthems: A review and update. J Am Acad Dermatol 1989;21:891.

Higgins PG, Waran RP: Hand-foot-mouth disease: A clinically recognizable virus infection seen mainly in children. Clin Pediatr 1967;6:373.

Lutzner MA: The human papillomaviruses: A review. Arch Dermatol 1983;119:631.

McSorley J, Shapiro L, Brownstein MH, Hsu K: Simplex and varicella-zoster: Comparative cases. Int J Dermatol 1974;13:69.

Mescon H, Gray M, Moretti G: Molluscum contagiosum. J Invest Dermatol 1954;23:293.

White DO: Viral infections of the skin (review). Aust J Dermatol 1970;11:5.

Fungal Diseases

Allen HB, Charles CR, Johnson BL: Hyperpigmented tinea versicolor. Arch Dermatol 1976;112:1110.

Brown JR: Human actinomycosis: A study of 181 subjects. Hum Pathol 1973;4:319.

Chapell TA, Gagliardi C, Nichols W: Congenital cutaneous candidiasis. J Am Acad Dermatol 1982;6:926.

Charles CR, Sire DJ, Johnson BL, et al.: Hypopigmented tinea versicolor: A histochemical and electron microscopic study. Int J Dermatol 1973;12:48.

Chu AC, Hay RJ, MacDonald DM: Cutaneous cryptococcosis. Br J Dermatol 1980;103:95.

Gottlieb GJ, Ackerman AB: The "sandwich sign" of dermatophytosis. Am J Dermatopathol 1986;8:347.

Grossman ME, Silvers DN, Walther RR: Cutaneous manifestations of disseminated candidiasis. J Am Acad Dermatol 1980;2:111.

Henchy FP III, Daniel CR III, Omura EF, et al.: North American blastomycosis. Arch Dermatol 1982;118:287.

Jorizzo JL: Chronic mucocutaneous candidiasis. Arch Dermatol 1982;118:963.

Lurie HL: Histopathology of sporotrichosis. Arch Pathol 1963;75:121.

McGinnis MR: Chromoblastomycosis and pehaehyphomycosis: New concepts, diagnosis and mycology. J Am Acad Dermatol 1983;8:1.

Perry HO, Weed LA, Kierland RR: South American blastomycosis. Arch Dermatol Syphilol 1954;70:477.

Rasmussen JE, Ahmed AR: Trichophyte reactions in children with tinea capitis. Arch Dermatol 1978;114:371.

Studdard JW, Sneed F, et al.: Cutaneous histoplasmosis. Am Rev Resp Dis 1976;113:689.

18

Reactions to Arthropod Bites, Parasitic Infestations, and Coelenterates

Contents

18-1 CERCARIAL DERMATITIS

CLINICAL DESCRIPTION

This self-limited dermatitis occurs mainly in Wisconsin and Michigan when humans become accidental hosts of cercariae of the *Schistosoma* genus.

Etiology and Incidence

This entity is seen on a limited basis due to its restriction to freshwater lakes in the north central United States. Schistosome eggs in the droppings from waterfowl and infested mammals hatch in these lakes. The next step in the ecological cycle requires the snail as an intermediate host. Cercariae are released into the water from the snail. The parasites finish their cycle in the blood system of waterfowl and rodents. Because humans are accidental hosts, the cercariae do not survive after penetration. The skin manifestations are caused by an immune response to the dead cercariae following repeated exposures.

Clinical Features

An urticarial reaction occurs after penetration of the cercariae. The host experiences a prickling sensation and soon thereafter develops pruritic papular lesions on uncovered areas of skin. The eruption subsides within two weeks.

Differential Diagnosis

Limited
Insect bites

HISTOLOGICAL DESCRIPTION

The histological features are similar to those seen in creeping eruption, scabies, and insect bite reaction. The cercariae can be found in burrows within the stratum corneum or at the

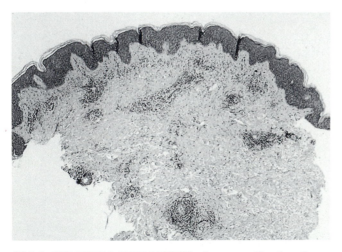

18-1-1 CERCARIAL DERMATITIS: Low magnification of cercarial dermatitis, showing a dense perivascular infiltrate. (40×)

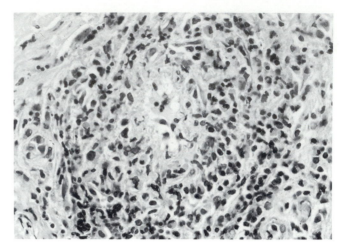

18-1-2 CERCARIAL DERMATITIS: Higher magnification shows the infiltrate containing large numbers of eosinophiles. (100×)

epidermal-stratum corneum junction. There is spongiosis and exocytosis of lymphocytes and eosinophils. In the dermis there is perivascular and diffuse infiltration with lymphocytes and eosinophils (Figures 18-1-1 and 18-1-2).

Differential Diagnosis

Scabies
Insect bite reaction

18-2 CUTANEOUS LARVA MIGRANS

CLINICAL DESCRIPTION

Geography plays an important role in this parasitic disorder. Most cases are seen along the shorelines of the Gulf of Mexico and the Atlantic coast from Florida to the Northeast.

Etiology and Incidence

Children playing at the shore, or in sandboxes or crawling under buildings are at greatest risk of invasion by the hookworm *Ancylostoma braziliense*. On occasion *Strongyloides stercoralis* causes a similar but more rapidly advancing eruption. Ova, deposited in the soil or sand via dog and cat excretions, hatch into larvae that penetrate the skin. The larvae frequently disappear within four weeks because the parasite cannot complete its life cycle in humans.

Clinical Features

The aimless migration of larval hookworms produces the classical pruritic serpiginous erythematous lesions of the skin, usually on the feet, hands, and buttocks (Plate 18-2-1).

Interesting patterns are produced by many larvae migrating simultaneously. Vesicles or bullae can occur along any portion of the tract. Older lesions become dry and crusted.

The *Strongyloides stercoralis* larva migrates rapidly, producing a tract 5 to 10 cm long in one hour, in contrast to 1 to 2 cm by *Ancylostoma braziliense*.

HISTOLOGICAL DESCRIPTION

Finding the organism on histological section is a fortuitous event; when found it is seen within the lower portion of the epidermis or in the epidermis just below the stratum corneum. The organism seen on cross section has a cuticular envelope with a crinkly surface, which surrounds the basophilic internal structures (Plate 18-2-2). The epidermis shows spongiosis and necrosis with exocytosis of lymphocytes and eosinophils. The dermal infiltrate consists of perivascular lymphocytes, histiocytes, and many eosinophils. In some instances neutrophils are seen in the infiltrate.

Differential Diagnosis
Scabies

18-3 INSECT BITES

CLINICAL DESCRIPTION

Children are vulnerable to a host of different insect bites because of their playing habits and love for pets.

Etiology and Incidence
Children living in the southeastern United States may suffer fire ant bites if they disturb an anthill inhabited by them. This pesky insect derives its name from the burning and pain caused by its venom. Bedbug bites occur infrequently in children. The insect resides in seams and tufts of mattresses, bed frames, springs, floor cracks, and wall surfaces and feeds on uncovered skin surfaces. Reactions occur following repeated bites and sensitization to the toxins and allergens contained in the bedbug's saliva. Bees, flies, and wasps produce their effects via the development of sensitivity to their infected venom.

Flea bites are second only to mosquito bites in producing problems for children. Because of the close relationship between children and their pets, dog and cat flea bites are most common. Fleas favor geographical regions with moderate temperatures and high humidity. The insect may live for two years and may survive for several months without a meal. Sensitization to flea bites occurs in a fashion similar to that of bedbug bites.

Mosquito bites are probably the most common insect bites in childhood. Children are bitten because they play in infested areas and their warm weather clothing leaves most skin surfaces exposed. Saliva containing toxins and allergens

produces its effects following sensitization from repeated bites. Once sensitized, an individual initially experiences a delayed reaction, with the papules appearing within twenty-four to forty-eight hours. Subsequently, wheals occur minutes after the bite, followed by the delayed reaction. Finally, the bite causes only an immediate wheal.

Clinical Features
Ant stings generally involve the lower extremities, but any part of the skin surface may be involved. Pain is felt immediately, followed by the development of a wheal. Sometimes bright red hemorrhagic puncta are seen. Several hours later a vesicle appears, followed by the development of umbilicated pustules with a surrounding red halo. This lesion persists for five days, crusts, and leaves a scar.

Since the bedbug feeds from multiple sites in close proximity, the lesions are grouped and frequently in a line. Exposed surfaces are usually involved. The lesions are papular or urticarial with a central hemorrhagic punctum. Bullae may be present. Papular urticaria also occurs.

Flies generally bite exposed areas. The erythematous papules generally disappear within a few hours. Bee or wasp stings occur on any body part. Local erythema and swelling generally subsides over a period of days. Systemic reactions occur, ranging from generalized urticaria to angioedema and hypotensive shock.

The distribution and grouping of lesions is valuable in making the diagnosis of flea bites. Exposed surfaces of skin and the hip and shoulder areas, where clothing fits snugly, are usually involved. Unlike mosquitoes, fleas feed at various sites during one meal. This results in grouped lesions in an irregular pattern. Pruritic urticarial or papular lesions are characteristic. Flea bites induce vesicular pustular or bullous reactions more often than any other insect bites (Figure 18-3-1).

Mosquito bites occur on exposed skin surfaces and are singular because the insect feeds at one spot until satisfied. The typical lesion is a pruritic wheal or papule. Severe local reactions may produce blisters or large areas of indurated erythema with central cyanosis. Papular urticaria and rarely an allergic lymphangitis is seen. Chronic papules and nodules occur in some children, which occasionally leads to skin biopsy.

Differential Diagnosis
Lymphoma
Drug reaction
Cellulitis

HISTOLOGICAL DESCRIPTION

In general, bites produce several types of reactions: acute necrosis (bees and wasps); urticarial response (mosquitoes, fleas, and bedbugs), lymphomatoid/granulomatous response

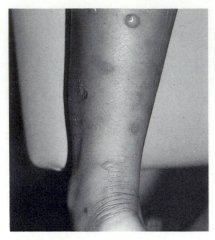

18-3-1 INSECT BITES: Bullous eruption secondary to flea bites. Looks very much like impetigo.

(ticks and the latter stages of bee and wasp bites). In the acute necrotic response bees and wasps produce the most superficial effect with focal areas of epidermal and superficial dermal necrosis. The ensuing inflammatory response is mixed with lymphocytes, histiocytes, and neutrophils seen early. As the reaction progresses eosinophils are seen in the inflammatory response and become the hallmark of bite reactions (Figure 18-3-2). In reactions secondary to arthropods, especially ticks, the reaction often shows a cellular infiltrate with many eosinophils and pseudogerminal follicles (Figure 18-3-3).

Flea and bedbug bites show a perivascular inflammatory infiltrate with lymphocytes and histiocytes. Eosinophils are found in a perivascular location as well as interstitially. The epidermis may show focal necrosis, parakeratosis, spongiosis, and exocytosis.

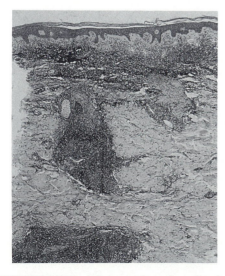

18-3-2 INSECT BITES: A dense perivascular collections of inflammatory cells, extending into the deep dermis. (40×)

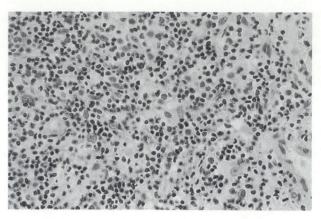

18-3-3 INSECT BITES: A higher magnification of Figure 18-3-2 showing a mixed infiltrate of lymphocytes, histiocytes and eosinophiles. (100×)

Differential Diagnosis
Urticaria
Drug eruption

18-4 COELENTERATES

CLINICAL DESCRIPTION

Itching and burning after a saltwater swim may indicate contact with a coelenterate, such as a Portuguese man-of-war or a jellyfish.

Etiology and Incidence
These marine creatures are found in tropical and subtropical waters. There are more than 9,000 different species, but only 100 of these produce skin changes in humans. These organisms have nematocysts, concentrated on their tentacles. Nematocysts contain a spirally coiled barb, which when fired introduce a toxin into the skin. Histamine, histamine-releasing agent, or serotonin is contained in the toxin.

Clinical Features
The venom produces a linear papular eruption accompanied by erythema and edema (Figure 18-4-1). Anaphylactic reactions may occur, as well as hemolysis and acute renal failure. The venom also contains neurotoxins and cardiotoxins.

Differential Diagnosis
Contact dermatitis

HISTOLOGICAL DESCRIPTION

Jellyfish stings produce urticarial responses with dermal edema, vascular dilatation, and an early infiltrate of lymphocytes and eosinophils. Portuguese man-of-war stings vary in

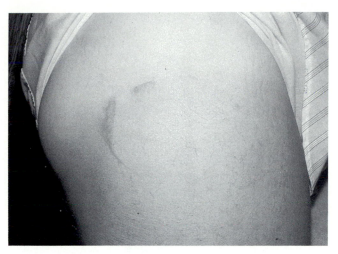

18-4-1 COELENTERATES: Jellyfish sting on a patient who was waterskiing. Note linear distribution.

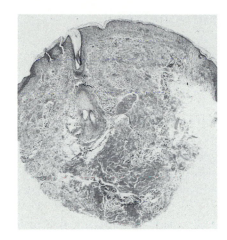

18-5-1 PAPULAR URTICARIA: Low-power view of papular urticaria. There is a modest perivascular infiltrate and perivascular edema. (20×)

response depending on the duration of contact with the tentacles (nematocysts) and the amount and duration of exposure to the toxin. Early biopsies of this condition can show the nematocyst within the stratum corneum. The dermis shows engorged, dilated blood vessels with discrete areas of hemorrhage. Later biopsies may show epidermal and dermal necrosis, and hemorrhage with a mixed inflammatory response consisting of lymphocytes, histiocytes, eosinophils, and neutrophils. Limited brief and minimal exposure will produce a urticarial response.

Differential Diagnosis
Urticaria
Burn

18-5 PAPULAR URTICARIA

CLINICAL DESCRIPTION
This clinical condition occurs following significant sensitization to a number of biting insects.

Etiology and Incidence
Papular urticaria is due to hypersensitivity to bites of fleas, gnats, mosquitoes, and bedbugs. Bedbugs probably cause more than 75% of cases in adults. In children, fleas and mosquitoes are the major offenders. Following sensitization, previous bite sites may flare.

Clinical Features
Any of the patterns produced by insect bites described in this chapter may occur.

Differential Diagnosis
Urticaria

HISTOLOGICAL DESCRIPTION
The histological features are not specific, with findings varying from subacute to chronic inflammation. In the more acute phase there is spongiosis with exocytosis. The inflammatory infiltrate consists of lymphocytes, histiocytes, and eosinophils (Figures 18-5-1 and 18-5-2). Later stages show less epidermal reaction, but the dermal infiltrate remains.

Differential Diagnosis
Drug eruption
Atopic dermatitis

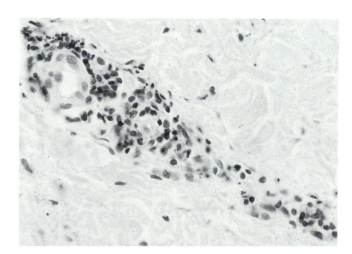

18-5-2 PAPULAR URTICARIA: Higher magnification shows a lymphocytic infiltrate admixed with scant eosinophils. (200×)

18-6 PEDICULOSIS

CLINICAL DESCRIPTION

There are three forms of lice that infest humans: head lice, body lice, and pubic lice.

Etiology and Incidence

The incidence of pediculosis, especially pediculosis capitis, is gradually increasing in the United States. The female louse can lay eggs at a rate of eight to twelve per day, producing large populations of lice within three to four months. Eggs (nits) are glued to hairs or fibers of clothing. Once hatched, the lice depend on blood meals for survival and, therefore, cannot exist for more than a few days away from humans. During feedings the toxins contained in the saliva produce small red or purpuric spots on the skin. Repeated bites induce sensitization and the formation of papules and wheals.

Head Lice

This is the major louse infestation that involves children. Children are more susceptible than adults, and females are more susceptible than males. Blacks are rarely infested. Infestation follows direct contact with an affected individual or indirectly via the hat, brush, or comb of an infested individual. The duration of infestation may be estimated by the distance of the nit on the hair shaft from the scalp surface: hair growth averages 0.35 mm per day.

Body Lice

Body lice live in clothing or bedding and are found on the body only when feeding. This is a rare infestation in children.

Pubic Lice

Transmission of pubic lice is usually venereal in adolescents and by close contact with infested adults in preadolescents.

Clinical Features

Head Lice

Secondary excoriations, usually behind the ears or on the occiput, and infection with cervical lymphadenopathy frequently occur from vigorous scratching.

Body Lice

Pressure points beneath the collar, belt, and underwear are the usual sites of bite marks. Frequently primary lesions are obliterated by scratching.

Pubic Lice

Pubic lice infest the hairs and skin of the genital area, lower abdomen, thighs, and, occasionally, axillae (Figure 18-6-1). Preadolescents may have organisms in their eyelashes, eye-

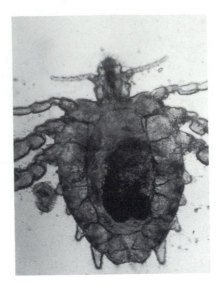

18-6-1 PUBICLOSIS: Phthirius pubis (crab louse). (20×)

brows, and scalp lines. Excoriations are frequently present. With severe infestations maculae cerulea (blue macules) can be seen on the thighs, abdomen, or thorax.

Differential Diagnosis

Seborrheic dermatitis
Atopic dermatitis
Blepharitis
Impetigo
Dandruff

HISTOLOGICAL DESCRIPTION

The histological features of pediculosis are not specific. There may be an eczematous reaction that shows the changes of an acute to subacute inflammatory response with spongiosis and exocytosis. Eosinophilia in the infiltrate is variable.

Differential Diagnosis

Acute and subacute dermatoses
Atopic dermatitis

18-7 SCABIES

CLINICAL DESCRIPTION

One of the more difficult entities to diagnose is the dermatitis caused by the mite *Sarcoptes scabiei.*

Etiology and Incidence

Fertile females burrow into the stratum corneum, laying several eggs per day during a one to two month life span. Within two weeks the ova become adults. Pruritus occurs one month after infestation, indicating sensitization to the mite protein. *Sarcoptes scabiei* completes its life cycle in humans and may, therefore, persist indefinitely.

Mites cannot live off the human host for more than twenty-four to forty-eight hours. The viability of ova is one to two weeks. Transmission of the mite requires close contact. An incidental handshake is unlikely to spread the mite, as are fomites. Family members and caretakers often have skin lesions and pruritus.

Epidemics occur in thirty year cycles, each lasting fifteen years with a fifteen year gap before the next. Cases continue to occur during this gap, but not at a significant rate.

Clinical Features

Despite diffuse involvement, these lesions are concentrated on the skin of the hands and feet (including the palms and soles in infants and young children) and in the folds of the body (axillae, groin, and especially the fingerwebs). Infants, in contrast to adolescents and adults, frequently have involvement of the skin of their face and head.

Skin lesions consist of papules, pustules, vesicles (especially in infants), and nodules. Burrows occur in 10% of patients and are frequently distorted by vigorous scratching and eczematization. Persistent erythematous or reddish brown nodules (Plate 18-7-1) may develop. Norwegian scabies is seen in institutionalized, retarded, or immunologically deficient individuals. This form of scabies produces thick, crusted lesions teeming with mites.

Differential Diagnosis

Atopic eczema
Contact dermatitis
Seborrheic dermatitis
Papular urticaria

HISTOLOGICAL DESCRIPTION

Scabies can show several histological features, depending on the lesion biopsied. Papular lesions reveal a dense infiltrate in the dermis that consists of lymphocytes, histiocytes, and many eosinophils. The infiltrate extends into the lower dermis in a nodular fashion about blood vessels and eccrine glands. Eosinophils are seen in the infiltrate. The epidermis may show focal spongiosis and parakeratosis. If the leading edge of the burrow is biopsied, the organism may be seen at the stratum corneum-epidermal junction (Figure 18-7-1). In this space may be seen the female mite with eggs or only eggs or feces (scybala). The mite is seen in cross section with the internal parts covered by a refractile chitinous skeleton, which stains distinctly positive with periodic acid-Schiff technique. The inflammatory response in the dermis is the same as that seen in the papular lesion.

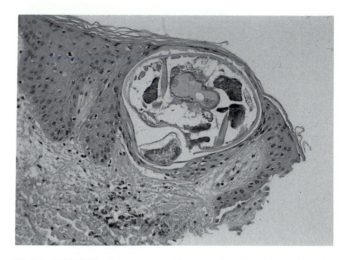

18-7-1 SCABIES: Subcorneal collection of scabies mites. (40×)

Differential Diagnosis
Creeping eruption

18-8 SPIDER BITES

CLINICAL DESCRIPTION

Brown recluse and black widow spiders cause most spider bites in the United States. It is the bite of the brown recluse that produces significant skin disease.

Etiology and Incidence

The brown recluse spider (*Loxosceles reclusus*) is indigenous to the Mississippi and Ohio River valleys but has been reported increasingly in other parts of the United States. The spider measures 8 to 10 mm long. A violin-shaped band is present over the dorsal cephalothorax. The spider introduces a venom containing necrotizing, hemolytic, and spreading factors with its bite.

Clinical Features

Any body part can be involved, but the distal extremities are most often affected. Several hours after the bite, a painful hemorrhagic blister forms. This is followed by necrosis and the formation of a gangrenous eschar. An ulcer can form, which continues to enlarge and takes many months to heal. Cutaneous reactions in addition to the local changes secondary to the bite include a maculopapular or scarlatiniform petechial eruption. Systemic symptoms may include nausea, vomiting, chills, myalgia, shock, and coma. Thrombocytopenia, hemolysis, and hemoglobinemia have been described. The hemoglobinuria may lead to renal failure.

Differential Diagnosis
Any condition producing necrosis

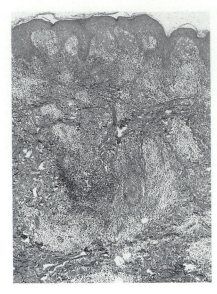

18-8-1 SPIDER BITES: Low magnification showing prominent papillary dermal edema and a brisk lympho-histiocytic infiltrate in the reticular dermis. Centrally there is a large collection of neutrophils. (40×)

HISTOLOGICAL DESCRIPTION

The bite of the brown recluse spider produces a significant skin reaction. The early reaction is epidermal and dermal necrosis, which may extend to the dermal subcutaneous junction. The adjacent papillary dermis is markedly edematous and there is an inflammatory infiltrate of neutrophils and lymphocytes (Figure 18-8-1). Dermal vessels show necrosis with fibrinoid. Necrosis can be seen in the dermis (Figure 18-8-2). Adjacent to the necrotic area, subepidermal blisters may develop secondary to epidermal necrosis and dermal epidermal separation. This intense reaction may extend to the subcutaneous tissue and produce panniculitis, which may be lobular as well as septal (Figure 18-8-3). As this process evolves, eosinophils can be seen in the inflammatory infiltrate. The panniculitis heals with fibrosis and scarring.

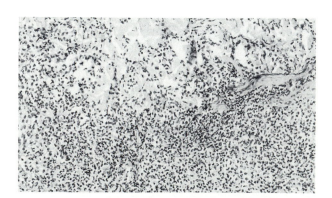

18-8-2 SPIDER BITES: A large collection of neutrophils surrounds partially necrotic collagen bundles. (100×)

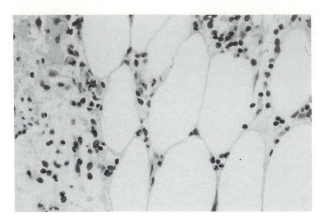

18-8-3 SPIDER BITES: The inflammation in a spider bite extends into the adipose tissue. Hemorrhage is also present. (200×)

Differential Diagnosis

Burn
Electrical injury
Vasculitis

18-9 TICK BITES (ERYTHEMA CHRONICUM MIGRANS)

Erythema chronicum migrans is a characteristic skin finding heralding Lyme disease.

CLINICAL DESCRIPTION

Etiology and Incidence

Erythema chronicum migrans which develops in 60% of patients is produced following a tick bite (e.g., *Ixodes scapularis* formerly known as Ixodes dammini on the east coast and Ixodes pacificus in the west) that introduces the spirochete *Borrelia burgdorferi*. Thirty percent of patients report having been bitten by a tick. The infection has been seen in forty-eight states in the United States and in many other countries. Indigenous areas in the United States include the northeast (from Massachusetts to Virginia) Wisconsin and Minnesota, northern California and Oregon. These areas account for more than 90% of the reported cases. The incidence in these areas is 0.15 to 4.4 cases per 1,000 population.

Clinical Features

Erythema chronicum migrans which frequently appears 8 to 9 days (range 2 to 28 days) after the tick bite usually occurs on a proximal extremity or the trunk. The lesion begins as a red macule or papule that gradually expands to various sized rings with a mean diameter of 15 cm (at times concentric) with clear centers (Figure 18-9-1). One-half of the patients have multiple secondary skin lesions usually smaller than the

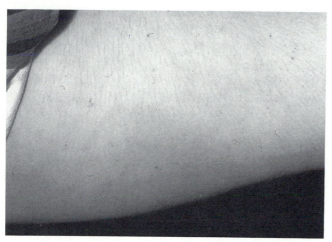

18-9-1 TICK BITES: This patient has a history of a tick bite and developed a ring of erythema (erythema migrans). Little central clearing has occurred.

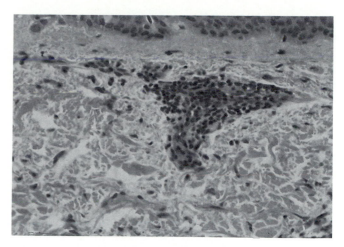

18-9-3 TICK BITES: A higher magnification shows lymphocytes and plasma cells about dermal vessels. (100×)

initial lesion. Scaling is not prominent. The rash gradually resolves over three weeks, but evanescent flares with arthritis can occur later. One half of patients have fever, malaise, chills, headache and stiff neck. Erythema chronicum migrans may herald the later manifestations of Lyme disease: arthritis (weeks to months after onset of the rash); neurologic complications, including aseptic meningitis, Bell's palsy, and neuritis (at any time); and cardiac abnormalities (weeks to months after introduction of the spirochete).

Differential Diagnosis
Cellulitis
Erythema marginatum
Erythema multiforme

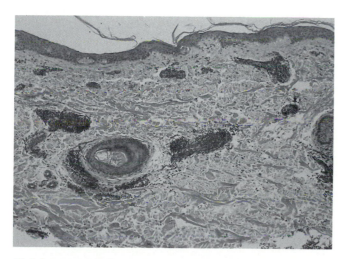

18-9-2 TICK BITES: Tightly cuffed perivascular lymphocytic and plasma cell infiltrate as seen in erythema chronicum migrans. (40×)

HISTOLOGICAL DESCRIPTION

Reactions on the skin secondary to tick bites are erythema chronicum migrans and persistent papular nodules. The distinctive histological feature in erythema chronicum migrans is a striking sheathing of dermal vessels by lymphocytes (Figures 18-9-2 and 18-9-3). The epidermis is essentially unaffected and there may be dermal edema. Eosinophilia is uncommon.

Tick bites also produce persistent lymphoid granulomatous reactions. In acute reactions there is papillary dermal edema, spongiosis, and exocytosis. In some instances tick parts can be seen in the dermis as a yellow-brown homogenous material with surrounding mixed inflammation (lymphocytes, neutrophils, histiocytes, foreign body giant cells, and eosinophils). The tick parts are doubly refractile and can be viewed with polarized light. The epidermis at this point may be ulcerated or acanthotic.

In chronic reactions, dense dermal nodules of inflammation may extend from the papillary dermis to the dermal subcutaneous junction. These nodules consist of aggregates of lymphocytes, histiocytes, and eosinophils. Eosinophils are also seen in the interstitial dermis. Some of the inflammatory nodules may be organized into pseudolymphoid follicles.

Differential Diagnosis
Lymphocytic infiltration of the skin
Cutaneous lymphoma

REFERENCES

Swimmer's Itch
Kirschenbaum MB: Swimmer's itch: a review and case report. Cutis 1979;23:212.

Cutaneous Larva Migrans

Katz R, Ziegler J, Blank H: The natural course of creeping eruption and treatment with thiabendazole. Arch Dermatol 1965;91:420.

Sulica VJ, Berberian B, Ko GF: Histopathologic findings in cutaneous larva migrans (ABSTR). J Cutan Pathol 1988;15:346.

Insect Bites

Burnett JW, Calton GJ, Morgan RJ: Bedbugs. Cutis 1985;40:20.

DeShazo RD, Butcher BT, Banks WA: Reactions to the stings of the imported fire ant. N Engl J Med 1990;7:462.

Honig PJ: Arthropod bites, stings, infestations: Their prevention and treatment. Pediatr Dermatol 1986;3:189.

Coelenterates

Bengston K, Nicholas MM, Schradig V, et al.: Sudden death in a child following envenomation by chiropsalmus quadrumicenus. JAMA 1991;266:1404.

Gruess HA, Soniteer PL, Morris CR: Hemolysis and renal failure following a Portuguese man-of-war sting. Pediatrics 1982;70:979.

Ioannides G, Davis JH: Portuguese man of war stinging. Arch Dermatol 1965;91:448.

Papular Urticaria

Heng MCY, Kloss SG, Haberfelde GC: Pathogenesis of papular urticaria. J Am Acad Dermatol 1989;10:1030.

Shaffer B, Jacobsen C, Berman H: Histopathologic correlation of the lesions of papular urticaria and positive skin test reaction to insect antigens. Arch Dermatol 1954;74:437.

Pediculosis

Rasmussen JE: Pediculosis and the pediatrician. Pediatr Dermatol 1984;2:74.

Scabies

Fernandez N, Torres A, Ackerman AB: Pathological findings in human scabies. Arch Dermatol 1977;113:320.

Honig PJ: Arthropod bites, stings, infestations: Their prevention and treatment. Pediatr Dermatol 1986;3:189.

Spiders

Pucevich MV, Chesney TM: Histopathologic analysis of human bites by the brown recluse spider. Arch Dermatol 1983;119:851.

Russell FE: A confusion of spiders. Emerg Med 1986;18:8.

Tick Bites

Abek DC, Anders KH: The many faces and phases of borreliosis I Lyme disease. J Am Acad Dermatol 1990;73:117.

Shapiro ED, Gerber MA, Holabird NB, et al.: A controlled trial of antimicrobial prophylaxis for Lyme disease after deer-tick bites. N Engl J Med 1992;327:1769.

Spach DH, Liles WC, Campbell LL, et al.: Tick-borne diseases in the United States. NEJM 1993;329:936.

Tobias N: Tick bite granuloma. J Invest Dermatol 1949;12:255.

19

Lymphoproliferative Disorders

Contents

19-1 ACQUIRED IMMUNODEFICIENCY SYNDROME

CLINICAL DESCRIPTION

Acquired immunodeficiency syndrome (AIDS) is a retrovirus-associated disease. Although most often reported in adults, it has been recognized in children since 1982.

Etiology and Incidence

Acquired immunodeficiency syndrome is caused by human T cell lymphotropic virus type III, also known as human immunodeficiency virus (HIV), a small RNA virus with the capability of replicating in its human host using the enzyme reverse transcriptase. The enzyme permits transcription of RNA into proviral DNA, which is then incorporated into the host's DNA. The result of viral infection is impaired immunity. This manifests as increased susceptibility to opportunistic infections and rare cancers.

Most children with AIDS acquire it through transplacental passage of the virus from HIV-infected mothers (83%). The remainder have received blood products contaminated with the virus (10%) or are hemophiliacs who were infected during therapy (5%).

Clinical Features

The papular or papulosquamous eruption of seroconversion with HIV infection has not been described in children as it has been in adults. This may be due to acquisition of the infection in utero in most cases as well as the prevalence of assorted viral exanthems in children, which are not traced as to cause.

The most frequent type of skin involvement is related to infectious etiologies and correlates with the degree of impairment of immunity. In particular, severity of infection can be related to counts of T helper lymphocytes. When T4 cell counts fall below 200 per mm^3 patients experience severe infections, often with multiple agents, and respond poorly to conventional therapies.

In particular, infections with bacteria (folliculitis, cellulitis, furuncles), fungi (mucocutaneous candidiasis, tinea corporis, tinea capitis), deep fungi (histoplasmosis, cryptococcosis, sporotrichosis), viruses (herpes simplex, herpes zoster, warts, molluscum contagiosum), and parasites (scabies) have all been reported in children. Of note, the incidence of persistent mucocutaneous candidiasis increases with increasing impairment of immunity. Another mucosal process, oral hairy leukoplakia, harbors Epstein-Barr virus in verrucous-appearing oral plaques, but is rare in children.

Various inflammatory disorders may present de novo or be exacerbated with HIV infection. These include atopic and seborrheic dermatitis, psoriasis, vasculitis, and nutritional disorders. Acquired ichthyosis has been reported as well. Drug eruptions are common, especially to trimethoprim-sulfamethoxazole, and may evolve into toxic epidermal necrolysis.

Kaposi's sarcoma, a common neoplastic disorder in adult patients, is rare in children and may be confined to lymph nodes. Assorted other findings range from hypertrichosis of the eyelashes and alopecia to eruptive dysplastic nevi.

A constellation of clinical findings indicative of immunosuppression suggests the possibility of AIDS. Serologic studies for antibodies to HIV antigens allow separation of AIDS from other possible causes of immunosuppression in children.

Differential Diagnosis

Severe combined immunodeficiency
Congenital thymic aplasia
Thymic hypoplasia
Wiskott-Aldrich syndrome
Chronic candidiasis with or without endocrinopathy

HISTOLOGICAL DESCRIPTION

No single finding on skin biopsy is diagnostic of AIDS. Rather, the histological features reflect the diminished resistance to infectious diseases and aberrant proliferative states. Occasionally, more than one process can be seen in the same biopsy specimen, therefore increased vigilance is necessary in cases of suspected AIDS.

With infectious diseases, each invading organism retains its usual morphological features in tissue sections, but may be present in larger numbers than in non-HIV-infected hosts. Thus, scabetic, fungal, or mycobacterial organisms are found in the usual locations in sections but are more easily detectable in routine or specially stained sections. Viral changes are often pronounced: large numbers of eosinophilic brick-shaped inclusions are seen in keratinocytes with molluscum contagiosum infection. Organisms of *Cryptococcus neoformans* can be seen in dermal stroma within or outside of histiocytes, surrounded by a small number of lymphocytes. The inflammatory response to invading organisms reflects the host's capability to fight infection.

Inflammatory disorders, such as seborrheic and atopic dermatitis, appear in sections similar to their non-AIDS-related counterparts. They are discussed in Chapter 14.

Two lesions seen in association with AIDS not discussed elsewhere in this text are oral hairy leukoplakia and Kaposi's sarcoma. The verrucous plaques of oral hairy leukoplakia histologically show a ridged, markedly hyperparakeratotic surface within which *Candida* organisms usually proliferate. The superficial layers of mucosal epithelium show ballooning degeneration and perinuclear halo formation (koilocytosis). Nuclei of keratinocytes show basophilia and peripheral displacement of chromatin. In aggregate, these changes indicate viral cytopathic effects. Immunohistochemical stains for human papilloma virus are frequently positive, and Epstein-Barr virus antigens can be detected as well.

Kaposi's sarcoma in its early phases appears as a subtle proliferation of spindle-shaped cells that use preexisting dermal structures as a scaffolding. There is a hint of increased cellularity to the dermal stroma, and rare erythrocytes can be seen outside of endothelial spaces. As lesions progress from patches to plaques and then nodules, spindle cells progressively replace the collagenous dermal stroma (Plate 19-1-1). The spindle cells show mild cellular pleomorphism and occasional mitotic figures. Erythrocytes are situated among these cells and appear to lie in slitlike spaces. Hemosiderin and eosinophilic droplets indicate breakdown of erythrocytes within this stroma. At the periphery, lymphocytes and plasma cells are seen.

Differential Diagnosis
See individual disorders

19-2 GRAFT VERSUS HOST DISEASE

CLINICAL DESCRIPTION

This disorder occurs when lymphocytes in a donor graft recognize the host, or recipient of the graft, as being immunologically foreign and produce a destructive inflammatory response.

Etiology and Incidence
Graft versus host disease occurs in a host with a congenital, radiation-induced, or chemotherapy-induced immunologic deficit who receives a graft in which donor lymphocytes recognize it (the host or graft recipient) as being "nonself." This process is thought to be mediated by cytotoxic T lymphocytes. Target organs in this disorder are the liver, gastrointestinal tract, and skin. It occurs in 30% to 70% of patients receiving allogeneic bone marrow transplants and in 20% to 50% of marrow transplants from siblings who are HLA-identical.

Clinical Features
Graft versus host disease may be acute or chronic. The acute type occurs within one to two weeks of transplantation but not later than 100 days. This variety most often occurs in patients who differ at the HLA-D locus from the donor blood or bone marrow. Characteristic early signs of acute graft versus host disease include pruritus, discomfort with pressure of palms and soles, and erythema of the pinnae of the ears and the nailfolds. The intensity of disease is graded according to the degree of organ involvement: grade 1 (mild) shows a maculopapular eruption involving less than 50% of the body,

serum bilirubin of 2 to 3 mg/dl, no diarrhea or change in physical activity; grade 4 (severe) shows erythroderma with blistering and desquamation that mimics toxic epidermal necrolysis, bilirubin levels in excess of 15 mg/dl, diarrhea of 1.5 l or more per day, fever, toxicity, and decreased activity.

Chronic graft versus host disease occurs 100 days to two years after transplantation with or without antecedent acute disease. It takes the form of either a lichenoid process reminiscent of lichen planus or a sclerodermoid process in which there is localized or diffuse hardening and thickening of the skin. The lichenoid form preferentially affects the distal extremities, palms, and soles. The sclerodermoid form is associated with contractures, variable hyper- and hypopigmentation, and hair loss (Plate 19-2-1). The prognosis varies with the intensity and extent of involvement.

Differential Diagnosis
Acute

Drug reaction

Infection

Toxic epidermal necrolysis

Chronic

Lichen planus

Scleroderma

Sjögren's syndrome

Eosinophilic fasciitis

Systemic lupus erythematosus

HISTOLOGICAL DESCRIPTION

Acute graft versus host disease is characterized by a sparse mononuclear infiltrate that approximates the dermal-epidermal and dermal-follicular interfaces, causing vacuolar alterations of basilar keratinocytes. In addition, inflammatory cells are present in the epithelium surrounding individual keratinocytes, causing cell death. The latter finding has been called satellite necrosis (Figure 19-2-1) and is commonly (but not exclusively) seen in graft versus host disease. As the process intensifies (grades 3 to 4), subepidermal separation and blistering may occur.

Chronic lichenoid graft versus host disease shows epidermal changes reminiscent of lichen planus: hyperorthokeratosis, hypergranulosis, acanthosis, vacuolar changes of the basilar layer, and mild sawtoothing of the dermal-epidermal junction. The dermis contains a sparse perivascular and interstitial infiltrate of mononuclear cells (lymphocytes, macrophages, and plasma cells). The sparsity of inflammation distinguishes lichenoid graft versus host disease from classical lichen planus.

Chronic sclerodermoid graft versus host disease is histologically similar to morphea and scleroderma (Figure 19-2-2): there is thickening and decreased cellularity of reticular

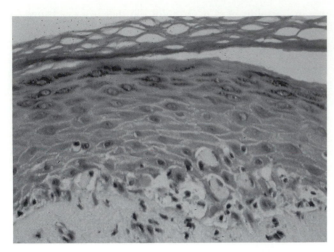

19-2-1 LICHENOID GRAFT VERSUS HOST DISEASE:
Effacement of the rete ridge pattern and necrosis of individual
keratinocytes. The amorphous eosinophilic keratinocytes are
focally approximated by lymphocytes ("satellite necrosis"). (200×)

dermal collagen bundles, blurring of the papillary and reticular dermal-stromal interface, and trapping and atrophy of eccrine coils and hair follicles within the dense stroma. As the
process proceeds, there is loss of eccrine glands and hair follicles. The overlying epidermis is variably atrophic or acanthotic, has a thickened granular layer, and is surmounted by
compact hyperkeratotic scale. A sparse mononuclear infiltrate
accompanies these changes but is not present at the depths of
the dermis where it joins the panniculus, as is characteristically seen in morphea and scleroderma.

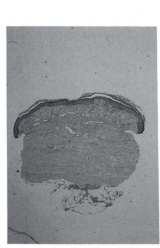
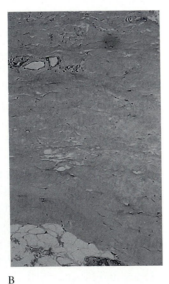

A   B

19-2-2 SCLERODERMOID GRAFT VERSUS HOST DISEASE:
Low-power view of a "squared-off" punch biopsy shows dermal
fibrosis and loss of appendages. (40×) (B) Sclerotic eosinophilic
collagen bundles impinging on the panniculus. Note the absence
of appendages. (200×)

Differential Diagnosis
Acute
Drug reactions
Lupus erythematosus
Dermatomyositis
Chemotherapy-induced drug reaction

Chronic
Lichen planus
Scleroderma
Morphea

19-3 LYMPHOCYTOMA CUTIS

CLINICAL DESCRIPTION

Lymphocytoma cutis represents a spectrum of cutaneous lesions that clinically and histologically can mimic malignant
lymphoma. These lesions have also been described as pseudo-
lymphoma, lymphadenosis benigna cutis, and cutaneous lymphoid hyperplasia.

Etiology and Incidence
In many instances the cause of lymphocytoma cutis has been
traced to antigens such as drugs, spirochetes, and insect bites.
The cause in many other instances remains unknown.

Clinical Features
Lymphocytoma cutis presents as solitary or multiple, deeply
erythematous to violaceous papules, plaques, or nodules
(Plate 19-3-1) with smooth, nonulcerated surfaces. They occur most often on the head and neck but may involve the
trunk and extremities as well. Since lesions can persist on the
skin for variably long periods of time, they often come to the
attention of parents and pediatricians. Such lesions tend to
involute spontaneously, but some may recur. In instances
where lesions progressively enlarge over time or fail to respond to conservative therapy, it is important to rule out the
possibility of cutaneous lymphoma with routine histological
study and cell marker analysis.

Differential Diagnosis
Pyogenic granuloma
Spitz nevus
Lymphoma cutis

HISTOLOGICAL DESCRIPTION

The unifying feature of the various lesions of lymphocytoma
cutis is a dense mononuclear infiltrate. The architecture and
composition is variable. At times the intensity of such infiltrates is alarming, and the pattern of permeation of the stroma

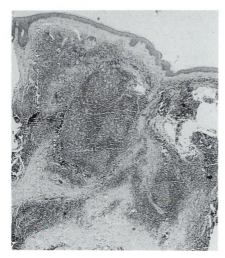

19-3-1 LYMPHOCYTOMA CUTIS: Nodular aggregates of mononuclear cells within the dermis. The infiltrate is more pronounced in the upper reticular dermis. (20×)

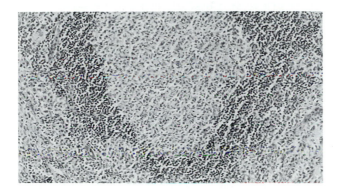

19-3-2 LYMPHOCYTOMA CUTIS: Germinal centerlike areas. The central pale-staining areas contain B lymphocytes; the mantles surrounding them are composed of T lymphocytes. (40×)

may simulate lymphoma. In general, infiltrates concentrated in the upper dermis (Figure 19-3-1) that respect preexisting appendageal structures tend to behave in a benign fashion. By contrast, those concentrated in the lower dermis (bottom-heavy infiltrates) that infiltrate and/or destroy preexisting adnexal structures behave in a malignant fashion.

Since pattern alone may be insufficient to separate such lesions, immunohistochemical markers are often employed to analyze cell populations present in these processes. Polymorphous rather than monomorphous composition and expression of normal phenotypes are in keeping with benign reactive infiltrates. Several patterns of lymphocytoma have been discerned based on immunohistochemical studies: (1) a dense superficial lymphocytic infiltrate with a band-like configuration composed of T lymphocytes; (2) a dense superficial and middermal T lymphocytic infiltrate arranged in nodules; and (3) dermal nodules composed of clusters of B lymphocytes surrounded by cuffs of T lymphocytes (Figures 19-3-1 to 19-3-6) with or without a dendritic cell component. In the latter instance, when dendritic cells are present, the pattern mimics germinal centers such as those seen in lymph nodes. Occasionally a small population of aberrant lymphocytes may be obscured by a bulky reactive infiltrate. In such cases, if suspicion of malignancy exists, gene rearrangement studies may discern a malignant population within the infiltrate.

Differential Diagnosis
Lymphoma cutis
Persistent insect bite

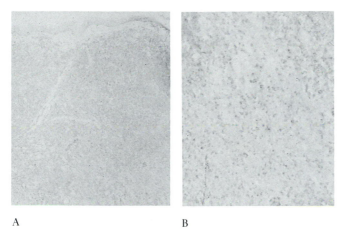

A   B

19-3-3 LYMPHOCYTOMA CUTIS: Immunohistochemical staining pattern with CD5 (left panel; 20×) and CD3 (right panel; 100×). Most cells display pan-T cell maturation markers on their surfaces. Note circumscribed central zones where reactivity is not noted (see Figure 19-3-5 for reactivity of these cells).

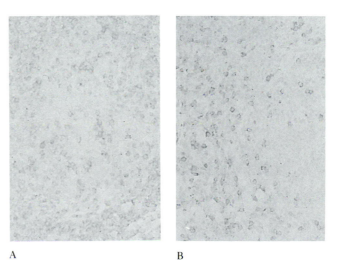

A   B

19-3-4 LYMPHOCYTOMA CUTIS: The cells marking in Figure 19-3-2 show a CD4 (left panel, helper cell; 200×) to CD8 (right panel, suppressor cell; 200×) ratio of 3:1.

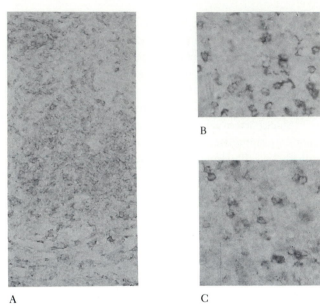

A   C

19-3-5 LYMPHOCYTOMA CUTIS: The lucent areas seen in Figure 19-3-3 react with B cell marker CD 19 (A; 200×). Both kappa- (B; 400×) and lambda- (C; 400×) producing B cells are present in these areas.

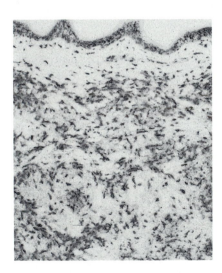

19-3-6 LYMPHOCYTOMA CUTIS: Dendritic cells (CD1) are seen in the dermis, in areas surrounding B cell areas. These features recapitulate the architectural organization of germinal centers in lymphoid tissue. (100×)

19-4 LYMPHOMATOID PAPULOSIS

CLINICAL DESCRIPTION

This disorder has some features in common with pityriasis lichenoides et varioliformis acute (PLEVA), and therefore must be distinguished from it.

Etiology and Incidence

The etiology of this disorder is unknown. It has rarely been reported in children; it is more common in the adult population.

Clinical Features

Lymphomatoid papulosis is characterized by recurrent crops of eruptive papules (Figure 19-4-1) or, occasionally nodules, which may initially appear vesicular. The smaller lesions become hemorrhagic and acquire a crust before involuting, while the larger ones become ulcerated and necrotic before resolving. Scarring may follow involution.

Although rare, cases of lymphomatoid papulosis have been associated with lymphoreticular malignancies, including Hodgkin's disease and cutaneous T cell lymphoma. Therefore, long-term follow-up study of patients is important.

Differential Diagnosis

Insect bite
Pityriasis lichenoides et varioliformis acuta (PLEVA)
Eruptive keratoacanthoma (nodular lesion)
Cutaneous lymphoma

HISTOLOGICAL DESCRIPTION

The histological feature of lymphomatoid papulosis, similar to that of PLEVA and insect bite reactions, is a wedge-shaped dermal inflammatory infiltrate (Figure 19-4-2). The broad base of the wedge extends along the dermal-epidermal interface and the apex extends into the reticular dermis. The infiltrate is composed of mononuclear cells in a perivascular distribution in the deep dermis and interstitial distribution in the superficial dermis. These cells infiltrate the epidermis along with extravasated erythrocytes. The epidermis can be spongiotic and show zones of necrosis. The key histological feature is the presence of large atypical mononuclear cells with prominent nucleoli (Figure 19-4-3; Plate 19-4-1). Occasional cells may be binucleate, reminiscent of Reed-Sternberg cells as seen in Hodgkin's disease. Mitotic activity of mononuclear cells may be present as well. Immunohistochemical markers show positive staining of the large atypical cells with

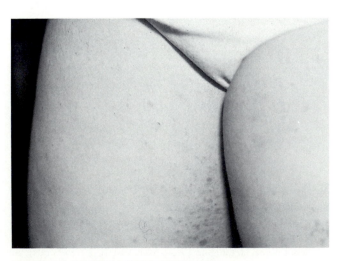

19-4-1 LYMPHOMATOID PAPULOSIS

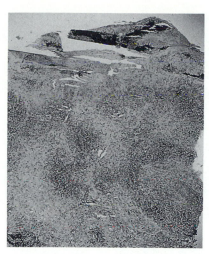

19-4-2 LYMPHOMATOID PAPULOSIS: Low-power view of an ulcerated lesion with a roughly wedge-shaped architecture. (20×)

CD 30 or Ki-1, the Reed-Sternberg-associated antigen, as well as TAC, the interleukin-2 receptor (Plate 19-4-1).

Lack of eosinophils in the infiltrate allows separation of these lesions from insect bite reactions, while the presence of atypical mononuclear cells permits separation of lymphomatoid papulosis from PLEVA. There may be some overlap of lymphomatoid papulosis, especially the large ulceronodular variant, with regressing atypical histiocytiosis. Both entities have been found to have gene rearrangements in the infiltrating cell populations and occasionally protracted clinical courses. Clinicopathologic correlation may be necessary to separate such cases.

Differential Diagnosis
Insect bite
Pityriasis lichenoides et varioliformis acuta (PLEVA)
Regressing atypical histiocytosis

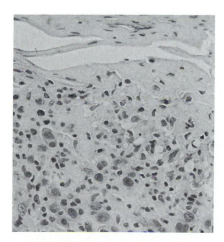

19-4-3 LYMPHOMATOID PAPULOSIS: The mononuclear cell component of this infiltrate has large hyperchromatic nuclei, nuclear pleomorphism, and occasional binucleation. (400×)

19-5 LANGERHANS' CELL HISTIOCYTOSIS (HISTIOCYTOSIS X)

CLINICAL DESCRIPTION
This term is given to a group of proliferative disorders of Langerhans' cell origin. It includes Hand-Schüller-Christian disease, Letterer-Siwe disease, and eosinophilic granuloma as well as many overlapping forms.

Etiology and Incidence
These disorders are caused by an abnormal proliferation of Langerhans' cells, which may affect one or multiple organs. The cause is as yet unknown. This group of diseases does not fulfill all the criteria of malignancy. Different presentations affect different age groups, as addressed below.

Clinical Features
Letterer-Siwe Disease
Of all these disorders, Letterer-Siwe is the most serious. It generally occurs in children younger than two years of age and is noted as a rash resembling seborrheic dermatitis. The scalp (Plate 19-5-1), face, ears, axillae, and inguinal and perianal regions are sites of involvement. Vesicular lesions in association with crusted papules may be found during the neonatal period. Later, the character of lesions is more variable: erythematous macules and papules blend with greasy-appearing, scaly, reddish brown or purpuric papules. The more typical skin changes consist of crops of scaling yellow-brown papules with a purpuric component. Ulcerations may occur in the mouth as well as the postauricular, inguinal, and perineal regions. Premature loss of deciduous teeth (by five years) as well as permanent teeth may occur due to erosion of the lamina dura. Involvement of the lungs may result in pulmonary failure.

If the process is limited to the skin the prognosis is good; if there is visceral involvement the prognosis is guarded. Occasionally, spontaneous remissions have been reported. Children with onset of disease before two years of age with visceral organ dysfunction have the poorest prognosis.

Hand-Schüller-Christian Disease
This disorder usually affects children between the ages of two and five years. The classic triad of skull defects, diabetes insipidus, and exophthalmos is rarely seen. Skin changes are seen in up to 50% of patients. Pulmonary involvement may occur in up to 30% of patients.

The distribution of lesions and skin changes are much the same as in Letterer-Siwe disease except the hemorrhagic component is generally absent and lesions are less destructive. Tumors of the mucosa may arise and ulcerate.

Eosinophilic Granuloma

This is a disorder of older children and adolescents characterized by solitary or multiple bony lesions. Symptoms are first noted between four and seven years of age. Skin lesions are rare; when present they are similar to those found in Letterer-Siwe or Hand-Schüller-Christian disease. Rarely, kindreds with Letterer-Siwe disease have been described.

Congenital Self-Healing Histiocytosis

This disorder, described by Hashimoto and Pritzker in 1973, presents as solitary or multiple firm, red-brown nodules with or without ulceration at birth or in early infancy. Such lesions may have a generalized distribution. They may increase in size and number for several weeks before they spontaneously involute over course of several weeks to months. This disorder is limited to the skin, thus associated systemic findings are rare.

Differential Diagnosis

Solitary Lesions

Reticulohistiocytoma
Juvenile xanthogranuloma
Mastocytoma

Multiple/Generalized Lesions

Atopic dermatitis
Seborrheic dermatitis
Bone cysts (other causes)
Nonhistiocytosis X disorders

HISTOLOGICAL DESCRIPTION

In general, in histiocytosis X there is infiltration of the dermis and epidermis by a population of monotonous-appearing cells with abundant eosinophilic cytoplasms and gently infolded nuclei. The cells may have nuclei with a central linear crease, an appearance likened to coffee beans. The cells display an affinity for stratified squamous epithelium (epidermis and adnexal epithelium), the normal location of Langerhans' cells (Figure 19-5-1). The infiltrate is often accompanied by eosinophils. If the infiltrate is intense, it may cause dermal-epidermal separation, which results in clinically perceptible bullous lesions.

In Letterer-Siwe disease Langerhans'-type cells fill an edematous papillary dermis and infiltrate the overlying spongiotic epidermis, where they may aggregate in nests. In Hand-Schüller-Christian disease the dermal infiltrate appears polymorphous: Langerhans'-type cells are accompanied by eosinophils, neutrophils, multinucleated histiocytes, plasma cells, and lymphocytes. Although the epidermis appears thinned and less spongiotic, exocytosis is present. In congenital self-healing histiocytosis the dermis contains an infiltrate composed of lymphocytes, eosinophils, and large histiocytes with single or multiple nuclei and "ground glass" eosinophilic

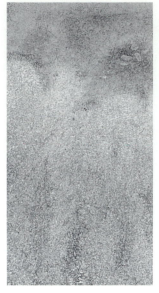 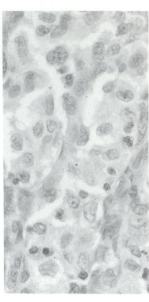

A   B

19-5-1 HISTIOCYTOSIS X: (top) An ulcerated nodule. (20×) (bottom) The dermis is permeated by a population of cells with abundant eosinophilic cytoplasms and gently infolded nuclei accompanied by large numbers of eosinophils. (400×) The affinity of these cells for epithelium is apparent as they infiltrate eccrine ductal epithelium.

cytoplasms. The infiltrate is usually localized to the reticular dermis but may occasionally involve the papillary dermis as well (Plate 19-5-2; Figure 19-5-2).

A presumptive diagnosis of Langerhans' cell histiocytosis can be made based on routine sections but should be confirmed by staining of paraffin sections with S-100 (Plate 19-5-2) or peanut agglutinin. If fresh frozen tissue is available,

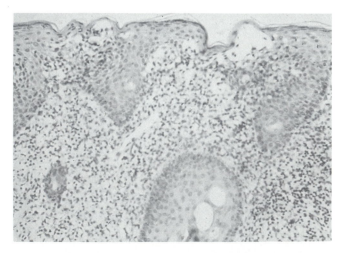

19-5-2 CONGENITAL SELF-HEALING HISTIOCYTOSIS: There is a brisk polymorphous infiltrate within the dermis. Nested mononuclear cells can be seen within the overlying epidermis. (40×)

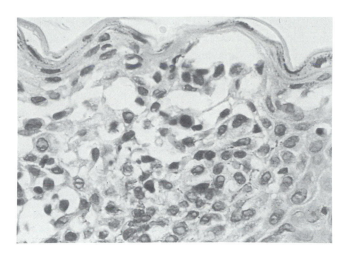

19-5-3 CONGENITAL SELF-HEALING HISTIOCYTOSIS: Mononuclear cells form variably sized nests within the epidermis. (200×)

confirmatory stains include ATPase and/or alpha-mannosidase. A definitive diagnosis can be made if infiltrating cells show CD1 positivity on frozen sections or contain intracytoplasmic rodlike inclusions with vesicular ends (Birbeck's granules) by electron microscopy (Plate 19-5-2). In congenital self-healing histiocytosis only a small percentage of cells show positivity with S-100 stains (Figure 19-5-4) and contain Birbeck's granules within their cytoplasms. The prognosis of this group of disorders cannot be gauged by histological study but is based on clinical presentation.

Differential Diagnosis

Mastocytosis
Juvenile xanthogranuloma
Reticulohistiocytoma
Cutaneous T cell lymphoma

19-6 NON-HISTIOCYTOSIS X DISORDERS

CLINICAL DESCRIPTION

Etiology and Incidence

Benign cephalic histiocytosis and malignant histiocytosis, two non-histiocytosis X disorders, are caused by an aberrant proliferation of cells of monocyte-macrophage lineage. These disorders are rare.

Clinical Features

Malignant Histiocytosis

This disorder is characterized by the proliferation of atypical histiocytes throughout the reticuloendothelial system. It is accompanied by systemic symptoms with or without cutaneous lesions. When skin involvement occurs it is characterized by hemorrhagic papules, plaques, or nodules. Lesions may be single or multiple and may have ulcerated surfaces.

Benign Cephalic Histiocytosis

Children affected by this disorder have single (Figure 19-6-1) or multiple round to oval red-brown papules, most often on the face, neck, and ears (thus the term *cephalic*). The trunk and extremities are less often affected. These usually resolve spontaneously without scarring over the course of one to four years. Associated systemic abnormalities have not been reported.

Differential Diagnosis

Juvenile xanthogranuloma
Histiocytosis X

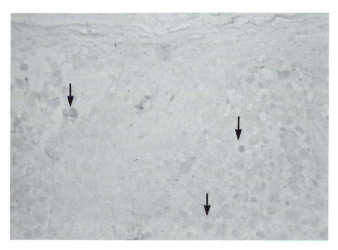

19-5-4 CONGENITAL SELF-HEALING HISTIOCYTOSIS: Only rare cells mark with S-100 stains. (100×)

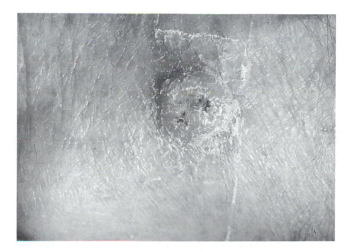

19-6-1 BENIGN CEPHALIC HISTIOCYTOSIS: A single scalp mass.

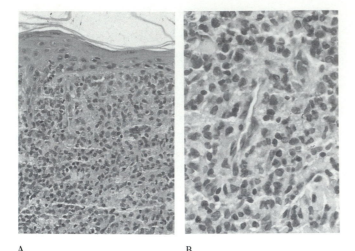

A   B

19-6-2 BENIGN CEPHALIC HISTIOCYTOSIS: (A) Large cells surrounded by a population of small lymphocytes. There is no zone of papillary dermal sparing (Grenz zone) in this lesion. (100×) (B) The large cells have basophilic nuclei and abundant eosinophilic cytoplasms. These cells separate and obscure dermal collagen bundles. (400×)

HISTOLOGICAL DESCRIPTION

Malignant Histiocytosis

Within the dermis there are large numbers of histiocytic-type cells with nuclear pleomorphism and abundant eosinophilic cytoplasms. Mitotic figures are abundant. The pattern of infiltration of dermal stroma simulates that seen in leukemic infiltration of skin. The infiltrate does not involve the papillary dermis or epidermis but may extend into subcutaneous adipose tissue. Of note, the histiocytic cells may show cellular debris within their cytoplasms from ingestion of erythrocytes, leukocytes, or platelets.

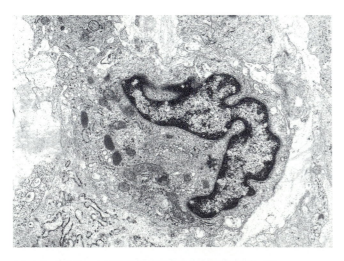

19-6-3 BENIGN CEPHALIC HISTIOCYTOSIS: Electron micrograph of infiltrating cell. Note the lack of Birbeck granules within the cytoplasm. (1200×)

Special stains and ultrastructural studies help confirm the diagnosis; nonspecific esterase is positive, alpha-1 antichymotrypsin is variable, S-100 is negative, and electron microscopy shows primary and secondary lysosomes. Birbeck's granules are absent in these cells.

Benign Cephalic Histiocytosis

Histiocytes with pale cytoplasms and indistinct cell borders are present within the superficial dermis and may infiltrate the epidermis (Plate 19-6-1; Figure 19-6-2). Eosinophils and lymphocytes are scarce. S-100 stains are negative, and ultrastructural studies show large numbers of 500 to 1500 nm coated vesicles; Birbeck's granules are not found (Figure 19-6-3).

Differential Diagnosis

Histiocytic cytophagic panniculitis
Juvenile xanthogranuloma
Histiocytosis X

19-7 LEUKEMIA CUTIS

CLINICAL DESCRIPTION

Leukemia is the most common form of cancer in children. It occurs with higher than expected frequency in patients with congenital and acquired immunodeficiencies as well as those with chromosomal abnormalities or chromosomal fragility. Cutaneous lesions associated with leukemia are subdivided into specific and nonspecific ones. Specific lesions contain the abnormal population of leukocytes, while nonspecific lesions result from tumor-induced aberrations (e.g., purpura). The latter type of lesion is not addressed in this chapter.

Etiology and Incidence

Leukemia cutis is the infiltration of skin by neoplastic leukocytes. It is a specific lesion that indicates dissemination of the disease. It usually occurs late in the course of leukemia and may herald progression leading to death within months to a year. An exception to this appears to be granulocytic sarcoma or the infiltration of skin by neoplastic leukocytes in acute or chronic myelogenous leukemia. In this instance cutaneous lesions do not appear to have the same prognostic value. Only rarely is leukemia cutis the initial presentation of leukemia.

The incidence of leukemia cutis varies with the type, occurring in less than 2% of patients with acute lymphocytic leukemia to up to 50% of patients with monocytic leukemia.

Clinical Features

In instances where the diagnosis of leukemia is known, the appearance of multiple, deeply erythematous to violaceous

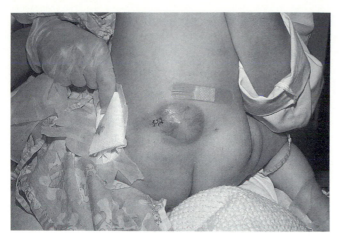

19-7-1 LEUKEMIA CUTIS: This child presented with a large plaque over the lower back. The biopsy showed skin involvement with acute myelomonocytic leukemia.

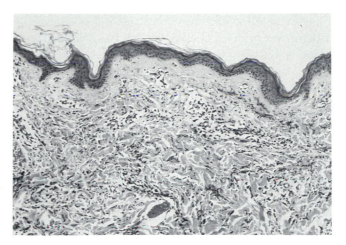

19-7-2 LEUKEMIA CUTIS: The dermis is infiltrated by extravasated erythrocytes and inflammatory cells. The inflammatory cells are present in a perivascular and interstitial distribution, which is unusual in benign reactive infiltrates. (100×)

papules, nodules, or plaques (Figure 19-7-1) should raise suspicions of leukemia cutis. Infection or sepsis should be excluded. In many instances the morphologic features of leukemia cutis are not characteristic. For example, deep-seated subcutaneous nodules may be flesh-colored and mimic erythema nodosum. When associated with extravasation of erythrocytes leukemia cutis may appear as ecchymoses or palpable purpura. It may form blisters or ulcers. The mucosa may show a variety of lesions, including gingival hypertrophy. Leukemia cutis may mimic reactive cutaneous lesions, ranging from urticaria and sarcoidosis to eczematous eruptions and urticaria pigmentosa. Although some types of lesions occur with greater frequency in some leukemias than others (e.g., gingival swelling with acute monocytic or myelomonocytic leukemia), none is pathognomonic for any given disease.

In instances where leukemia is not suspected, careful systemic workup, including bone marrow and peripheral smear examination, is necessary. With chemotherapy lesions of leukemia cutis may regress but do not necessarily do so.

Differential Diagnosis

Lymphoma cutis
Urticaria
Erythema nodosum
Drug eruption
Pyogenic granuloma
Phenytoin-induced hypertrophy
Various reactive-appearing cutaneous lesions

HISTOLOGICAL DESCRIPTION

Histological sections show diffuse permeation of the dermis or mucosa by monotonous-appearing cells. Neoplastic leukocytes may permeate the subcutis as well. The infiltrate is not confined to perivascular locations, as is characteristic of reac-

tive infiltrates, but rather has an interstitial pattern as cells weave among collagen bundles (Figures 19-7-2 and 19-7-3). Depending on the intensity of the infiltrate, these cells may occasionally outline collagen bundles. Cells infiltrating the skin reflect the type of leukemia: lymphoblasts are seen in acute lymphoblastic leukemia, predominantly immature granulocytes are seen in acute and chronic myelogenous leukemias, and monocytes are seen in acute myelogenous leukemia. The cytology of the infiltrating cells may show artifactual alterations, which precludes accurate typing of leukemias in skin. Morphologic and immunohistochemical studies of bone marrow and peripheral smears are essential in the accurate diagnosis of the type of leukemia.

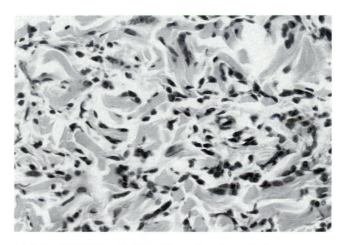

19-7-3 LEUKEMIA CUTIS: The infiltrating cells have a monotonous appearance and cytologic atypia. These are findings of leukemia cutis. The myelomonocytic type was determined by bone marrow examination. (400×)

In instances where leukemia cutis is the first manifestation of the disease, special stains (such as chloracetate esterase for cells of the granulocytic series) and cell marker analysis may be helpful in establishing the lineage of these cells.

Differential Diagnosis
Lymphoma cutis
Metastasis from other primary neoplasms

19-8 LYMPHOMA CUTIS

CLINICAL DESCRIPTION

Lymphoma cutis is the extension of neoplastic lymphocytes from affected lymph nodes into skin. It is important to distinguish lymphoma cutis from primary lymphoma of the skin and from leukemia metastatic to skin.

Etiology and Incidence
Lymphoma cutis is a heterogeneous group of disorders. It occurs in association with Hodgkin's disease as well as non-Hodgkin's lymphomas. The incidence of lymphoma cutis is addressed under clinical features of the individual subtypes.

Clinical Features
Hodgkin's Disease
Although Hodgkin's disease accounts for approximately one-fourth of malignant lymphomas in children, infiltration of the skin is seen infrequently. In addition, as patients are treated earlier, cutaneous lesions are even more rare.

There are scarce reports in the literature of Hodgkin's disease occuring in the skin first without evidence of visceral disease. Doubt exists as to the validity of the correct diagnoses of these cases, thus a diagnosis of primary cutaneous Hodgkin's disease should be viewed with skepticism. Usually, cutaneous involvement with Hodgkin's disease occurs late in the course of the disease. Similar to leukemia cutis, it indicates dissemination of the process and frequently is

thought to indicate a poor prognosis. Examples in the literature indicate that this is not uniformly true.

Cutaneous lesions of Hodgkin's disease are red-brown to violaceous papules or nodules, which may coalesce to form plaques. If lesions ulcerate, they tend to heal poorly. Rarely ulcers may also result from direct extension of the process to skin from an involved underlying node. More often, lesions occur distal to affected lymph nodes. This may occur via retrograde lymphatic flow secondary to tumor obstruction.

Non-Hodgkin's Lymphoma
Non-Hodgkin's lymphomas represent a heterogeneous group of diseases. They are often classified according to the cell of origin as B cell, T cell, pre-B cell, or null cell. Overall, these disorders present with painless adenopathy and behave in a biologically aggressive manner. Cutaneous extension of these lymphomas in children is rare and indicates an extremely poor prognosis.

Clinical lesions occur with greatest frequency on the head and neck. They may be single or multiple macules, papules (Figure 19-8-1), nodules, or plaques with a deep red to violaceous hue. They may be indistinguishable from lesions of leukemia cutis or Hodgkin's disease.

Ki-1 Lymphoma
Ki-1 lymphomas represent a subset of non-Hodgkin's lymphomas in which tissue sections show the presence of large anaplastic-appearing cells that express the Reed-Sternberg cell-associated antigen Ki-1. Knowledge about the clinical characteristics and biologic behavior of this lymphoma is still evolving. It is known that this disease may affect skin exclusively (primary cutaneous), lymph nodes exclusively, or both skin and lymph nodes, or it may evolve to infiltrate other viscera. Localization of the infiltrates in such lymphomas may determine their behavior: cutaneous disease alone often remains localized to skin for long periods of time, while primary lymph node disease usually spreads rapidly to other nodes and viscera.

Cutaneous lesions appear as rapidly growing erythematous exophytic nodules, which may mimic pyogenic granulomas or keratoacanthomas. They may spontaneously regress, causing confusion in the diagnosis. In the past, such clinical presentations have carried the mislabel of regressing atypical histiocytosis. Since the original report of Flynn et al., it has been shown that the cellular proliferation is not of histiocytic but of T lymphocytic lineage. Lesions may mimic ulcerative lesions of lymphomatoid papulosis clinically and histologically, thus some authors speculate that these two disorders may represent variations of the same disorder. The onset of lymphadenopathy or systemic symptoms with cutaneous lesions may herald disease progression. Close clinical follow-up study of affected patients is therefore necessary. The disease course is variable but may eventuate in death.

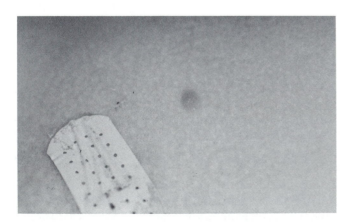

19-8-1 LYMPHOMA CUTIS: Red-brown papule.

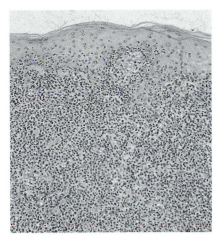

19-8-2 NON-HODGKIN'S LYMPHOMA: Low power shows that the dermis is permeated by a dense infiltrate. (100×)

Differential Diagnosis

Lymphocytoma cutis
Leukemia cutis
Lymphomatoid papulosis
Mycosis fungoides
Primary cutaneous (peripheral) lymphoma

HISTOLOGICAL DESCRIPTION

Hodgkin's Disease

Skin biopsy shows a dense polymorphous infiltrate within the dermis and/or subcutis. It is composed of lymphocytes, histiocytes, and eosinophils admixed with variable numbers of atypical cells with two "mirror image" nuclei and prominent nucleoli (Reed-Sternberg cells). Surrounding fibrosis may be evident. As with leukemia cutis, specific typing of Hodgkin's disease must be based on lymph node biopsy.

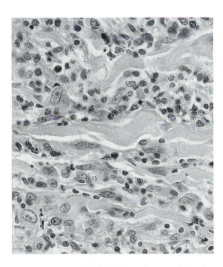

19-8-3 NON-HODGKIN'S LYMPHOMA: High magnification shows an atypical lymphoreticular infiltrate dissecting collagen bundles. (400×)

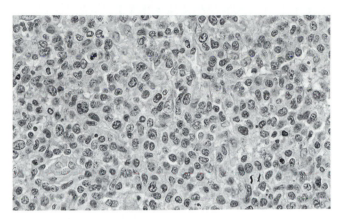

19-8-4 NON-HODGKIN'S LYMPHOMA: Another area shows the monotonous infiltrate of lymphoma cutis: there is focal necrosis and evidence of mitotic activity. (400×)

Non-Hodgkin's Lymphoma

The histological characteristic is sheets of monomorphous cells diffusely permeating the dermis (Figure 19-8-2) and/or subcutis. They dissect collagen bundles (Figure 19-8-2 and 19-8-3) and infiltrate preexisting appendageal structures. The papillary dermis and overlying epidermis are usually spared. Nuclear atypia of infiltrating cells is often prominent. Mitotic figures are frequent and areas of necrosis may be evident (Figure 19-8-4). Of note, epidermal changes are minimal. When the histological findings are less striking and the diagnosis of lymphocytoma cutis is in question, cell marker analysis is helpful in ascertaining the cell population(s) present in the infiltrate. On rare occasion, the malignant cells may be obscured by a bulky reactive component, making the diagnosis of lymphoma cutis difficult. In such cases gene rearrangement studies may detect clonal rearrangements indicative of neoplastically transformed cells.

Ki-1 Lymphoma

Histological sections of skin show permeation of dermal stroma by large, bizarre mononuclear cells. Binucleated cells reminiscent of Reed-Sternberg cells and multinucleated cells may be seen. Mitotic figures are usually present. A reactive lymphocytic infiltrate surrounds and permeates this process. Of note, the epidermis may be hyperplastic and/or ulcerted, but it is not infiltrated by the anaplastic cells.

Cell marker analysis often shows these cells to be of T cell lineage. In addition, such cells express CD30 or Ki-1 on their surfaces. Gene rearrangement studies show T cell receptor rearrangements.

Differential Diagnosis

Leukemia cutis
Lymphocytoma
Lymphomatoid papulosis
Regressing atypical histiocytosis
Ki-1 lymphoma

19-9 CUTANEOUS T CELL LYMPHOMA (MYCOSIS FUNGOIDES)

CLINICAL DESCRIPTION

Cutaneous T cell lymphoma usually occurs in middle-aged or older patients and is extremely uncommon in children.

Etiology and Incidence

Cutaneous T cell lymphoma (CTCL) is the proliferation of an aberrant clone of T lymphocytes primarily involving the skin. Although a role for retrovirus infection and chronic antigenic stimulation in the evolution of this process has been speculated, the exact cause of this disease is unknown. In various reports of CTCL the percentage of patients with disease onset prior to twenty years of age is small, usually less than 6% of all patients with this disorder. Because of the rarity of CTCL in children, there is a low index of suspicion of such lesions and hesitation to biopsy such lesions.

Clinical Features

Clinically, CTCL starts as scaly, erythematous patches that can progressively evolve into plaques and tumor nodules. The earliest lesions may clinically appear as eczematous patches (Figure 19-9-1) that respond poorly to conventional therapy. Such lesions may be labeled as parapsoriasis en plaques on biopsy study. When such lesions have mottled pigmentation and atrophy, they are labeled poikiloderma vasculare atrophicans. Localized cutaneous involvement by CTCL is known as Woringer-Kolopp disease.

As the lesions evolve into plaques and tumors they may be accompanied by lymphadenopathy. If tumor cells are not detectable in clinically affected lymph nodes the presentation is called dermatopathic lymphadenopathy. For the most

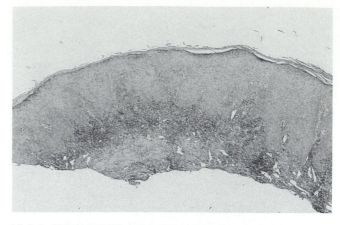

19-9-2 CUTANEOUS CELL LYMPHOMA: The most infiltrated area shows a bandlike infiltrate of inflammatory cells arranged beneath a hyperplastic epidermis. (25×)

part, this disease has a prolonged, indolent course. Extracutaneous disease does occur, however, and in such instances suggests a poor prognosis.

Differential Diagnosis

Eczematous eruptions (early lesions)
Lymphoma cutis
Leukemia cutis

HISTOLOGICAL DESCRIPTION

Criteria for the distinction between parapsoriasis and patch-stage CTCL (mycosis fungoides) are not universally agreed upon. In general, the earliest lesions of CTCL show a sparse lymphocytic infiltrate within a sclerotic and expanded papillary dermis. Individual lymphocytes can be seen infiltrating the overlying nonspongiotic epidermis. Lesions labeled as parapsoriasis usually lack cytologic atypia of lymphocytes. When such an infiltrate is seen in the context of an atrophic epidermis (effaced rete ridge pattern and thinned epidermis) and prominent superficial dermal vascular ectasia, the possibility of poikiloderma vasculare atrophicans is raised.

As the process evolves, the infiltrate is more brisk: a bandlike infiltrate of lymphocytes may be seen in the superficial dermis (Figure 19-9-2 and 19-9-3) and larger numbers of lymphocytes enter the overlying epidermis (epidermotropism). Lymphocytes begin to show atypia, with enlargement and hyperconvolution of their nuclei. Such cells are known as Sézary cells. Nests of such cells in the epidermis are known as Pautrier's microabscesses (Figure 19-9-4). Because of the intraepidermal disturbance, parakeratotic scale is often formed. The epidermis itself may be hyperplastic, unaltered, or thinned.

As CTCL progresses into tumor stage, atypical mononuclear cells no longer infiltrate the epidermis as avidly as before. They congregate within the dermis, where they are

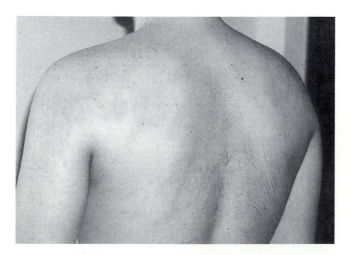

19-9-1 CUTANEOUS T CELL LYMPHOMA: Large eczematous patches on the back of an adolescent with mycosis fungoides.

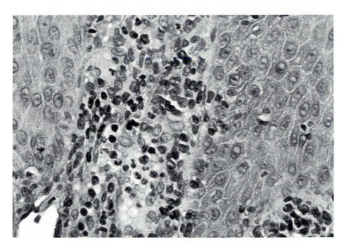

19-9-3 CUTANEOUS T CELL LYMPHOMA: Higher magnification shows the presence of large numbers of atypical mononuclear cells with hyperconvoluted nuclear contours within the papillary dermis and infiltrating the overlying epithelium. (400×)

present as a dermal nodule. In such instances it may be difficult to distinguish nonepidermotropic CTCL from lymphoma cutis. The overlying epidermis is usually atrophic and may be ulcerated.

Cell marker analysis shows various aberrations depending on the stage of the disease: they are most subtle in parapsoriasis and patch-stage CTCL and most pronounced in tumor-stage CTCL. These changes include loss of maturation antigens that normal lymphocytes bear on their surfaces (CD2, CD3, CD5). The aberrant cell population is usually helper T lymphocytic (CD4+) and thus ratios of helper to suppressor cells in tissue are skewed in favor of CD4+ cells (CD4 to CD8 ratio is usually greater than 6:1).

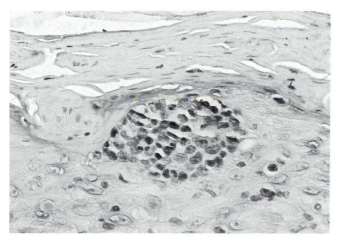

19-9-4 CUTANEOUS T CELL LYMPHOMA: Within the epidermis these cells form nests, known as Pautrier's microabscesses. Note the formation of parakeratotic scale. (400×)

When the diagnosis of CTCL is in question and histological findings equivocal, gene rearrangement studies may add diagnostic information. Finding a monoclonal population of T lymphocytes with rearrangements in the T cell receptor helps to confirm a diagnosis of CTCL.

Differential Diagnosis
Nonspecific dermatitis (early lesions)
Chronic eczematous dermatitis
Lymphoma cutis (late lesions)

REFERENCES

Acquired Immunodeficiency Syndrome
Casanova JM, Puig T, Rubio M: Hypertrichosis of the eyelashes in acquired immune deficiency syndrome. Arch Dermatol 1987; 123:1599.

Duvic M, Lowe L, Rapini RP, et al.: Eruptive dysplastic nevi associated with human immunodeficiency virus infection. Arch Dermatol 1989; 123:397.

Greenspan JS, Mastrucci TM, Leggott PL, et al: Hairy leukoplakia in a child. AIDS 1988; 2:143.

Lim W, Sadick N, Gupta A, et al. Skin diseases in children with HIV infection and their association with degree of immunosuppression. Int J Dermatol 1990; 29:24.

Pierard GE, Pierard-Franchimont C, Estrada JA, et al.: Cutaneous mixed infections in AIDS. Am J Dermatopathol 1990; 12:63.

Prose NS: HIV infection in children. J Am Acad Dermatol 1990; 22:1223.

Prose NS: Mucocutaneous disease in pediatric human immunodeficiency virus infection. Ped Clin North Am 1991; 38:977.

Graft versus Host Disease
Farmer ER: The histopathology of graft-versus-host disease. Adv Dermatol 1986; 1:173.

Hood AF, Farmer ER: Interface dermatitis. In Farmer ER, Hood AF, eds: Pathology of the skin. Norwalk, CT: Appleton & Lange, 1990; 122.

Kleigman RM: Transplantation medicine. In Behrman RE, Kleigman RM, Nelson WE, et al., eds.: Nelson textbook of pediatrics, 14th ed. Philadelphia: W.B. Saunders, 1992; 238.

Santo GW, Hess AD, Vogelsang GB: Graft-versus-host reactions and disease. Immunol Rev 1985; 88:169.

Lymphocytoma Cutis
Kerl H, Ackerman AB: Cutaneous pseudolymphomas. In Fitzpatrick TB, Eisen AZ, Wolff K, Austen KF, eds.: Dermatology in general medicine. New York: McGraw-Hill, 1987: 1118.

Smolle J, Torne R, Soyer HP, et al.: Immunohistochemical classification of cutaneous pseudolymphomas: Delineation of distinct patterns. J Cutan Pathol 1990; 17:149.

Lymphomatoid Papulosis

Ashworth J, Paterson WD, MacKie RM: Lymphomatoid papulosis/pityriasis lichenoides in two children. Pediatr Dermatol 1987; 4:238.

Cerio R, Black MM: Regressing atypical histiocytosis and lymphomatoid papulosis: Variants of the same disorder? Br J Dermatol 1990; 123:515.

Hellman J, Phelps RG, Baral J, et al.: Lymphomatoid papulosis with antigen deletion and clonal rearrangement in a 4-year-old boy. Pediatr Dermatol 1990; 7:42.

Sina B, Burnett JW: Lymphomatoid papulosis: Case reports and literature review. Arch Dermatol 1983; 119:189.

Langerhans' Cell Histiocytosis (Histiocytosis X)

Esterly NB, Maurer HS, Gonzales-Crussi F. Histiocytosis X: A seven year experience at a children's hospital. J Am Acad Dermatol 1985; 13:383.

Malone M: The histiocytoses of childhood. Histopathol 1991; 19:105.

van der Valk P, Meijer CJLM: Cutaneous histiocytic proliferations. Dermatol Clin North Am 1985; 3:705.

Non-Histiocytosis X Disorders

Malignant Histiocytosis

Warnke RA, Kim H, Dorfman RF: Malignant histiocytosis (histiocytic medullary reticulosis): I. Clinicopathologic study of 29 cases. Cancer 1975; 35:215.

Wick MR, Sanchez NP, Crotty CP, et al.: Cutaneous malignant histiocytosis: A clinical and histopathologic study of eight cases, with immunohistochemical analysis. J Am Acad Dermatol 1983; 8:50.

Congenital Self-Healing Histiocytosis

Berger TG, Lane AT, Headington JT, et al.: A solitary variant of congenital self-healing reticulohistiocytosis: Solitary Hashimoto-Pritzker disease. Pediatr Dermatol 1986; 3:230.

Hashimoto K, Pritzker MS: Electron microscopic study of reticulohistiocytoma: An unusual case of congenital, self-healing reticulohistiocytosis. Arch Dermatol 1973; 107:263.

Kapila PK, Grant-Kels JM, Allred C, et al.: Congenital, spontaneously regressing histiocytosis: Case report and review of the literature. Pediatr Dermatol 1985; 2:312.

Benign Cephalic Histiocytosis

Gianotti F, Caputo R, Ermacora E, et al.: Benign cephalic histiocytosis. Arch Dermatol 1986; 122:1038.

Leukemia Cutis

Krause JR: Granulocytic sarcoma preceding acute leukemia. Cancer 1979; 44:1017.

McCune A, Cohen BA: Urticarial skin eruption in a child. Arch Dermatol 1990; 126:1497.

Stawiski MA: Skin manifestations of leukemias and lymphomas. Cutis 1978; 21:814.

Su WPD, Buechner SA, Li CY: Clinicopathologic correlations in leukemia cutis. J Am Acad Dermatol 1984; 11:121.

Lymphoma Cutis

Hodgkin's Disease

Gordon RA, Lookingbill DP, Abt AB: Skin infiltration in Hodgkin's disease. Arch Dermatol 1980; 116:1038.

Hayes TG, Rabin VR, Rosen T, et al.: Hodgkin's disease presenting in the skin: Case report and review of the literature. J Am Acad Dermatol 1990; 22:944.

Smith JL, Butler JJ: Skin involvement in Hodgkin's disease. Cancer 1980; 45:354.

White RM, Patterson JW: Cutaneous involvement in Hodgkin's disease. Cancer 1984; 55:1136.

Non-Hodgkin's Lymphoma

Murphy SB: Classification, staging and end results of treatment of childhood non-Hodgkin's lymphoma: Dissimilarities from lymphomas in adults. Semin Oncol 1980; 7:332.

Zaatari GS, Chan WC, Kin TH, et al.: Malignant lymphoma in the skin of children. Cancer 1987; 59:1040.

Ki-1 Lymphoma

Cerio R, Black MM: Regressing atypical histiocytosis and lymphomatoid papulosis: Variants of the same disorder? Br J Dermatol 1990; 123:515.

Flynn KJ, Dehner LP, Gajl-Peczalska KJ, et al.: Regressing atypical histiocytosis: A cutaneous proliferation of atypical neoplastic histiocytes with unexpectedly indolent behavior. Cancer 1982; 49:959.

Headington JT, Roth MS, Ginsburg D, et al.: T-cell receptor gene rearrangement in regressing atypical histiocytosis. Arch Dermatol 1987; 123:1183.

Kadin ME, Sako D, Berliner N, et al.: Childhood Ki-1 lymphoma presenting with skin lesions and peripheral lymphadenopathy. Blood 1986; 68:1042.

Kaudewitz P, Stein H, Dallenbach F, et al.: Primary and secondary cutaneous Ki-1+ (CD30+) anaplastic large cell lymphomas: Morphological, immunohistologic, and clinical characteristics. Am J Pathol 1989; 135:359.

Oka K, Mori N, Kojima M, et al.: Childhood Ki-1 lymphoma. Arch Pathjol Lab Med 1989; 113:998.

Schnitzer B, Roth MS, Hyder DM, et al.: Ki-1 lymphomas in children. Cancer 1988; 61:1213.

Cutaneous T Cell Lymphoma (Mycosis Fungoides)

Koch SE, Zackheim HS, Williams ML, et al.: Mycosis fungoides beginning in childhood and adolescence. J Am Acad Dermatol 1987; 17:563.

Peters MS, Thibodeau SN, White JW, et al.: Mycosis fungoides in children and adolescents. J Am Acad Dermatol 1990; 22:1011.

Wilson AGM, Cotter FE, Lowe DG, et al.: Mycosis fungoides in childhood: An unusual presentation. J Am Acad Dermatol 1991; 25:370.

20

Disorders of Pigmentation

Contents

20-1 EPHELIS

CLINICAL DESCRIPTION

Etiology and Incidence

Freckles (ephelides) are hyperpigmented macules that occur in children around the age of two years. They are inherited as an autosomal dominant trait.

Clinical Features

Freckles are hyperpigmented macules 2 to 5 mm in diameter. They are more prominent in the summer months because they darken with sun exposure. They are most prevalent over the nose and cheeks. Children who have freckles are usually of a fair complexion. There are no systemic conditions associated with ephelides.

Differential Diagnosis

Lentigines

HISTOLOGICAL DESCRIPTION

The distinguishing histological feature in ephelis is basal cell hyperpigmentation with associated rete ridge hyperplasia. Sections stained by the dopa technique show that there is an actual decrease in the number of melanocytes when compared to adjacent uninvolved skin. Cytologically the melanocytes in the ephelis are larger and produce large melanosomes that are well-melanized and unpackaged.

Differential Diagnosis

Café-au-lait spot
Normal skin

20-2 CAFÉ-AU-LAIT SPOTS

CLINICAL DESCRIPTION

Etiology and Incidence

Café-au-lait spots are the hallmark of neurofibromatosis, occurring in over 95% of the cases, although they occur as isolated lesions in 15% of individuals without neurofibromatosis. They can also be seen with McCune-Albright syndrome and a variety of other disorders. Café-au-lait spots may be present at birth, but more often appear between ages 2 and 16.

Clinical Features

Café-au-lait spots are hyperpigmented yellow-brown macules that usually vary in size from 1 to 3 cm (Plate 20-2-1). They can be as large as 30 cm. Their color is uniform, although the borders may be slightly darker than the central portion. They are visible at all times and not induced by sunlight as are ephelides, although they do darken after sun exposure. The diagnosis of neurofibromatosis is indicated by six or more café-au-lait spots of greater than 0.5 cm of surface area in prepubertal children or 1.5 cm in postpubertal children and adults. Axillary freckling is another sign of this disorder. There is no clinical difference in the quality of café-au-lait spots found in neurofibromatosis and those in normal individuals. The only difference is in number and volume.

Differential Diagnosis

Ephelides
Lentigines

HISTOLOGICAL DESCRIPTION

The epidermis shows well-defined retes with moderate hyperplasia. The pigmentary change within the basal layer may be very subtle when compared to adjacent normal skin. There is an increase in basal cell pigmentation and presence of clear cells in the basal layer. On hematoxylin and eosin-stained sections there is the impression of more clear cells in the basal layer than would be expected. Dopa-stained sections show more melanocytes per square millimeter in café-au-lait spots than in normal adjacent areas. Melanocytes within most café-au-lait spots produce macromelanosomes (giant melanin granules, Figure 20-2-1). Macromelanosomes can be demonstrated in thinly cut (1 to 2 μm) hematoxylin and eosin-stained sections. The inflammatory response is not significant and there is no dermal change.

Differential Diagnosis

Ephelides
Normal skin
Lentigenes

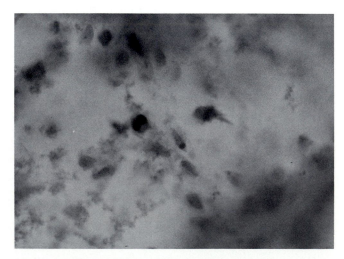

20-2-1 CAFÉ-AU-LAIT SPOTS: Macromelanosomes in melanocytes of a patient with neurofibromatosis. (400×)

20-3 LENTIGINES SYNDROME

CLINICAL DESCRIPTION

Etiology and Incidence

Lentigines are a normal skin finding in most children. They may also be part of syndromes when present in excessive numbers or a particular distribution. Examples of syndromes associated with lentigenes are Peutz-Jeghers syndrome (autosomal dominant periorificial and mucosal, and bowel polyps) and the LEOPARD (*l*entigenes, *E*CG abnormalities, *o*cular hypertelorism, *p*ulmonic stenosis, *a*bnormal genitalia, *r*etardation of growth, and *d*eafness).

Clinical Features

Lentigines are macular areas of pigmentation. They are brown-black and darker than freckles or café-au-lait spots. Lentigines are about the size of freckles (2 to 6 mm) and usually first appear during school age (Plate 20-2-2) but may be congenital when they are part of a syndrome. They may occur on most cutaneous surfaces but are concentrated on the face, neck, and upper trunk.

Differential Diagnosis

Blue nevus

HISTOLOGICAL DESCRIPTION

Lentigolike lesions are seen in several cutaneous syndromes, all of which show similar, if not identical, histological features. There is epidermal hyperplasia in the form of elongated rete ridges. A striking feature is hypermelanosis of the epidermis, especially at the basal cell layer and at the sides of the elongated rete (Figure 20-3-1). There may be associated dermal melanophage pigmentation in lentigo simplex as well as an occasional nest of nevus cells. Multiple lentigines syndrome has lentiginous changes with epidermal hyperpigmentation. Junctional nevus cell nests have also been reported in this condition. Peutz-Jeghers syndrome has lentiginous hyperplasia with melanocyte hyperactivity, and there is an apparent increase in the number of melanocytes.

Differential Diagnosis

Ephelis
Solar lentigo
Café-au-lait spot

20-4 BECKER'S NEVUS

CLINICAL DESCRIPTION

Etiology and Incidence

Described in 1949 by S. W. Becker as an area of macular hyperpigmentation that occurs most commonly in males, this nevus is found most often on the upper trunk (shoulders, chest, and scapular areas). It is usually manifested at puberty but may be seen in early childhood.

Clinical Features

Becker's nevi consist of area of grayish brown pigmentation on the upper chest, arm, or back that measure approximately 10 to 20 cm in diameter. The lesion is sharply demarcated from normal skin. After puberty, coarse, dark hairs may be seen growing from the lesion (Figure 20-4-1). In later stages, the

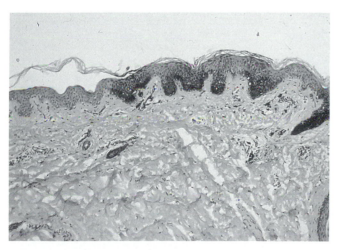

20-3-1 LENTIGINES SYNDROME: Sharply circumscribed elongation and hyperpigmentation of the rete ridges. These changes are characteristic of lentigenes and are seen in LEOPARD syndrome (40×)

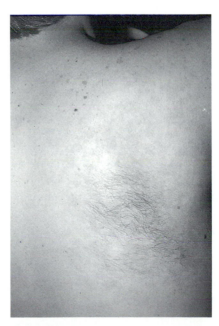

20-4-1 BECKER'S NEVUS: Hyperpigmentation, dark coarse hair. (Courtesy of Allen Gaisin, M.D.)

hair in this pigmentary process may be the most conspicuous feature.

Differential Diagnosis
Congenital hairy nevus
Ito's nevus

HISTOLOGICAL DESCRIPTION

Becker's pigmented hairy nevus is essentially a lentiginous process. There is acanthosis with elongation of the rete ridges and hyperpigmentation of the basal cell layer. Melanophage pigmentation occurs in the dermis. There is disagreement as to the melanocytic increase in this condition. Dopa-stained sections often show increased melanocytes in the epidermis in Becker's nevus when compared to uninvolved adjacent skin. Electron microscopic studies have shown increased melanosome production and retention of melanosomes within keratinocytes. Hair can be seen within this melanocytic process and appears normal. Occasionally associated with Becker's nevi are smooth muscle hamartomas found deep to the epidermal proliferative changes.

Differential Diagnosis
Lentigines
Nevus (nevocelluar nevus)

20-5 POSTINFLAMMATORY HYPERPIGMENTATION

CLINICAL DESCRIPTION

Etiology and Incidence
Postinflammatory hyperpigmentation can occur after any inflammatory episode. It does not occur after each episode and predicting its occurrence is difficult, although more severe inflammatory events tend to produce hyperpigmentation. Postinflammatory hyperpigmentation is very common in black skin.

Clinical Features
Hyperpigmented macules, patches, or plaques occur at the sites of inflammation (Figure 20-5-1) and are sharply separated from surrounding skin. Postinflammatory hyperpigmentation is most common in black skin but occurs in others to a lesser degree. The inflammatory event initiating postinflammatory hyperpigmentation may be external (chemicals, medications, or injury) or secondary to infection (bacterial or fungal) or a systemic eruption (lichen planus, lupus erythematosus, or systemic medications).

Differential Diagnosis
Congenital nevus

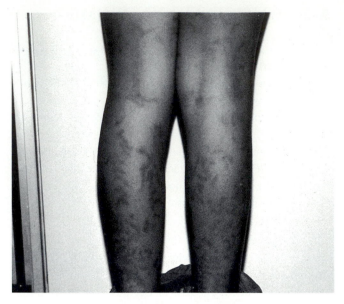

20-5-1 POSTINFLAMMATORY HYPERPIGMENTATION: Posterior aspects of a child's legs with irregular areas of hyperpigmentation, secondary to dermatitis.

HISTOLOGICAL DESCRIPTION

Postinflammatory hyperpigmentation can be epidermal, dermal, or both. The dermal pigmentation is in melanophages and can be quite dense (Figure 20-5-2). This finding is commonly seen following lichen planus and lichen planus-like drug eruptions and is marked in black patients. When dermal pigmentation is intense, the clinical coloration of the patient is blue-black rather than brown.

If the primary process was a disease such as lichen planus or lupus erythematosus, histological features of that process may also be seen. However, in most cases, residual hyperpigmentation is the only manifestation of the preceding process. The inflammatory infiltrate associated with this

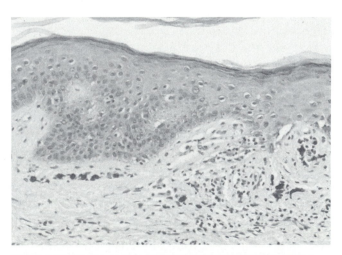

20-5-2 POSTINFLAMMATORY HYPERPIGMENTATION: The papillary dermis contains large numbers of melanophages and lymphocytes. (100×)

condition consists of perivascular lymphocytes, histiocytes, and many melanophages within the dermis.

Differential Diagnosis
Blue nevus
Tattoo

20-6 INCONTINENTIA PIGMENTI (see Chapter 4)

20-7 VITILIGO

CLINICAL DESCRIPTION

Etiology and Incidence
Vitiligo is an acquired disorder of depigmentation of uncertain etiology, but in many cases appears to be inherited in an autosomal dominant pattern with variable expressivity. It affects 2% to 3% of the world's population and has been associated with autoimmune disorders that include thyroiditis, diabetes, Addison's disease, pernicious anemia, and uveitis. Mucocutaneous candidiasis and Down's Syndrome may also be associated with vitiligo.

Clinical Features
Vitiligo should be distinguished from piebaldism in which there is a *congenital* absence of melanocytes and melanin. Piebaldism is associated with mutations in the c-Kit oncogene. The Waardenburg syndrome (sensorineural hearing loss, dystopia canthorum) and piebaldism is now associated with defects in the PAX3 gene.

Vitiligo develops as symmetrical hypopigmented then depigmented patches of varying sizes and shapes (Plate 20-7-1). It can be found at any location but periocular, perioral, and genital sites and the feet, elbows, and knees are common sites of occurrence. The hairs within these areas are also usually depigmented. The course of vitiligo is unpredictable. Many areas may spontaneously repigment, or the condition may proceed to almost complete loss of color. Vitiligo is striking in black skin where there is a sharp transition from the normal to the vitiliginous areas. Dramatic changes are less apparent in light Caucasians. Vitiligo may occur in a dermatomal or zosteriform distribution but has not been associated with viral infections.

Differential Diagnosis
Leprosy
Postinflammatory hypopigmentation
Lichen sclerosis et atrophicus

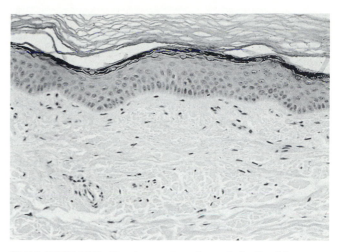

20-7-1 VITILIGO: Routine sections show a lack of striking changes. (100×)

Morphea
Piebaldism

HISTOLOGICAL DESCRIPTION

The histological features of vitiligo in hematoxylin and eosin-stained sections are not diagnostic (Figure 20-7-1). There can be loss of pigmentation and a decrease or absence of melanocytes at the basal cell zone. The inflammatory infiltrate, when present, is lymphocytic and perivascular in location and exocytotic to the epidermis, suggesting lymphocyte destruction of melanocytes. Sections stained with Dopa, or S-100 in established cases of vitiligo reveal an absence of melanocytes in the vitiliginous areas (Plate 20-7-2). At the junction of the areas of vitiligo and normal skin, melanocytes may be large and atypical. Electron microscopy demonstrates absence of or nonfunctional melanocytes. These histological features are similar to those of piebaldism and Vogt-Koyanagi-Harada syndrome.

Differential Diagnosis
Normal skin
Vogt-Koyanagi-Harada syndrome
Albinism
Piebaldism

20-8 ALBINISM

CLINICAL DESCRIPTION

Etiology and Incidence
Albinism is a heterogeneous group of congenital pigmentary disorders manifested by the absence or decrease in pigment of the eyes, hair, and skin. Albinism occurs in oculocutaneous and ocular forms. The ocular form is more rare and may be

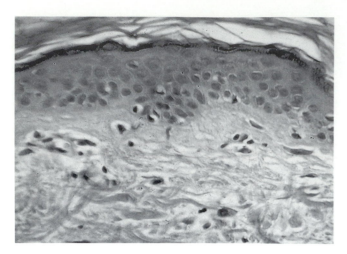

20-8-1 ALBINISM: Although melanocytes are present in the basalar layer, they are hypo- or nonfunctional. (200×)

inherited as an X-linked, autosomal recessive, or as an autosomal dominant entity associated with lentigenes and deafness. Oculocutaneous forms are more common and are almost always inherited as autosomal recessives, affecting males and females of all races. To date, defects in at least two distinct genes have been implicated in human oculocutaneous albinism (tyrosinase-chromosome 11g; the P gene-chromosome 15g.). Other syndromes associated albinism include the Chédiak-Higashi syndrome, Hermansky-Pudlak syndrome and the Cross-McKusick-Breen syndrome.

Clinical Features

Albinos have little or no pigment of their hair, irises, fundi and skin (Plate 20-8-1). They have decreased visual acuity, nystagmus, and marked photophobia with foveal hypoplasia and frequently, iris transillumination. Their skin is subject to ultraviolet exposure, and albinos are especially prone to squamous cell carcinomas (more than basal cell carcinoma and melanoma). Skin color varies from pale, milk-white to straw-yellow. The melanocytes in a population of albino patients may show reactivity to incubation with tyrosinase (usually measured in hair bulbs) (tyrosinase-positive albinos); others do not react to incubation with tyrosinase (tyrosinase-negative). Tyrosinase-positive patients usually have straw-yellow hair and may have pigmented nevi.

Differential Diagnosis
Vitiligo
Leprosy

HISTOLOGICAL DESCRIPTION

The histological features in albinism are those of skin with absent or decreased pigment, but with melanocytes present. In an isolated biopsy specimen without a history, a diagnosis

of albinism is tenuous. On hematoxylin and eosin-stained sections poorly functional melanocytes are seen in the basal layer (Figure 20-8-1). Sections incubated with Dopa demonstrate melanocytes in tyrosinase-positive patients but not in tyrosinase-negative patients. Electron microscopy demonstrates melanocytes in both classes of patients, but they contain fewer mature (stage II and IV) melanosomes. In X-linked ocular albinism, Nettleship Falls type, melanin macroglobules (giant pigment granules) are a prominent finding in affected males and many carrier females.

Differential Diagnosis
Histologically normal skin

20-9 HYPOMELANOSIS OF ITO
(see Chapter 4)

20-10 POSTINFLAMMATORY HYPOPIGMENTATION

CLINICAL DESCRIPTION

Etiology and Incidence
Postinflammatory hypopigmentation follows inflammatory events. It does not occur with all inflammatory episodes. Pigmented skin is more susceptible to postinflammatory hypopigmentation than nonpigmented skin.

Clinical Features

Hypopigmented or depigmented areas develop in the sites of previous inflammatory changes, such as atopic eczema, chickenpox, and pityriasis rosea. The area of pigment loss corresponds to the size and shape of the preceding inflammatory event. The prognosis is excellent for repigmentation following resolution of the inflammatory event.

HISTOLOGICAL DESCRIPTION

There is diminished pigment at the basal cell zone. Basal cells may show vacuolar degeneration. The dermis has a perivascular lymphohistiocytic inflammatory response. Melanocytes can be demonstrated in the epidermis with special stains (Dopa, S-100) and with electron microscopy. This condition is one of melanocyte hypofunction. In severe cases there is melanocyte destruction.

Differential Diagnosis
Vitiligo

REFERENCES

Café-au-Lait Spots

Johnson BL, Charneco DR: Café-au-lait spots in neurofibromatosis and in normal individuals. Arch Dermatol 1970; 102:442.

Lentigines

Nordlund JJ, Learner AB, Braveman IM, et al.: The multiple lentigines syndrome. Arch Dermatol 1973; 107:259.

Becker's Nevus

Becker SW: Concurrent melanosis and hypertrichosis in the distribution of nevus unis lateris. Arch Dermatol 1949; 60:155.

Tate PR, Hodges J, Owen LG: A quantitative study of melanocytes and Becker's nevus. J Cutan Pathol 1980; 7:404.

Urbanek RW, Johnson WC: Smooth muscle hamartoma associated with Becker's nevus. Arch Dermatol 1978; 114:98.

Vitiligo

Lerner AB: Vitiligo. J Invest Dermatol 1959; 32.285.

Albinism

Kugelman TP, Van Scott EJ: Tyrosinase activity in melanocytes of human albinos. J Invest Dermatol 1961; 37:73.

King RA, Summers CG: Albinism. Dermatologic Clinics 1988; 6:217.

Halaban R, Moellmann G: White mutants in mice, shedding light on humans. J Invest Dermatol 1993; 100:1765.

21

Unclassified Disorders

Contents

21-1 ACANTHOSIS NIGRICANS

CLINICAL DESCRIPTION

This disorder is categorized into four types: benign acanthosis nigricans, pseudo-acanthosis nigricans, syndromal acanthosis nigricans, and acanthosis nigricans associated with malignancy in childhood. The last is so rare that it will not be discussed.

Etiology and Incidence

True benign acanthosis nigricans is an extremely rare inherited disorder (autosomal dominant). It presents at birth or anytime during childhood. The most common form is pseudo-acanthosis nigricans, associated with obesity. Next most common is syndromal acanthosis nigricans (insulin-resistant diabetes, Reed's syndrome, Bloom's syndrome, lipodystrophy, etc.). The cause is unknown. Steroids, diethylstilbesterol, and niacin have been known to induce the problem.

Clinical Features

Brown to black discoloration appears on the neck, axillae, and groin (Plate 21-1-1). Verrucous, papillomatous, elevated lesions also can appear on the knuckles, flexor surfaces, lower abdomen and umbilicus, face, thigh, and breasts.

Differential Diagnosis
Dirt
Hyperpigmentation associated with Addison's disease
Ichthyosis hystrix
Other epithelial nevi

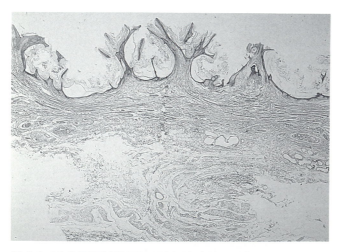

21-1-1 ACANTHOSIS NIGRICANS: The epidermis has a prominent papillomatous architecture. The overlying scale is orthokeratotic. (20×)

HISTOLOGICAL DESCRIPTION

Acanthosis nigricans, whether due to obesity or malignancy, has identical histological features. Most interesting is that it is neither acanthotic nor nigricans (pigmented). There are discrete fingerlike elongations of the rete, without basalar pigmentation (unless the patient is pigmented). There is papillomatosis and a sparse perivascular infiltrate of lymphocytes (Figure 21-1-1). The initial impression is of normal, but papillomatous, skin.

Differential Diagnosis
Normal skin
Epidermal nevus
Papilloma

21-2 ANETODERMA AND ATROPHODERMA

CLINICAL DESCRIPTION

These terms describe idiopathic atrophy of the skin.

Etiology and Incidence

Anetoderma may be primary (develop from normal skin) or secondary (form following an inflammatory process of the skin). The inflammatory process may include such disorders as viral exanthems, lupus, and acne vulgaris.

Atrophoderma, the cause of which also unknown, is a rare disorder of the skin. Some believe it is a variant of morphea.

Clinical Features

In anetoderma there are hypopigmented oval lesions with thin, wrinkled, skin that measure approximately 1 cm in diameter (Plate 21-2-1). At times there is outpouching of the underlying tissue. Atrophoderma differs from anetoderma in the size (1 to 12 cm) and color (slate gray to brown) of the lesions. Whereas anetoderma usually appears on the face and upper trunk, atrophoderma is more likely to be seen on the trunk and lower extremities. However, any body surface may be involved.

Differential Diagnosis
Morphea
Any condition producing atrophy of the skin
Scarring
LSA (lichen sclerosis at atrophicus)

HISTOLOGICAL DESCRIPTION

Anetoderma may show only minimal histological features. Early lesions of the inflammatory type show inflammatory features that include a lymphocytic perivascular infiltrate (Figure 21-2-1). In some instances the infiltrate contains

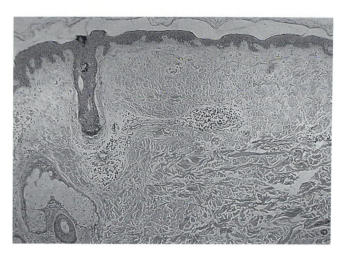

21-2-1 ANETODERMA: Anetoderma with a middermal perivascular inflammatory infiltrate without accompanying collagen alterations. (40×)

neutrophils and the vascular response may be leukocytoclastic. The usual features seen are those of the end-stage reaction. There is minimal inflammation and the changes do not appear to be significant.

Elastic tissue stains show loss of elastic tissue in the central portion of the specimen (Plate 21-2-2). Anetodermas secondary to significant cutaneous inflammation (syphilis, acne, viral exanthems, and so on) show the histological features of the initiating condition.

Atrophoderma, sampled simultaneously with normal skin of the same site, shows a normal or thinned epidermis covering a depression. The deep dermal collagen may show mild thickening and scant angiocentric lymphocytic infiltrates without associated loss of collagen or elastin.

Differential Diagnosis
Normal skin

21-3 CHEILITIS GRANULOMATOSA (MELKERSSON-ROSENTHAL SYNDROME)

CLINICAL DESCRIPTION

Melkersson-Rosenthal syndrome consists of facial palsy, swelling of the upper lip, and a fissured tongue.

Etiology and Incidence
Although the etiology of this condition is unknown, infection, allergy, neurologic dysfunction, and genetic predisposition have been postulated. Over 250 cases have been reported.

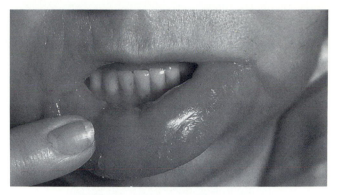

21-3-1 CHEILITIS GRANULOMATOSA: Swollen, infiltrated lip.

The disorder begins between two and seventy years of age, with 45% of patients manifesting the disorder before twenty years. There is a female predominance in those with the disorder who are younger than twenty years.

Clinical Features
The disorder may manifest any of the three components listed above. Most commonly, the swelling involves the upper lip, lasting up to one week and then disappearing. The swelling is asymptomatic and the overlying skin may be reddish brown (Figure 21-3-1). Eventually, brawny induration of the lip remains. The facial paralysis is partial or complete and unilateral or bilateral. It tends to occur on the same side as the swelling. A furrowed tongue occurs in one-half of patients.

Differential Diagnosis
Congenital lymphangioma
Hemangioma
Heerfordt's disease
Ascher's syndrome

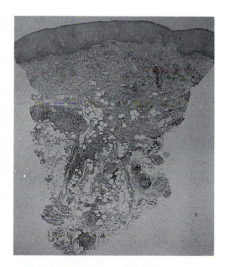

21-3-2 CHEILITIS GRANULOMATOSA: Characteristic submucosal lymphocytic inflammatory infiltrates. (20×)

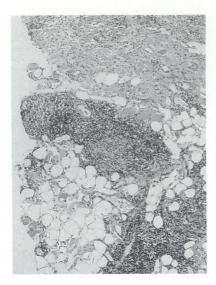

21-3-3 CHEILITIS GRANULOMATOSA: Clusters of epithelioid histiocytes surrounded by a brisk lymphocytic infiltrate. This process extends into the subcutaneous fat. (100×)

HISTOLOGICAL DESCRIPTION

The histological features are mucosal epithelium with a granulomatous dermal infiltrate. The granulomas are composed of epithelioid histiocytes in nodules, surrounded by plasma cells and lymphocytes. The infiltrate can be found at all levels of the dermis and extend into the subcutaneous fat (Figures 21-3-2 and 21-3-3).

Differential Diagnosis
Sarcoidosis
Tuberculosis

21-4 CUTANEOUS REACTIONS TO COLD

CLINICAL DESCRIPTION

Two important reactions to cold are frostbite and pernio (chilblain).

Etiology and Incidence
Frostbite follows exposure to extreme cold. Many factors influence its occurrence, including wind velocity and length of exposure. The injury is a result of the production of ice crystals and injured circulation.

Perniosis occurs in susceptible individuals when cold temperatures produce an exaggerated vasoconstriction, leading to tissue anoxia.

Clinical Features
In both conditions, those parts of the body exposed to cold temperatures are most susceptible (Plates 21-4-1 and 21-4-2). Children with frostbite manifest erythema or cyanosis edema and hemorrhagic vesicles or bullae. Gangrene and skin necrosis may follow with severe injury.

Blanching followed by infiltrated pink to violaceous macules characterizes perniosis. Edematous nodules or plaques of erythema or cyanosis may occur later in the course of events. Numbness and tingling may be experienced.

Differential Diagnosis
Vasculitis associated with collagen vascular disease

HISTOLOGICAL DESCRIPTION

Frostbite
Severe cold injury to the skin produces epidermal and dermal necrosis. The epidermis shows vacuolation of epidermal cells with epidermal death and necrosis. The dermis shows noninflammatory necrosis. Frequently there is a hemorrhagic subepidermal bulla. Milder cold injury produces less severe epidermal and dermal reactions.

Pernio
Pernio shows a less intense and severe reaction than that seen in frostbite. There is a dense perivascular infiltrate of lymphocytes associated with dermal edema. The dermal vessels have swollen endothelial cells. There is no occlusive vasculitis.

Differential Diagnosis
Frostbite
Thermal injury
Venom necrosis
Disseminated intravascular coagulation

Pernio
Polymorphous light reaction
Persistent erythema

21-5 CHILD BATTERING

CLINICAL DESCRIPTION

Child abuse is a complex phenomena that can be divided into four categories: physical abuse, sexual abuse, emotional abuse, and neglect. The first two conditions are most likely to be seen by the dermatologist.

Etiology and Incidence
It is believed that 10% of children younger than five years brought to an emergency room because of traumatic injury have been abused. Up to 4 million children are abused each year, 65% of them physically abused. More than 2,000 deaths per year are due to abuse. The incidence of sexual abuse is 100,000 cases per year. The dynamics involved in abuse are complex and not within the scope of this book. Many references are available to those who are interested.

Clinical Features

The major body organ injured is the skin. Bruises are seen most frequently, in various stages of healing and concentrated in a central distribution (truncal). New bruises are red to red-blue in color. Those one to four days old are more likely to be dark blue or purple; within one week they become green to yellow-green; finally, a yellow-brown tint appears. Often the appearance of the injury reflects the weapon used: loop-shaped marks reflect the use of an electric cord or wire; linear marks indicate a belt or paddle; circular lesions around the wrists, ankles, neck indicate rope burns; hand prints indicate slapping; tooth marks indicate biting; circular scars indicate cigarette burns (Plate 21-5-1). Immersion in scalding water may also produce burns. Traction alopecia may be a sign of abuse. Signs of sexual abuse include bruising of the genitalia, vaginal lacerations, and rectal lacerations.

Differential Diagnosis

Accidental trauma
Spooning, cupping, or coining (cultural phenomena used in other countries that may be considered abuse in the United States)
Lichen sclerosis et atrophicus

HISTOLOGICAL DESCRIPTION

The histological features are those of skin trauma. The most frequent finding is noninflammatory purpura. Blunt trauma usually produces purpura. Old lesions will show fibrosis and hemosiderin pigmentation. Trauma due to burns will show polarization of epidermal cells, necrosis, and dermal coagulation necrosis. There is no inflammatory response.

Differential Diagnosis

Trauma of any cause

21-6 EOSINOPHILIC FASCIITIS (see Chapter 16)

21-7 GRANULOMA ANNULARE

CLINICAL DESCRIPTION

This disorder is frequently misdiagnosed by the inexperienced observer.

Etiology and Incidence

Granuloma annulare is seen often in pediatric patients: 40% of cases occur in this age group. Although 75% of lesions disappear spontaneously over the course of two years, 40% of children have recurrences.

Trauma is thought to play an important role, a theory supported by the distribution of lesions. Patients claim that lesions have occurred following insect bites.

Clinical Features

The lesions occur most frequently on the extensor surfaces of the distal extremities (especially those areas most susceptible to trauma). However, any area may be involved.

Flesh-colored to violaceous papules or nodules appear in a circle. These indurated lesions may coalesce to form a continuous elevated circinate border. Individual papules or nodules may clear centrally, forming a ring (Plate 21-7-1). The rings may expand to form lesions 5 cm or more in diameter. Multiple lesions are not uncommon.

Differential Diagnosis

Tinea corporis
Nummular eczema
Rheumatoid nodule

HISTOLOGICAL DESCRIPTION

The histological findings are multiple, varying sized foci of necrobiotic collagen surrounded by an infiltrate that varies from only lymphocytes to histiocytes, giant cells, and eosinophils. The earliest change is discrete foci of lymphocytes in the collagen. Within this area there is increased ground substance (hyaluronic acid) without distinct necrobiosis. The process progresses from this point to distinct necrobiosis with the characteristic granulomatous infiltrate (Figure 21-7-1). The necrobiotic area, although usually superficial, can extend into the subcutis (deep granuloma annulare); this form tends to have a greater infiltrate of eosinophils.

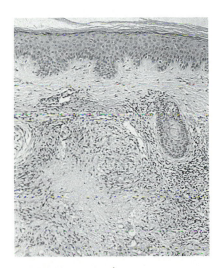

21-7-1 GRANULOMA ANNULARE: Acellular collagen of the middermis is outlined by a palisaded array of lymphocytes and histiocytes. (40×)

Differential Diagnosis
Necrobiosis lipoidica
Foreign body granuloma

21-8 GRANULOMA GLUTEALE INFANTUM

CLINICAL DESCRIPTION

This benign condition can cause much consternation due to its ominous appearance.

Etiology and Incidence
The exact incidence of granulomata gluteale infantum is unknown, but infrequent referrals indicate the condition is uncommon. Many hypotheses as to the etiology have been suggested; most believe the condition is a granulomatous response secondary to a foreign material (e.g., talc, steroids, or infection with *Candida albicans*).

Clinical Features
Reddish blue to purple nodules varying in size from less than 1 cm to 4 cm or more occur in the diaper area (Plate 21-8-1). These lesions are very firm and are elevated above the skin surface. Other intertriginous areas can be involved.

Differential Diagnosis
Kaposi's sarcoma
Lymphoma
Foreign body granuloma

HISTOLOGICAL DESCRIPTION
There is a hyper- and parakeratosis and acanthosis (in some cases to the point of pseudoepitheliomatous hyperplasia) with scattered exocytosis of lymphocytes. In the dermis there is a dense infiltration of lymphocytes, histiocytes, neutrophils, eosinophils, plasma cells, and hemorrhage. There is vascular proliferation of the type seen in pyogenic granulomas.

Differential Diagnosis
Pyogenic granuloma
Infection

21-9 LICHEN SCLEROSIS ET ATROPHICUS

CLINICAL DESCRIPTION

This disorder is not difficult to diagnose when the perineum is involved.

Etiology and Incidence
The cause of lichen sclerosis et atrophicus is unknown. The disorder is seen at any age, and 85% of patients are female.

Seventy-five percent of patients have anogenital involvement. When extragenital sites are involved the genital area should be examined because of its frequent involvement (42%) in these cases. Pruritus is present in 50% of patients and a vaginal discharge in 20%.

Clinical Features
The most consistent feature is an hourglass distribution of inflammation and hypopigmentation about the vagina and anus (Plate 21-9-1). Lesions are usually hypopigmented and atrophic, with sharp borders. The plaques frequently have central depressions. On occasion, flat-topped papules (hypopigmented) appear early in the course of the disease. Petechiae, purpura, hemorrhage, and skin denudation may be present.

When not found in the perineum, lesions are usually distributed in a symmetric fashion over the neck, upper trunk (Plate 21-9-2), and axillae.

Differential Diagnosis
Morphea
Lichen planus
Vitiligo
Infection
Vulvovaginitis
Postinflammatory hypopigmentation
Sexual abuse

HISTOLOGICAL DESCRIPTION
Hyperkeratosis, epidermal atrophy, liquefaction degeneration of the basal cell layer, papillary dermal homogenization, and an underlying lymphocytic infiltrate are the classic features of lichen sclerosis et atrophicus (Plate 21-9-3). There is often telangiectasia of the papillary dermal vessels. Purpura can be significant in some lesions due to the fragility of the vessels. Subepidermal bullae arise because of the basal layer degeneration. When the infiltrate has decreased and the homogenization is the most conspicuous feature, differentiation from morphea is difficult. However, the cellular infiltrate in morphea is at the dermal subcutaneous junction, which is not the case in lichen sclerosis.

Differential Diagnosis
Morphea
Lupus erythematosus

21-10 SCLEREDEMA (BUSCHKE'S DISEASE)

CLINICAL DESCRIPTION

Symmetrical cutaneous induration suggests the diagnosis of scleredema.

Etiology and Incidence

Scleredema has its onset in childhood in 50% of cases. The mechanisms leading to the skin changes in this disorder are unknown. Postinfectious and metabolic disorders have been associated with the clinical findings (e.g., poststreptococcal, viral, diabetes mellitus).

Clinical Features

Brawny induration of the skin appears suddenly on the posterior neck and shoulders. Extension to other parts of the upper body ensues. The lower trunk and extremities are less frequently involved. Maximum progression occurs within six weeks. Most of the induration disappears within six months to two years.

Differential Diagnosis

Scleroderma
Eosinophilic fasciitis

HISTOLOGICAL DESCRIPTION

Viewed at low magnifications, histological sections do not show striking findings (Figure 21-10-1). The characteristic features are a significantly thicker dermis and separation of the collagen bundles (Figure 21-10-2). There is an increase in ground substance (hyaluronic acid) at the dermal subcutaneous junction and throughout the dermis in the areas of separation. Adnexae are preserved, in contrast to scleroderma, in which they atrophy and are lost. Inflammatory cells are sparse in this condition.

Differential Diagnosis

Morphea
Scleroderma

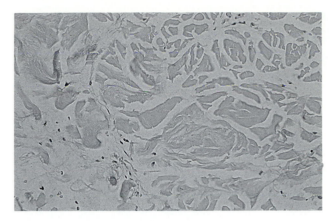

21-10-2 SCLEREDEMA: High magnification shows separation (fenestration) of collagen bundles. (200 ×)

21-11 DERMAL HEMATOPOIESIS

CLINICAL DESCRIPTION

Etiology and Incidence

Dermal hematopoiesis is a normal occurrence in the developing embryo and usually ends by the fifth gestational month. When this condition persists and is found at birth it is frequently secondary to intrauterine infection. The more common infections implicated are rubella and cytomegalovirus.

Clinical Features

Affected infants present with blue-red macules or papulonodules (Plate 21-11-1). The lesions are often generalized but with a preference for the head and neck. They vary in size from 1 to 9 mm. There is progressive resolution of the lesions; within about two months only residual red-brown macules remain. Because of the multiple blue-red papulonodules present at birth these children have been labeled "blueberry muffin babies."

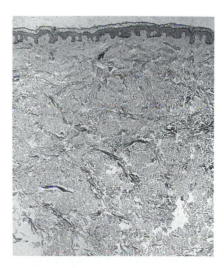

21-10-1 SCLEREDEMA: Low magnification shows no specific change. (20 ×)

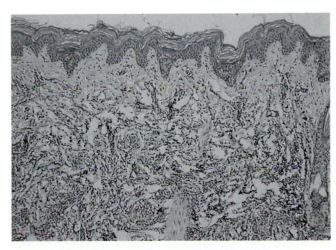

21-11-1 DERMAL HEMATOPOIESIS: A dense interstitial infiltrate outlines collagen bundles and adnexal structures. (40 ×)

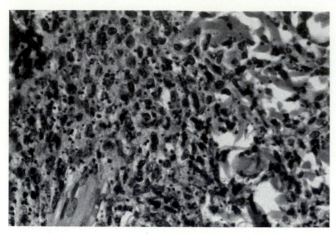

21-11-2 DERMAL HEMATOPOIESIS: The infiltrate contains nucleated erythrocytes and immature myeloid cells. (200×)

Differential Diagnosis
Purpura
Infection
Drug eruption
Angioma

HISTOLOGICAL DESCRIPTION

The histological features are a rather dense, diffuse infiltrate of nucleated red blood cells (Figure 21-11-1) and areas of myxoid degeneration in the dermis. Admixed with the nucleated red cells are immature myeloid cells (Figure 21-11-2).

Differential Diagnosis
Leukemia

21-12 EOSINOPHILIC PUSTULAR FOLLICULITIS

CLINICAL DESCRIPTION

Etiology and Incidence
First reported by Ofuji, eosinophilic pustular folliculitis is a condition of unknown cause. It has been found with frequency in HIV-positive individuals. In reported cases in children there has not been this linkage. Cases have been seen worldwide, although the first cases were from Japan.

This condition affects females to a greater extent than males. Although it is seen in children, the peak age is thirty years.

Clinical Features
Patients develop recurrent crops of erythematous follicular papules that become rapidly pustular on the scalp. The face, chest, back, and extensor aspects of the extremities can be affected (Figures 21-12-1 and 21-12-2). The mucosa is not

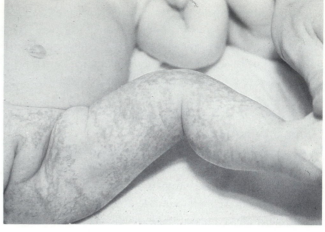

21-12-1 EOSINOPHILIC PUSTULAR FOLLICULITIS: Erythematous papulopustular lesions in a child's groin and on the thigh and leg. (Courtesy of G. Darmstadt, M.D.)

affected. The folliculopustules resolve with scaling and, ultimately, postinflammatory hyperpigmentation. The only consistent systemic finding is peripheral eosinophilia.

Differential Diagnosis
Erythema toxicum neonatorum
Acropustulosis
Transient neonatal melanosis
Incontinentia pigmenti

HISTOLOGICAL DESCRIPTION

The significant feature is a follicular pustule filled with eosinophils. There is overlying follicular hyper- and parakeratosis (Figure 21-12-3). The dermis shows a dense infiltrate of

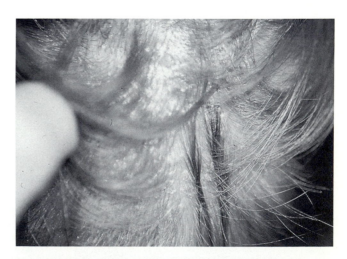

21-12-2 EOSINOPHILIC PUSTULAR FOLLICULITIS: Numerous pustules in a child's scalp. Patient also had lesions scattered on trunk. These pustules contained eosinophils.

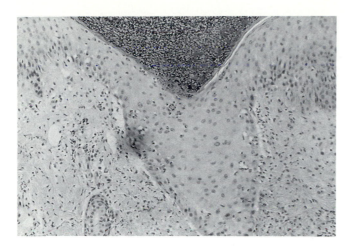

21-12-3 EOSINOPHILIC PUSTULAR FOLLICULITIS: A follicular pustule with eosinophilic exocytosis. Many eosinophils are seen in the dermis. (100×) (Courtesy G. Darmstadt, M.D.)

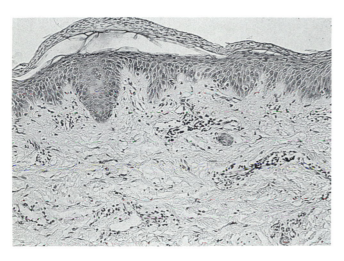

21-12-4 EOSINOPHILIC PUSTULAR FOLLICULITIS: A late lesion, showing parakeratosis, basilar layer pigmentation, and a perivascular infiltrate of lymphocytes (40×) (Courtesy of G. Darmstadt, M.D.)

cells composed almost entirely of eosinophils which are exocytotic to an edematous and infiltrated follicular epithelium (Plate 21-12-1). The end stage shows only spotty parakeratosis and a chronic perivascular infiltrate (Figure 21-12-4).

Differential Diagnosis
Erythema toxicum

REFERENCES

Acanthosis Nigricans
Brown J, Winkelmann RK: Acanthosis nigricans: A study of 90 cases (review). Medicine (Baltimore) 1968; 47:33.

Anetoderma
Miller WM, Ruggles CW, Rist TE: Anetoderma. Int J Dermatol 1979; 18:43.

Chelitis Granulomatosa
Klaus SN, Brunsting LA: Melkerson syndrome (persistent swelling of the face, recurrent facial paralysis and lingua plicata): Report of a case. Proc Mayo Clin 1959; 34:365.

Cutaneous Reactions to Cold
Lewis RB: Local cold injury-frostbite. Military Surg 1951; 110:25.
Wall LM, Smith NP: Perniosis: A histolopathological review. Clin Exp Dermatol 1981; 6:263.

Granuloma Annulare
Muhlbauer JE: Granuloma annulare. J Am Acad Dermatol 1980; 3:217.
Thyresson HN, Doyle JA, Winkelmann RK: Granuloma annulare: Histopathologic and direct immunofluoresence study. Acta Derma Venerol (Stockh) 1980; 60:261.

Child Abuse
George JE: Spare the rod: A survey of the battered-child syndrome. Forensic Sci 1973; 2:129.
Helfer RE, Pollock CB: The battered child syndrome. Adv Pediatr 1968; 15:9.
Lauer B, Broek E, Grossman M: Battered child syndrome: Review of 130 patients with controls. Pediatr 1974; 54:67.
Margrain SA: Review: Battered children, their parents, treatment and prevention. Child Care Health Dev 1977; 3:49.

Granuloma Gluteal Infantum
Bluestein J, Furner BB, Philips D: Granuloma gluteal infantum. Pediatr Dermatol 1990; 7:196.
Valli F, Della-Morte MA, Meschi V, Tadini G: Infantile gluteal granuloma: A case report. Pediatr Med E Chir 1985; 7:137.

Lichen Sclerosis et Atrophicus
Bergfeld WF, Lesowitz SA: Lichen sclerosis et atrophicus. Arch Dermatol 1990; 101:247.
DiSilverio A, Serri F: Generalized bullous and hemorrhagic lichen sclerosis et atrophicus. Br J Dermatol 1975; 93:215.
Jenny C, Kirby P, Fuguay D: Genital lichen sclerosis mistaken for sexual abuse. Pediatr 1981; 83:597.

Scleredema
Greenberg LM, Geppert C, Worthen HG, et al.: Scleredema "adultorum" in children. Pediatrics 1963; 32:1044.

Holubark K, Mach KW: Sclededema (Buschke). Acta Derm Venereol (Stockh) 1967; 47:102.

Dermal Hematopoiesis

Argyle JC, Zone JJ: Dermal erythropoiesis in a neonate. Arch Dermatol 1981; 117:492.

Bowden JB, Herbert AA, Rapini R: Dermal hematopoiesis in neonates: Report of five cases. J Am Acad Dermatol 1989; 20:1104.

Eosinophilic Pustular Folliculitis

Darmstadt GL, Tunnessen WW Jr, Sweren RJ: Eosinophilic pustular folliculitis. Pediatrics 1992. 89:1095.

Lucky AW, Esterly NB, Heskel N, et al.: Eosinophilic pustular folliculitis in infancy. Pediatr Dermatol 1984; 1:202.

Ofuji S: Eosinophilic pustular folliculitis. Dermatologica 1987; 174:53.

Index

Page numbers followed by *t* and *f* indicate tables and figures, respectively.